Chirality in Drug Design and Synthesis

To Mary, Bea and Sam,
who did all the real work

Chirality in Drug Design and Synthesis

Edited by

C. BROWN

Smith Kline Beecham Pharmaceuticals,
Welwyn, Hertfordshire, UK

ACADEMIC PRESS

Harcourt Brace Jovanovich Publishers

London   San Diego   New York
Boston   Sydney   Tokyo   Toronto

ACADEMIC PRESS LIMITED
24/28 Oval Road
LONDON NW1 7DX

United States Edition published by
ACADEMIC PRESS INC.
San Diego, CA 92101

British Library Cataloguing in Publication Data
Chirality in drug design & synthesis.
1. Organic drugs. Synthesis
I. Brown, C.
615.3
ISBN 0-12-136670-7

Typeset by EJS Chemical Composition, Bath, Avon
Printed in Great Britain by TJ Press, Padstow, Cornwall

Contributors

E. J. Ariens Institute of Pharmacology, University of Nijmegen, Groenewoodseweg 45, 6524 TP Nijmegen, The Netherlands

C. Brown Department of Physical and Organic Chemistry, Smith Kline Beecham, The Frythe, Welwyn, Hertfordshire A16 9AR, UK

J. P. L. Cox Cambridge Centre for Molecular Recognition, University Chemical Laboratory, Lensfield Road, Cambridge CB2 1EW, UK

D. S. Davies Department of Clinical Pharmacology, Royal Postgraduate Medical School, London W12 0NN, UK

S. G. Davies The Dyson Perrins Laboratory, University of Oxford, South Parks Road, Oxford OX1 3QY, UK

J. Dent Research and Development, Smith Kline Beecham Pharmaceuticals, 709 Swedeland Road, King of Prussia, Pennsylvania 19406-2799, USA

A. J. Doig Cambridge Centre for Molecular Recognition, University Chemical Laboratory, Lensfield Road, Cambridge CB2 1EW, UK

D. K. Donald Fisons Pharmaceuticals PLC, Bakewell Road, Loughborough, LE11 0RH, UK

M. Gardner Cambridge Centre for Molecular Recognition, University Chemical Laboratory, Lensfield Road, Cambridge CB2 1EW, UK

U. Hacksell Department of Organic Pharmaceutical Chemistry, Uppsala Biomedical Centre, Uppsala University, S-751 23 Uppsala, Sweden

J. B. Hook Research and Development, Smith Kline Beecham Pharmaceuticals, 709 Swedeland Road, King of Prussia, Pennsylvania 19406-2799, USA

M. Hyneck   Research and Development, Smith Kline Beecham Pharmaceuticals, 709 Swedeland Road, King of Prussia, Pennsylvania 19406-2799, USA

A. M. Johansson   Department of Organic Pharmaceutical Chemistry, Uppsala Biomedical Centre, Uppsala University, S-751 23 Uppsala, Sweden

A. Karlén   Department of Organic Pharmaceutical Chemistry, Uppsala Biomedical Centre, Uppsala University, S-751 23 Uppsala, Sweden

P. Kocienski   Department of Chemistry, The University, Southampton, SO9 5NH, UK

I. Lantos   Chemical Development, Smith Kline Beecham Pharmaceuticals, Research and Development, P.O. Box 1539, King of Prussia, Pennsylvania 19406, USA

K. Luthman   Department of Organic Pharmaceutical Chemistry, Uppsala Biomedical Centre, Uppsala University, S-751 23 Uppsala, Sweden

C. Mellin   Department of Organic Pharmaceutical Chemistry, Uppsala Biomedical Centre, Uppsala University, S-751 23 Uppsala, Sweden

I. A. Nicholls   Cambridge Centre for Molecular Recognition, University Chemical Laboratory, Lensfield Road, Cambridge CB2 1EW, UK

W. Oppolzer   Department of Organic Chemistry, University of Geneva, 30 Quai Ernest-Ansermet, CH-1211 Geneva 4, Switzerland

V. Novack   Chemical Development, Smith Kline Beecham Pharmaceuticals, Research and Development, P.O. Box 1539, King of Prussia, Pennsylvania 19406, USA

S. M. Roberts   Department of Chemistry, University of Exeter, Stocker Road, Exeter EX4 4QD, UK

M. Stocks   Department of Chemistry, The University, Southampton, SO9 5NH, UK

J. M. Stoddart   Department of Chemistry, The University, Sheffield S3 7HF, UK

D. H. Williams   Cambridge Centre for Molecular Recognition, University Chemical Laboratory, Lensfield Road, Cambridge CB2 1EW, UK

Foreword

Scientists today are exposed to a plethora of conferences, and it is not easy to decide in advance which ones are going to be really worthwhile, and to merit detailed record in a book like this. Specialized, sharply focussed meetings are fairly reliable, but it is harder to succeed with those of broader scope which span more than one discipline. If these do work, however, they can be truly valuable, and even memorable, as was the 1990 Smith Kline & French Research Symposium on Chirality in Drug Design and Synthesis.

A conference on this theme could hardly have been more timely and, as it progressed, it became even more so. Whilst chirality has long been a major feature of the structural and synthetic chemistry of natural products, its full significance in medicinal chemistry has emerged only more recently, with the general recognition that the enantiomers of chiral drug molecules (which constitute over half of the 1800 or so in clinical use) are different chemical species, and should be treated as such. The problems and the challenge arise, of course, because of the subtlety of the difference.

How sensible, then, of the Organizing Committee to take a broad view of this fundamental issue and, with the generous resources at their command, to assemble pharmacologists, toxicologists, medicinal chemists, and mechanistic and synthetic organic chemists to discuss it. The broad scope of the conference is immediately clear from the lecture titles. The speakers were very distinguished, including many of the leading international experts, and they, in turn, attracted a large and lively audience.

The various specialists interacted surprisingly well, to their mutual advantage, and the conference, and this volume, demonstrate the significant interdependence of the many sciences involved in the design, synthesis, pharmacology, metabolism, and toxicology of chiral drug molecules. Much has already been achieved, particularly in the elegant methods available for the synthesis of chiral molecules, and the scientific tools are in place for the next phase—the complete investigation of candidate compounds as single stereoisomers. If there were any lingering doubts about the importance (and the cost!) of this, and the scientific challenges it presents, they were certainly dispelled at this exciting conference.

C. W. REES

Contents

Introduction

This volume records the lectures delivered by a group of distinguished scientists at the 4th Smith Kline and French Research Symposium on Chirality in Drug Design and Synthesis, held in Cambridge in March 1990. They brought together in one forum expertise in the pharmacology, toxicology, mechanism of action and chemical synthesis of chiral drugs and provided a unique opportunity for discussion and debate on these important issues. They thereby amply fulfilled the aim of the Symposium, which was organized with a view to examining firstly the very need for the preparation and study of pure enantiomers of chiral drug substances, secondly the mechanism of interaction of such species with enzymes and receptors, and methods for the study of such interactions and finally, and certainly not least importantly, methods for their synthesis in enantiomerically pure form.

Chiral molecules have intrigued scientists for more than 150 years, and it is interesting in the present context to note that it was a biologist, Pasteur, working before the structural theories of Kekulé, Van't Hoff and Le Bel had been formulated, who first separated a pair of enantiomers and distinguished among them and their 1:1 mixture or racemate. Interest in the separation of enantiomers from racemic reaction products and in the synthesis of pure enantiomers has continued ever since. However, enantiomerism has always been treated as a rather 'special' type of isomerism, probably because ostensibly the only difference between enantiomers is the manner in which they interact with polarized light. One enantiomer has therefore rarely been regarded as an 'impurity' when present in a sample of the other enantiomer, in contrast to, say, a mixture of two aromatic positional isomers or a mixture of (E)- and (Z)-alkenes. In fact, this lack of any difference other than optical activity only holds in a truly achiral situation: as soon as any chirality is introduced into the environment of a chiral molecule the enantiomers are differentiated. This will clearly be the case when a chiral drug interacts with an enzyme or receptor, as such biomolecules will typically represent a chiral environment.

The important difference between the way in which chiral and achiral drugs act on a chiral receptor can be effectively illustrated by analogy with a comparison of the game of baseball and the game of golf. Unlike a baseball bat, an achiral object with a variety of symmetry elements, a golf club lacks any element of symmetry and can therefore be made in either right- or left-handed form. A right-handed player (representing the receptor) may thus play to maximum effect only with a right-handed club (representing the drug) and not with a left-handed one. No such distinction arises in the case of the baseball bat (representing an achiral drug). The same is also true of a cricket bat, although it is important to note that in the hands of the player the two edges of the bat become inequivalent and, in use, probe quite different regions of space, the cricket bat being a prochiral object. On the face of it therefore, in the hands of a right-handed player (the receptor), a left-handed club (the 'wrong' enantiomer) will be of little more use than, say, a baseball bat representing a 'normal' impurity, and the analogy requires that the enantiomer of a drug be treated just as any impurity would. However, a closer acquaintance with the game of golf shows that the situation is not so clear cut. A left-handed one-iron, for example, could be used much more effectively by a right-handed player than could a left handed nine-iron. (Those totally familiar with the game will of course realize that certain putters have a plane of symmetry and are, therefore, prochiral, like the cricket bat.) We might therefore anticipate that drug molecules might behave similarly, with receptors being less enantioselective towards some drugs than to others.

This notion that differences in pharmacological effect of the two enantiomers of a chiral drug must be related to the degree of chirality or perhaps to the degree to which the chiral centre plays a crucial role in the mechanism of action of a particular drug is implicit in Pfeiffer's rule which equates large differences in pharmacological effect of the enantiomers of a chiral drug with low effective doses. It is important to realize, however, that we have to consider the possibility that our enantiomer may be more than just an ineffective version of its mirror image, and may have dramatically different (and potentially undesirable) pharmacological effects in its own right. Furthermore, processes such as drug absorption, distribution, excretion and metabolism are all potentially subject to enantioselection.

A proper understanding of the complex game of golf clearly requires a thorough understanding of the rules, of the finer points of the way in which it is played and of the structure of the clubs used. By analogy, drug research with chiral molecules requires a clear understanding of the regulatory requirements (the rules) the distribution, mechanism of action and metabolism of drug substances (the game itself) and their synthesis (club manufacture) before a clear cut decision can be made as to whether racemates may be considered acceptable or described as 50% impure. The contributors to this volume demonstrate clearly that the ever-increasing understanding of the mode of action of drug substances reveals a variety of situations with regard to the acceptability of using chiral drugs in racemic or enantiomerically pure form, and that elegant synthetic methodology is available to provide the latter where necessary.

1

Chirality: Pharmacological Action and Drug Development

MARTHA HYNECK, JOHN DENT
and JERRY B. HOOK
*Research and Development, Smith Kline Beecham
Pharmaceuticals, 709 Swedeland Road,
King of Prussia, Pennsylvania 19406–2799, USA*

Introduction

The field of stereochemistry has been developing since the early 1800s when Jean-Baptiste Biot, a French physicist, discovered optical activity in 1815. By the middle of the 19th century, Louis Pasteur had performed the first resolution of a racemic mixture, D- and L-tartaric acid. From this work Pasteur made the remarkable proposal that optical activity was caused by molecular asymmetry and that nonsuperimposable mirror-image structures resulted from this molecular asymmetry. Despite considerable scepticism within the community of chemists, scientists from several countries continued exploring this new field and with each new scientific contribution the relationship between optical activity and molecular asymmetry unfolded. By the end of the 18th century, Van't Hoff of Holland and Le Bel of France strengthened Pasteur's proposal by hypothesizing that the chiral nature of compounds was due to the fact that carbon constituents could have a non-planar spatial arrangement giving rise to nonsuperimposable mirror images (Drayer, 1988a).

Today we realize that most naturally occurring medicinal agents exist in their optically active or single isomer form, such as quinidine and quinine (Fig. 1), (−)-morphine and (+)-digitoxin. However, many synthetic chemicals are produced as the optically inactive racemate. According to a

CHIRALITY IN DRUG DESIGN AND SYNTHESIS
ISBN 0-12-136670-7

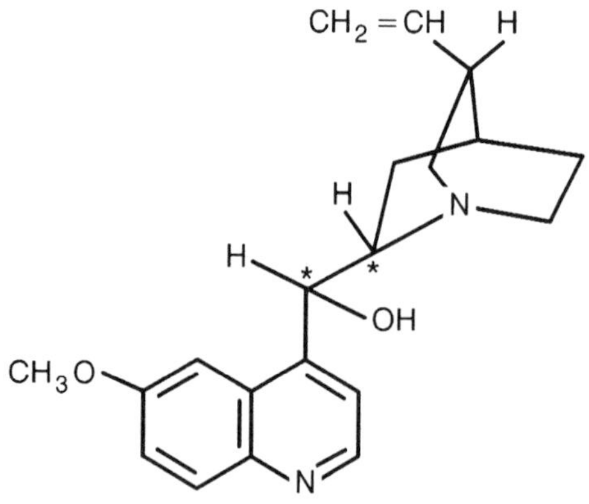

Fig. 1 Structure of quinidine and quinine.

survey reported in 1984, nearly 400 racemates were prescribed for patients in the 1970s and 1980s (Mason, 1984). The fact that so many drugs are administered as racemic mixtures has led to considerable concern and debate (Ariens, 1984; Caldwell *et al.*, 1988). Because of potential pharmacological, pharmacokinetic and toxicological issues, some scientists suggest that only single isomers should be considered for drug development and regulatory approval. In support of racemic drug development, proponents cite examples of racemic compounds that have been administered for years without untoward effects, and the technical difficulties associated with large-scale production of single isomers.

In the past few decades pharmacological and toxicological investigations have clearly demonstrated significant differences in the biological activity of some isomeric pairs. Recently, pharmacokinetic investigations into the disposition of enantiomers have enhanced our understanding of racemic drug action and have helped us to understand previously inexplicable pharmacodynamic outcomes following administration of racemates to patients.

2 Terminology

A myriad of terms in stereochemistry are used to define molecules and to describe the relationship between molecules and receptors in the body (Wainer and Marcotte, 1988; Caldwell *et al.*, 1988). This section is not meant to be an exhaustive review of the field, but to cover the major terms and concepts to be used.

Isomers are unique molecular entities composed of the same chemical constituents with common structural characteristics. *Stereoisomers* are those isomers whose atoms, or groups of atoms, differ with regard to spatial arrangement of the ligands. Stereoisomers can be either geometric or optical isomers. *Geometric isomers* are stereoisomers without optically active centres; for these compounds terminology such as *cis* or *Z* isomer (meaning together or same side), and *trans* or *E* isomer (meaning opposite side) are used to describe the spatial arrangement.

Optical isomers are a subset of stereoisomers, from which at least two isomers are optically active; these compounds are said to possess *chiral* or asymmetrical centres. The most common chiral centre is carbon, but phosphorus, sulphur and nitrogen can also form chiral centres. If the isomer and its mirror image are not superimposable, the pair are referred to as *enantiomers* or *optical antipodes*. A mixture of equal portions (50/50) of each enantiomer is called a *racemate*. Optical isomers that are not enantiomers are called *diastereoisomers* or *diastereomers*. One type of diastereomer is a molecule with two chiral centres; all four isomers of this diastereomer are not superimposable mirror images of each other. Whereas enantiomers have physically identical characteristics such as lipid solubility and melting/boiling points, diastereomers can have different chemical and physical characteristics.

The earliest method of differentiating one enantiomer from its antipode was to assign the D or (+) designation to stereoisomers which caused a clockwise rotation of a beam of polarized light, and L or (−) to stereoisomers which cause a counterclockwise rotation of the polarized light. Since this system did not describe the actual spatial arrangement, the Fischer convention was developed (Wichelhaus *et al.*, 1919; Freudenberg, 1966). In this system, the molecule had to be converted to a compound of known configuration, such as (+)-glyceraldehyde and then named accordingly. Due to the difficulty of the chemical transformation, the awkwardness of the convention in some situations (i.e. diastereomers) and the confusion between small and capital letter system (D and *d*), the convention has fallen into disfavour.

The Cahn–Ingold–Prelog convention is currently recommended for specifying the configuration of the isomers (Cahn *et al.*, 1966). In this method, the ligands around the chiral centre are 'sized' according to their atomic number (Fig. 2). The molecule is then positioned with the smallest ligand(s) away from the viewer ('into the page'). If the sequence of the remaining three ligands are arranged so that the largest (L) to the smallest (S) size is in a clockwise manner, the molecule is assigned the *R* or *rectus*; the counterclockwise sequencing is given the *S* or *sinister* designation.

Two other terms may be used to compare the pharmacological activity of two enantiomers. It has been proposed that the isomer imparting the desired activity be called the *eutomer* and that the 'inactive' or unwanted isomer

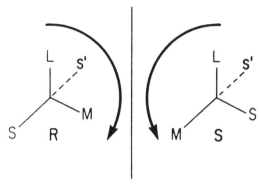

Fig. 2 The Cahn–Ingold-Prelog convention. Reprinted from Wainer and Marcotte (1988) by courtesy of Marcel Dekker Inc.

be labelled the *distomer* (Lehmann, 1986). From this comes the *eudismic ratio* which is the ratio of the potencies for the two enantiomers. These eudismic ratios can be used to describe *in vitro* or *in vivo* potency ratios, and there could potentially be more than one eudismic ratio for a racemate if the compound had more than one pharmacological action.

For further information on the rules and nomenclature used in stereochemistry, the reader should refer to the IUPAC publication on this topic (Anonymous, 1970).

3 Enantioselectivity in pharmacological activity

Traditionally, pharmacologists and physicians have assumed that the administration of a 'drug' would act as a 'single agent' and would produce a 'single action'. When pure enantiomers are administered, this may be the outcome. But this is frequently not the case when racemic mixtures are given since several different pharmacological outcomes are possible depending on the pharmacological action of each enantiomer and on the disposition of the enantiomers in the body.

Enantioselectivity in pharmacology following administration of a racemic xenobiotic has been recognized since the early part of this century. These differences were anticipated because of the diastereomeric relationship between asymmetrical molecules and asymmetrical receptors (enzymes plasma proteins and activity receptors) (Simonyi, 1984; Testa, 1989). It has only been within the past 10–20 years, however, that advances in analytical and preparative technology have allowed researchers to separate and study individual enantiomers. This has allowed us to begin to understand the differences in activity of enantiomers and identify factors that alter the expected pharmacodynamic response under therapeutic conditions. With these new tools in hand, investigators have been able to carefully describe the differences in pharmacological activity in drug enantiomers and been able to relate these differences to clinical and toxicological findings.

Pharmacological assessment of chiral compounds in an early research phase can lead to the selection of a single isomer for development. This selection process can maximize the potential for specific activity and minimize the potential for side-effects. For various reasons, however, many racemates have been developed and for these compounds the pharmacological picture is considerably more complex than the single enantiomer activity picture.

3.1   Pharmacological activity is, or appears to be, due to one isomer

When racemates are administered, the overall pharmacological effect may portray *single-isomer-activity* if;

(1) all activity resides in one of the isomers, with the antipode being inactive;
(2) both isomers are equal in activity; or
(3) both isomers have the same qualitative activity but differ in potencies.

Careful analysis of isomeric data in the last category may reveal the real differences in activity of the isomers.

3.1.1   All pharmacological activity mimics one isomer; other isomer(s) 'inactive'

It may be highly desirable to have all the activity in one enantiomer so as to avoid the unwanted activity and/or toxicity that may reside in the antipode, but examples where this has been proven to be true are uncommon. Usually the 'inactive' isomer possesses some demonstrable biological activity, even if it is not the desired effect. In other cases, the potency of each isomer to elicit the *desired* clinical reponse is evaluated during preclinical development; the 'inactive' antipode is then dropped and may not be screened for other than the desired effect or for toxicity. Therefore, whether the non-selected isomer is truely 'inactive' is uncertain.

The antihypertensive agent α-methyldopa is an example of a compound in which all the desired antihypertensive activity is reported to be confined to one optical isomer (Gillespie *et al.*, 1962). The pharmacological selectivity for the L isomer *in vivo* has been confirmed in studies demonstrating that there is both stereoselective metabolism of the L isomer to the active metabolite and that there is stereoselective affinity of this active metabolite for the central-acting adrenergic receptor (Baldwin and Abrams, 1988). Consequently, methyldopa was developed as a single isomer.

SB is currently developing a compound that fits into this category. SK&F 104353 (Fig. 3) is a novel, highly specific, peptidoleukotriene receptor antagonist. Results of preliminary Phase IIA studies suggest that the compound will be effective in the chronic prophylactic treatment of asthma. SK&F 104353 has two chiral carbons as indicated below.

Initial *in vitro* studies indicated that the 2*S*,3*R* diastereomer was approximately 100-fold more active than the 2*R*,3*S* configuration in competing for LTD_4 binding sites in guinea-pig lung membranes and for inhibiting LTD_4-induced contractions of guinea-pig trachea (Smith *et al.*, 1989). Due to the relative inactivity of the 2*R*,3*S* isomer we are currently developing only the 2*S*,3*R* form (SK&F 104353). The novel synthesis of SK&F 104353 is described in Chapter 9. As preparative technology improves, the isomer potency screening and selection process which took place with SK&F 104353 may become more common across the industry. However, until large-scale production of isomers is more economical and technically feasible, selection of active moieties may be of interest scientifically, but will have practical limitations.

3.1.2 Both enantiomers have similar activity and potency

It is rare that both enantiomers have similar qualitative and quantitative activity. This is not unexpected since receptors and enzymes should react selectively to configurational differences in xenobiotic structure. However, it has been reported that the two isomers of promethazine have equal activity and toxicity with regard to antihistaminic activity (Powell *et al.*, 1988). In addition, although one action of a compound may be

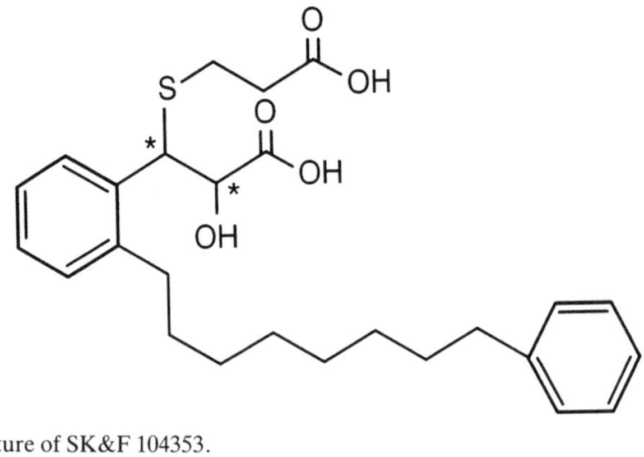

Fig. 3 Structure of SK&F 104353.

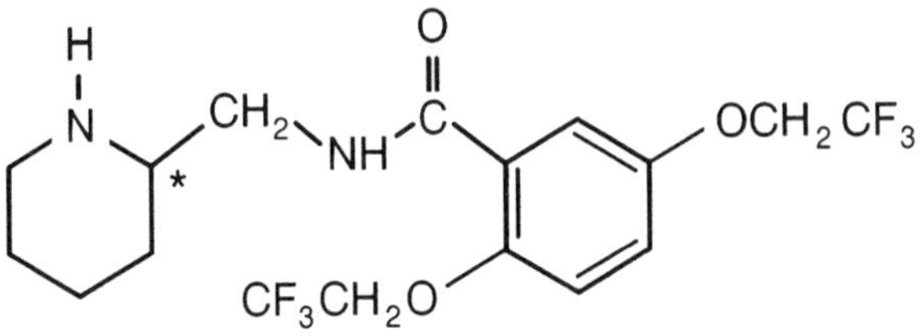

Fig. 4 Structure of flecainide.

stereoselective, other effects may not be. For example, the β-receptor blocking ability of propranolol is highly stereoselective, but the effect on insulin secretion is not selective.

Flecainide (Fig. 4), a new antiarrhythmic agent, may be another racemate in this category. The *in vitro* pharmacological activity of flecainide and the isomeric differences in steady-state plasma concentrations of flecainide following long-term therapy in 13 patients have been described (Kroemer *et al.*, 1989a). By assessing the effect of each isomer on the action potential characteristics in canine cardiac Purkinje fibres, these investigators concluded that the two enantiomers of flecainide exert very similar electrophysiological effects. The steady-state plasma concentration data indicated that the disposition of flecainide was only modestly enantioselective. Although no mention was made as to whether the observed side-effects of flecainide (e.g. depression of left ventricular function) are enantioselective, these authors concluded that 'at this point, administration of a single enantiomer appears to offer no advantage over the racemic mixture'.

3.1.3   *Enantiomers have similar activities but potencies differ*
In contrast to the examples above, it is quite common for enantiomers to have similar qualitative pharmacological activity, but to differ in their potencies. This would not represent a therapeutic dilemma if each enantiomer possessed only one pharmacological (and/or toxicological) activity. However, since drugs frequently have more than one pharmacological effect and enantioselectivity in drug disposition is often observed, achieving a predictable therapeutic outcome can be complex with racemates having this activity profile. If the pharmacokinetic disposition of the isomers is different, the pharmacodynamic effect can vary between patients, and even within the same patient over the course of one dosing interval. In addition, the response of patients with renal and/or hepatic disease may vary greatly from the response in normal volunteers. Factors that can alter the expected pharmacodynamic response are discussed in more detail later in this chapter.

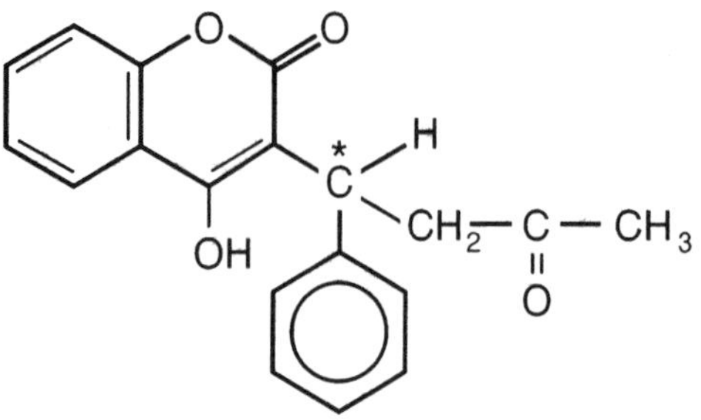

8   **Martha Hyneck** *et al.*

Fig. 5 Structure of warfarin.

Warfarin and propranolol (Figs 5 and 6) are perhaps classic examples of racemates whose isomers have similar qualitative activity but differ in quantitative activity. The potency of $S(-)$-warfarin, *in vivo*, is from two- to five-fold greater than $R(+)$-warfarin (O'Reilly, 1974). This difference in potency, however, is coincidentally offset by a two- to five-fold greater plasma clearance of $S(-)$-warfarin (Breckenridge *et al.*, 1974). These apparently off-setting properties are only part of the complex pharmacokinetic–pharmacodynamic profile of warfarin. Difficulties arise when racemic warfarin is used therapeutically. Warfarin is stereoselectively bound to plasma proteins, undergoes stereoselective metabolism and can interact stereoselectively with other drugs (Powell *et al.*, 1988; Tucker and Lennard, 1990). Clinical reports have shown that when the disposition of warfarin is altered, serious side-effects can occur. These factors are discussed in greater detail later in this chapter.

It has been shown that all β-blocking drugs, including propranolol (Fig. 6), stereoselectively bind to β-receptors and that it is the $S(-)$ enantiomer that imparts the β-blocking activity for all of these drugs (Walle *et al.*, 1988).

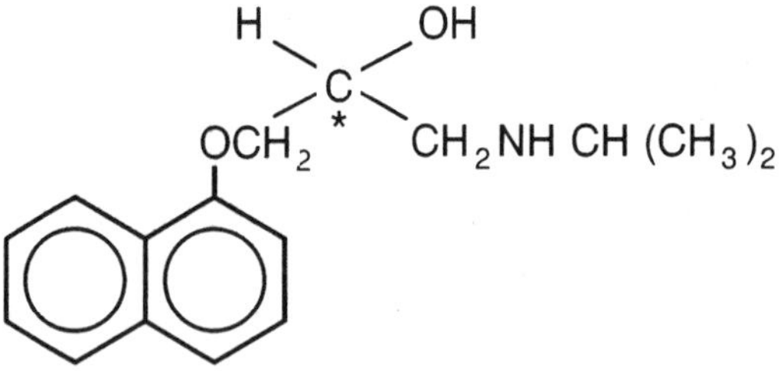

Fig. 6 Structure of propranolol.

However, the *in vitro* eudismic (affinity binding) ratio varies widely within this class of compounds depending on the structure. For example, this ratio $(-/+)$ is 100 for propranolol whereas for atenolol it is 10 and for pindolol it is 1000. Studies have shown, however, that propranolol possesses several pharmacological actions and, for some of these actions, stereoselectivity is either not evident (Hartling, 1981) or is due to the activity of the $R(+)$ isomer (Campbell *et al.*, 1981). In addition, like warfarin, propranolol is stereoselectively protein bound in plasma $(R > S)$ and is stereoselectively metabolized at different clearance rates $(R > S)$. Therefore, the pharmacodynamic outcome can vary between patients (who may have different P_{450} compositions) and with the route of administration (Walle *et al.*, 1988; Tucker and Lennard, 1990).

Another example in this category is verapamil (Fig. 7), a calcium channel blocker that is used as an antianginal agent and for the treatment of supraventricular tachyarrhythymias. Both $R(+)$ and $S(-)$-verapamil have been shown to increase cardiac blood flow through coronary vasodilation and to have cardiodepressant effects. Although both isomers are equipotent with regard to their coronary vasodilatory effects, the $R(+)$ isomer is approximately eight- to ten-fold less potent as a cardiodepressant compared with the $S(-)$ isomer (Echizen *et al.*, 1985). Again, because of differences in pharmacokinetic disposition (first-pass metabolism and systemic clearance), the ratio of the plasma concentrations of $R:S$ varies with the route of administration and the time after dosing (Eichelbaum *et al.*, 1984). These intra- and inter-patient variations could lead to significant therapeutic problems. Selective development of the $R(+)$ enantiomer as an antianginal agent may have circumvented these difficulties.

Thus, even when isomers have similar qualitative pharmacological activity, quantitative differences in activity and/or pharmacokinetic disposition can significantly influence the overall pharmacodynamic response. The variable or unpredictable nature of these effects increases the opportunity for therapeutic problems that could put patients at risk.

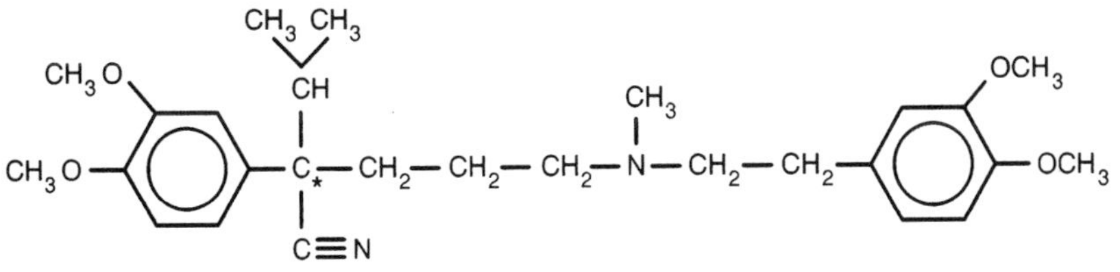

Fig. 7   Structure of verapamil.

3.2   Pharmacological activity differs qualitatively and quantitatively in each isomer

Racemates of this type provide the greatest opportunity for rational selection of an isomer for drug development. Since the desired activity resides primarily with one of the isomers, the antipode is likely to cause either unnecessary or unwanted effects. There are examples, however, where the combined activities of the isomers could be therapeutically useful, making the 'combination product' a rationale drug entity. Each isomer and racemic mixture should be evaluated on its own merits to assess the consequences of single isomer versus racemic mixture on therapy.

3.2.1   Single enantiomer developed because of activity in antipode

L-Dopa, α-dextropropoxyphene and S(−)-timolol are commercially available drugs that are marketed as single enantiomers because the antipode produced unwanted side-effects. For L-dopa, it was noted during early development that many of the serious side-effects, such as granulocytopenia, were due to the D isomer; the racemate is no longer used in humans (Cotzias *et al.*, 1969).

In contrast to flecainide where both enantiomers have been reported to have very similar activity, the isomers of propoxyphene appear to have completely different activities. D-Propoxyphene (Fig. 8) has analgesic properties, whereas its optical isomer L-propoxyphene has antitussive properties but is devoid of analgesic properties (Drayer, 1986). To reflect their mirror image relationship, Lilly gave them tradenames which are also mirror images of each other, Darvon® and Novrad®.

Timolol (Fig. 9) is the only β-blocking agent available as a pure enantiomer. Although the specificity of this class of compounds for the

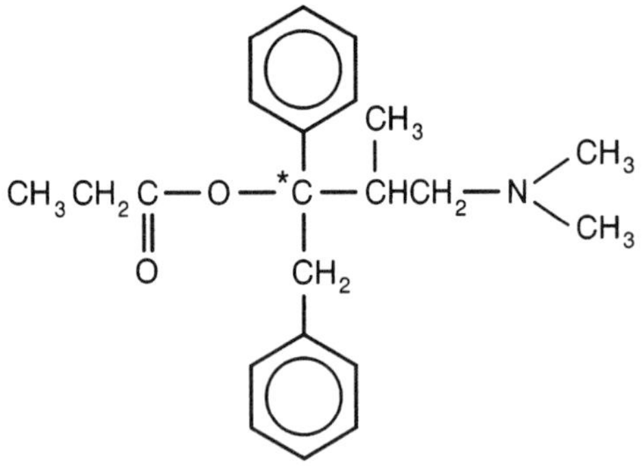

Fig. 8   Structure of propoxyphene.

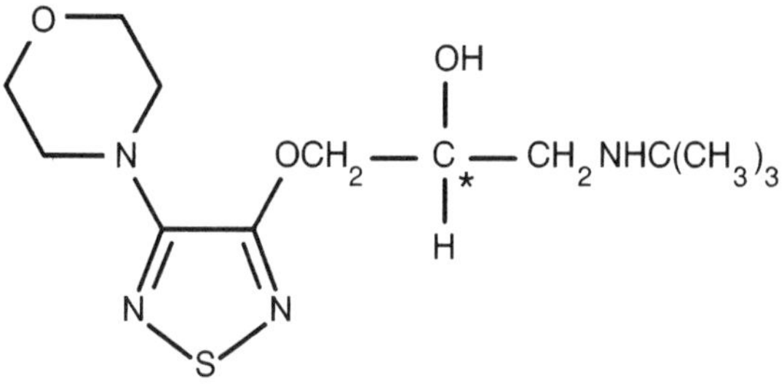

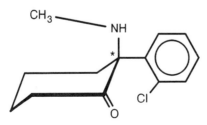

Fig. 9   Structure of timolol.

β-receptor is not absolute, the R/S affinity ratio for the receptor is 36 for timolol and is greater than 100 for propranolol (Baldwin and Abrams, 1988). Because the $R(+)$ enantiomer does have other pharmacological actions, the pure $S(-)$ enantiomer was selected for development. As Drayer has pointed out, however, the $R(+)$ enantiomer may have been the better isomer for patients being treated for glaucoma (Drayer, 1986). $S(-)$-Timolol can be absorbed systemically and has been reported to cause fatal β-blockade induced bronchoconstriction when applied topically to treat glaucoma. $R(+)$-Timolol, however, decreases intraocular pressure but is much less likely to induce β-blockade.

3.2.2   Racemate developed despite unwanted activity in antipode
Ketamine, disopyramide and cyclophosphamide are all marketed as racemic mixtures, and the enantiomers of each drug differ greatly in their pharmacological and toxicological profiles. Ketamine (Fig. 10) is a widely used anesthetic and analgesic agent that is chemically similar to phencyclidine, a drug of abuse. Post-anesthesia reactions to ketamine include hallucinations and agitation. When the effects of $S(+)$-ketamine were compared with $R(-)$-ketamine (Fig. 11), the potency ratio indicated that the $S(+)$ enantiomer had about 3 to 4 times the potency of the $R(-)$

Fig. 10   Structure of ketamine.

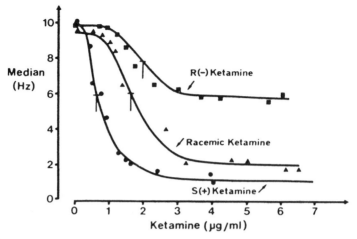

Fig. 11 Ketamine activity. From Schüttler *et al.*, 1987, with permission from Plenum Press.

enantiomer (White *et al.*, 1980; Schüttler *et al.*, 1987). The noted side-effects were overwhelmingly associated with the $R(-)$ antipode. This is a case where development of the more active enantiomer may have been warranted; this would have retained adequate potency and reduced the incidence of side-effects.

The therapeutic use of disopyramide (Fig. 12) as an antiarrhythmic is also somewhat limited because of the toxicological contributions of the less potent isomer. Recent *in vitro* studies have suggested that the beneficial antiarrhythmic properties of disopyramide are favoured in $S(+)$-disopyramide, while the negative inotropic effect predominates in the $R(-)$ isomer (Kidwell *et al.*, 1989). In addition, the pharmacokinetics (clearance and protein binding) of the enantiomers differ (Thibonnier *et al.*, 1984; Lima *et al.*, 1985; Giacomini *et al.*, 1986). For these reasons, selection of

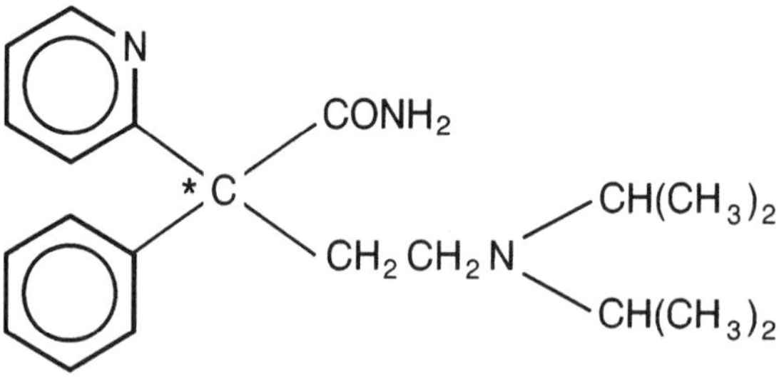

Fig. 12 Structure of disopyramide.

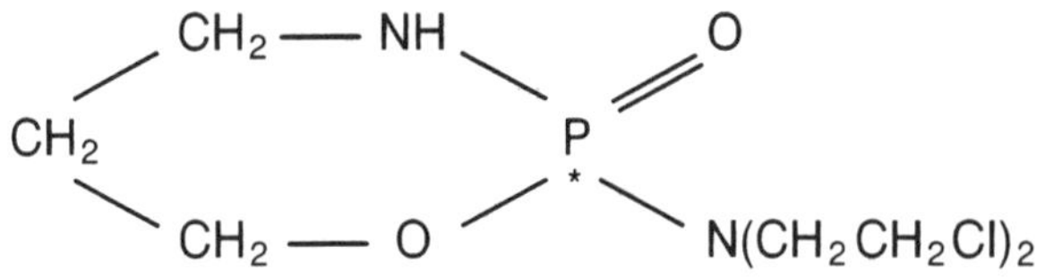

Fig. 13 Structure of cyclophosphamide.

the $S(+)$ isomer may have led to the development of a very effective drug with significantly fewer therapeutic problems.

Cyclophosphamide (Fig. 13) is a unique chiral compound in that its asymmetry is due to its chiral phosphorus atom rather than the usual carbon chiral centre. Cox and colleagues showed that $(-)$-cyclophosphamide was twice as effective as an antitumor agent but no more toxic than its $(+)$ antipode (Cox *et al.*, 1976). Development of the pure enantiomer rather than the racemate may have had some therapeutic advantages.

3.2.3 'Combination product' may have therapeutic advantages
Labetalol and indacrinone are racemic mixtures in which the isomers have very different pharmacological activities. In these instances the 'combination' product may be useful for a certain patient population. Labetalol is a diastereomer marketed as an equal mixture of all four stereoisomers. Labetalol (Fig. 14), an antihypertensive agent, has both α- and β-adrenoreceptor blocking properties. Brittain *et al.* (1982) reported that the R,R isomer conferred the non-specific β_1- and β_2-blocking properties, whereas the α_1-blocking activity resided in the S,R isomer. Many patients are benefiting from the combined effects of β-blockade and vasodilation. Therefore, to some extent the 'combination product' is useful. However, two of the isomers (S,S and R,S) are inactive and may be 'burdening' the body unnecessarily. Furthermore, for some patients the additional α-blockade is undesirable. Currently, the enantiomeric pure R,R isomer is being developed (dilevalol) for commercial use to address these issues.

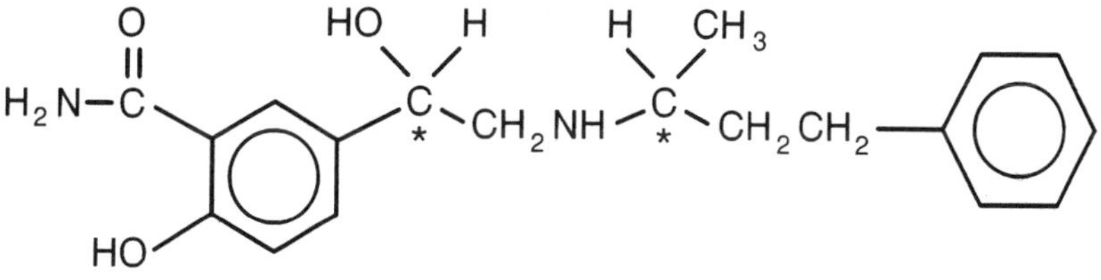

Fig. 14 Structure of labetalol.

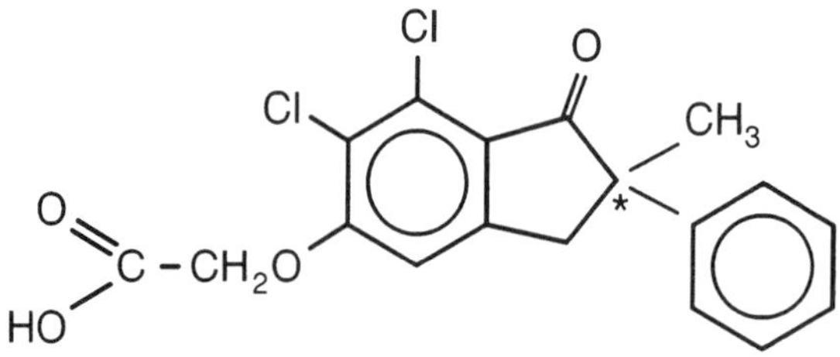

Fig. 15 Structure of indacrinone.

Indacrinone (Fig. 15) is an interesting investigational drug that has both diuretic and uricosuric activity. Preclinical and clinical studies have shown that $R(-)$-indacrinone and its active metabolite are responsible for the diuretic activity, whereas $S(-)$-indacrinone promotes uric acid excretion (Vlasses *et al.*, 1981). Each enantiomer seems to possess very little of the antipode's activity. Since many commercially available diuretics increase plasma uric acid concentration (e.g. furosemide and thiazides), and many hypertensive patients who need a diuretic are hyperuricemic, indacrinone as a racemate may be an ideal therapeutic agent for this population. However, because of the need to maintain the uricosuric activity of the $S(-)$ enantiomer during chronic administration when relative hypovolemia encourages uric acid reabsorption, the naturally occurring racemic ratio (50/50) may need to be altered (Tobert *et al.*, 1981; Vlasses *et al.*, 1984).

In summary, administration of isomers and racemates to patients can result in several different pharmacodynamic outcomes depending on qualitative and quantitative enantiomeric differences in activity, and on the differential disposition of these enantiomers in the body. In some cases these differences are subtle and, depending on the complexity and cost of large-scale production, the patient or the pharmaceutical manufacturer may benefit little from single-enantiomer development. In contrast, toxicity may be associated with the less potent isomer and dictate that a single enantiomer must be developed. Increased awareness of these enantiomeric differences in pharmacological and toxicological activity highlights the need to evaluate each isomer and the racemic mixture before deciding on the appropriate drug development programme.

4 Enantioselectivity in pharmacodynamics resulting from differences in the pharmacokinetics of the enantiomers

Enantioselectivity in pharmacodynamics can result not only from qualitative and quantitative differences in the activity of the enantiomers but also from differences in the pharmacokinetics of the enantiomers. Stereoselectivity in drug absorption, distribution, metabolism and excretion has been described in the literature and these dispositional factors must be understood to appreciate fully the pharmacological activity of a drug. Although a drug may be administered as a racemate, the clinical activity/toxicity of the drug will depend upon the *in vivo* unbound concentration of isomers at the site of action (e.g. brain or myocardium). The unbound concentration of the isomers can be significantly influenced not only by the pharmacokinetic disposition of each isomer but also by factors such as dose, route of administration, disease, concurrent drug administration and genetic phenotype.

4.1 Absorption

Drugs are absorbed, in general, by passive diffusion and, since enantiomers do not differ in their aqueous and lipid solubilities, absorption is not usually considered to be a stereoselective process. However, stereoselectivity has been described for drugs that are transported across the intestinal mucosa by a carrier-mediated process. For example, L-dopa is actively absorbed, whereas its antipode D isomer is absorbed by passive diffusion (Wade *et al.*, 1973). Similarly, L-methotrexate is well-absorbed by active transport but the D isomer, which is passively absorbed, has only 2.5% of the bioavailability of the L form (Hendel and Brodthagen, 1984).

Other mechanisms have also been suggested to account for differences in absorption. For instance, data recently presented suggest that (−)-terbutaline enhances the absorption of (+)-terbutaline (Fig. 16) by selectively promoting intestinal membrane permeability (Borgstrom *et al.*, 1989). Likewise, the bioavailability of $S(-)$-propranolol, the enantiomer with more potent β-blocking activity, is reduced when administered as a single enantiomer compared with its bioavailability when administered as a racemate, suggesting that the presence of $R(+)$-propranolol had a beneficial effect on the availability of $S(-)$-propranolol (Lindner *et al.*, 1989). In addition, differential effects of the isomers of bupivacaine on local blood

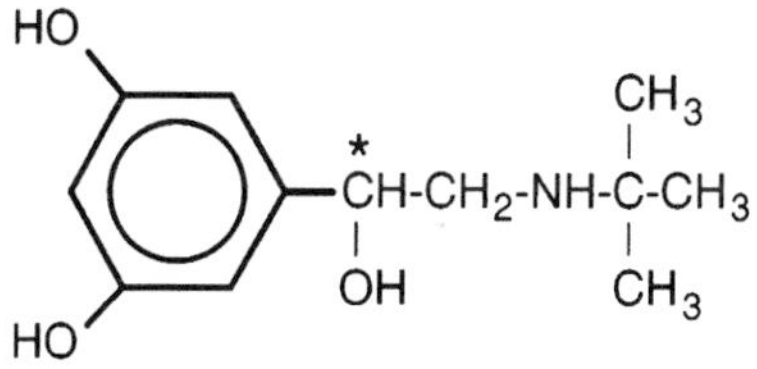

Fig. 16   Structure of terbutaline.

flow may account for differences in rates of absorption and, therefore, in duration of anesthesia (Aps and Reynolds, 1978).

4.2 Protein binding

Drug enantiomers can bind stereoselectively to plasma proteins; selectivity in binding to both albumin and α_1-acid glycoprotein (AAG) has been described in the literature (Table 1). It has been suggested, however, that pronounced 'stereospecific drug binding is rather the exception than the rule' when the large number of drugs that are protein bound are considered (Muller, 1988). When these differences in protein binding do occur, however, this factor can be critical to the dynamics of the racemic mixture since it is the concentration of the *unbound* isomer that triggers the receptor and is available for metabolism and excretion.

Acidic drugs commonly bind to human serum albumin (Table 1) in an enantioselective manner (Drayer, 1988b). Of the two binding sites on albumin, site I (the warfarin site) is usually less stereoselective than the

Table 1 Percentage of drug enantiomers unbound in human plasma

	Free fraction (%)		Ratio	
	(+)	(−)	(±)	Reference
Acids				
Indacrinone	0.3	0.9	0.3	Drayer (1988b)
Warfarin	1.2	0.9	1.3	Yacobi and Levy (1977)
Pentobarbital	36.6	26.5	1.4	Cook *et al.* (1987)
Phenprocoumon	1.07	0.72	1.5	Schmidt and Jahnchen (1978)
Bases				
Verapamil	6.4	11.5	0.6	Echizen *et al.* (1985)
Disopyramide	7.5	12.5	0.6	Le Corre *et al.* (1988)
Methadone	9.2	12.4	0.7	Romach *et al.* (1981)
Fenfluramine	2.8	2.9	1.0	Caccia *et al.* (1979)
Amphetamine	84	84	1.0	Wan *et al.* (1978)
Propoxyphene	1.8	1.8	1.0	Drayer (1988b)
Propranolol	20.3	17.6	1.0	Walle *et al.* (1988)
Terbutaline	20	20	1.0	Borgstrom *et al.* (1989)
Tocainide	83–89	86–91	1.0	Sedman *et al.* (1982)
Mexiletine	28.3	19.8	1.4	McErlane *et al.* (1987)
Moxalactam	0.47	0.32	1.5	Yamada *et al.* (1981)
Quinidine	8.9 (Quinidine)	9.5 (Quinine)	0.9	Notterman *et al.* (1986)

benzodiazepine/indole site (site II) (Fehske *et al.*, 1981). The classic example for this type of stereoselective binding is L-tryptophan, an essential amino acid. The binding of L-tryptophan to site II is 100 times greater than that of D-tryptophan (McMenamy and Oncley, 1958). Metabolites of oxazepam and diazepam are also stereoselectively bound at this site. In contrast to differences in affinity for a binding site, the *extent* of binding for the drug enantiomers that have been studied does not usually exceed 1.5, but exceptions to this have been reported. It has been suggested that binding to albumin may be used as an indicator of the extent of binding to receptors; so far the association between albumin and receptor binding appears to be too inconsistent to be of predictive use.

The binding of basic drugs, which usually bind to AAG, is relatively non-stereoselective (Table 1) (Drayer, 1988b; Muller, 1988). Noteworthy exceptions to this rule are verapamil, mexiletine and disopyramide.

Both enantiomers of warfarin, an acidic drug which binds to albumin, have hypoprothrombinemic activity. The inherent potency of unbound (S)-warfarin is about 6–8 times greater than (R)-warfarin (Wingard *et al.*, 1978; Toon and Trager, 1984). When assessed separately *in vivo*, however, (S)-warfarin is only 2–5 times more potent than (R)-warfarin (Breckenridge *et al.*, 1974; O'Reilly, 1974). The difference in *in vivo* activity is attributed to the fact that (S)-warfarin is more extensively bound than (R)-warfarin (99.1% vs. 98.8%, respectively) (Yacobi and Levy, 1977). This example demonstrates why the extent of protein binding must be taken into consideration in order to assess fully the potential pharmacodynamic impact of the isomer.

4.3 Metabolism

Enantioselective metabolism and clearance, whether presystemic or systemic metabolism, plays a major role in determining the pharmaco-dynamic effect of a drug (Table 2). A highly potent, rapidly cleared enantiomer may be of less clinical importance than its lower potency/slowly cleared antipode, depending on the resulting concentration of unbound enantiomer at the receptor. Drugs which undergo extensive pre-systemic clearance may never reach the site of action. Examples of differences in biotransformation and enantiomer clearance which affect the therapeutic use of the racemate are well documented in the literature (Jenner and Testa, 1973; Caldwell *et al.*, 1988; Eichelbaum, 1988; Testa, 1989).

(S)-Warfarin, for example, is eliminated mainly by 7-hydroxylation whereas (R)-warfarin is eliminated by ketone reduction and oxidation to 6-hydroxywarfarin and 8-hydroxywarfarin (Toon *et al.*, 1986; Hermans and

Table 2   Drug enantiomer average total body clearance

Drug	Enantiomer (+)	(−)	Ratio[a]	Reference
Hexobarbital	$1.9\,ml\,min^{-1}kg^{-1}$	$16.9\,ml\,min^{-1}kg^{-1}$	8.9	Chandler et al. (1988)
Verapamil	$800\,ml\,min^{-1}$	$1400\,ml\,min^{-1}$	1.8	Eichelbaum et al. (1984)
Warfarin	$234\,ml\,min^{-1}$	$333\,ml\,min^{-1}$	1.4	Toon et al. (1987)
Disopyramide	$13.4\,ml\,min^{-1}kg^{-1}$	$9.4\,ml\,min^{-1}kg^{-1}$	1.4	Kidwell et al. (1989)
Terbutaline	$0.186\,l\,h^{-1}kg^{-1}$	$0.125\,l\,h^{-1}kg^{-1}$	1.5	Borgstrom et al. (1989)
Propranolol	$1200\,ml\,min^{-1}$	$1000\,ml\,min^{-1}$	1.2	Walle et al. (1988)
Misonidazole	$48\,ml\,min^{-1}$	$41\,ml\,min^{-1}$	1.2	Williams (1984)
Pentobarbital	$40\,ml\,min^{-1}$	$32\,ml\,min^{-1}$	1.3	Cook et al. (1987)
Mexiletine	$8.1\,ml\,min^{-1}kg^{-1}$	$8.6\,ml\,min^{-1}kg^{-1}$	1.1	McErlane et al. (1987)

[a] More rapidly cleared enantiomer/less rapidly cleared enantiomer.

Thijssen, 1989). Similar differences in pathways of metabolism have been noted for propranolol. The metabolism of (R)-propranolol *in vivo* is due largely to oxidation of propranolol to 4-hydroxypropranolol, whereas glucuronidation favours (S)-propranolol (Silber *et al.*, 1980; Ward *et al.*, 1989). It is unclear whether the differences in these pathways fully accounts for the differences in systemic clearance, since enantioselective protein binding favours (S)-propranolol and may contribute to the slower elimination of this isomer.

Recently, the biotransformation of verapamil (Fig. 7) and its metabolites was investigated (Eichelbaum *et al.*, 1979; Eichelbaum, 1984). The enantio-selective differences in the systemic clearance have significant therapeutic implications. Verapamil is metabolized to more than 10 metabolites. In contrast to the lack of stereoselectivity for the N-dealkylation pathways, the formation of O-demethylation metabolites exhibits extensive enantioselectivity—a 30-fold higher clearance for $S(-)$-verapamil compared with $R(+)$-verapamil. Since results from these studies indicate that a greater percentage of $S(-)$-verapamil is unbound in the plasma, protein binding may be contributing to differences in intrinsic clearance to produce the substantial difference in systemic clearance of the two isomers. This enantioselectivity in clearance can perhaps explain the clinical therapeutic problems that had been noted for several years when verapamil was used to treat arrhythymia.

Clinicians had noted that there were large differences between the *intravenous* dose of verapamil and plasma concentrations that were necessary to achieve adequate PR prolongation compared with the *oral* dose and plasma concentrations that were necessary to achieve an equivalent therapeutic response. This inconsistency could be only partially accounted for by reduced bioavailability resulting from extensive first-pass metabolism (Eichelbaum, 1984). From an elegant series of experiments, it became obvious that these differences were due not only to the activity and potency of the two enantiomers, but also to the differences in clearance of the enantiomers. Therefore, after intravenous administration the $R:S$ isomers ratio was found to be about 2, whereas after oral administration the $R:S$ ratio was about 5. The higher relative concentrations of the $S(-)$ isomer, which has greater negative dromotropic activity, following intravenous therapy can account for much of the difference in effect seen following oral and intravenous administration.

In hepatic disease, the dispositional properties of verapamil are reported to change, not unexpectedly for a drug with high hepatic clearance. Eichelbaum and colleagues found that in patients with liver disease the stereoselectivity of first-pass metabolism was lost resulting in more of the active $S(-)$ isomer reaching the circulation (Eichelbaum, 1988). Therefore, the pharmacodynamics of verapamil in liver-failure patients would be expected to be quite different than the response in patients without liver disease.

In general, enantiomeric differences in metabolic clearance are more evident for drugs which undergo first-pass metabolism, such as verapamil and propranolol, following oral administration, when differences in protein binding and intrinsic clearances are highlighted (Wilkinson and Shand, 1975). For these drugs, pharmacological activity and pharmacokinetics from single, intravenous administration should not be used to predict activity or toxicity following oral administration. In addition, since the pathophysiology of disease may alter the pharmacokinetics of these drugs, patient and disease factors should be taken into consideration in dose selection and in predicting the pharmacological response.

4.4   Renal clearance

Stereoselectivity could, theoretically, occur with all aspects of renal clearance, (filtration, active secretion and active and passive reabsorption). However, selectivity is primarily associated with the intrinsic capacity of the renal tubules to secrete drugs. Selectivity in renal tubular reabsorption has been suggested to account for differences in the renal clearance of terbutaline (Borgstrom et al., 1989).

The most noteworthy example of stereoselectivity in renal clearance is that of the diastereomers quinidine and quinine (Fig. 1); quindine's renal clearance is more than four times that of quinine (Notterman et al., 1986). Pronounced stereoselectivity in the active tubular transport process is more apt to occur with diastereomers due to the greater spatial orientation differences between drug stereoisomers (Drayer, 1988b).

4.5 Drug interactions

The potential for drug interactions is greater when racemic mixtures are administered to humans than when achiral drugs are given. Drug interactions that are unique to racemates include drug-enantiomer and enantiomer–enantiomer interactions. The potential for these interactions should be explored during drug development since they can influence the efficacy and the side-effect profile of the compound.

Drug–enantiomer interactions include the possibility for enantioselective protein binding displacement, competition for receptor sites, and inhibition/induction of metabolism. Enantioselective interactions with warfarin have been described for several drugs. For example, when phenylbutazone and warfarin were given concomitantly, the anticoagulant effect of warfarin was augmented although the total plasma concentrations of warfarin did not change. Enantiospecific-pharmacokinetic analysis of the data revealed that there was inhibition of the clearance of the more active S isomer, consistent with the hypoprothrombinemia. Initial analysis suggested that there was induction of the clearance of the R isomer. However, calculation of the *unbound* clearance of (R)-warfarin showed the clearance of (R)-warfarin had also been inhibited (to a lesser degree than (S)-warfarin) and that protein-binding displacement of the R isomer had occurred, masking the inhibition (O'Reilly *et al.*, 1980; Banfield *et al.*, 1983).

Enantioselective effects on the metabolism of (S)-warfarin have also been reported when warfarin was given with sulphinpyrazone, trimethoprim-sulphamethoxazole and enoxacin (Toon *et al.*, 1986; O'Reilly, 1980). These interactions are important because the interaction predominates with the active enantiomer, is manifested as increased anticoagulation which could create therapeutic problems, and analysis of the data without assessing the impact on each enantiomer would have led to misinterpretation of the data.

In contrast to the above interactions with the S isomer, the interaction between cimetidine and warfarin involves the less potent R isomer (Toon *et al.*, 1987). We recently conducted a study to investigate the effect of dose on the interaction and found that the interaction was insignificant for both enantiomers at the low dose (100 mg four times a day). At the higher dose (200 mg four times a day), there was no significant change in the pharmacokinetics of (S)-warfarin but there was an 18% reduction in clearance of (R)-warfarin with a slight (< 10%) increase in anticoagulation (Burnham *et al.*, 1989).

These drug–enantiomer interactions with warfarin demonstrate that enantioselective, clinically meaningful interactions do occur but that each interaction must be evaluated stereoselectively and with pharmacodynamic assessment since some interaction may involve the inactive or less potent enantiomer.

Enantiomer–enantiomer interactions should also be anticipated since each enantiomer could be considered a separate drug. As previously mentioned, L-bupivacaine is reported to cause vasoconstriction and to delay the absorption of D-bupivacaine (Aps and Reynolds, 1978). Similarly, $S(-)$-propranolol is reported to cause vasoconstriction, reduce liver blood flow and, therefore, reduce the clearance of $R(+)$-propranolol (Branch et al., 1973). In contrast, $(-)$-terbutaline may enhance the absorption of $(+)$-terbutaline and improve its bioavailability (Borgstrom et al., 1989). There is also evidence that protein-binding displacement and competition for enzymatic binding sites exist (Tucker and Lennard, 1990). Only a limited number of studies have been done to explore these interactions.

4.6 Polymorphism

Genetic metabolizing capacity can be an important factor in the disposition of several drugs including some chiral compounds (Eichelbaum, 1988; Relling, 1989). Propafenone (Fig. 17) has been studied in extensive metabolizer (EM) phenotypes and poor metabolizer (PM) phenotypes based on the debrisoquine classification (Kroemer et al., 1989a,b).

In EM phenotypes a high degree of enantioselectivity in metabolism was observed (S/R ratio, 1.73). Although the concentration of the isomers was higher in the PM phenotypes, the S/R ratio was maintained in this population. In contrast, when a similar experiment was conducted using metoprolol, PM phenotypes lost the enantioselectivity in metabolism that was seen in the EM phenotypes (Lennard et al., 1983). These experiments highlight the need to assess each racemate and isomer individually and to understand the biotransformation pathway of each entity.

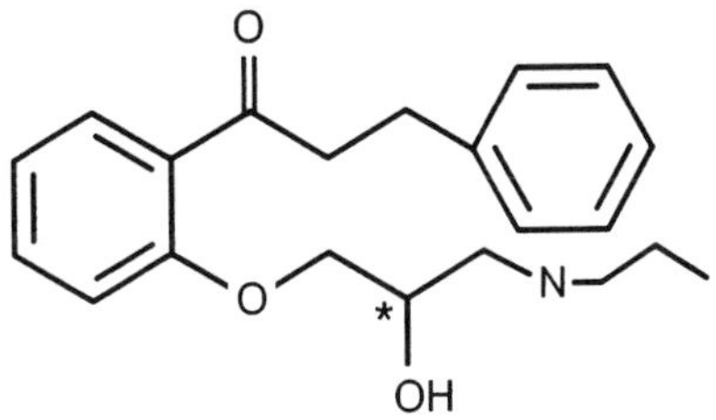

Fig. 17 Structure of propafenone.

4.7 In vivo *inversion*

Vital to our interpretation of the pharmacological action of single enantiomers is an appreciation for the degree of *in vivo* inversion that occurs with the administration of either the single enantiomer or the racemate (Hutt and Caldwell, 1984; Williams and Lee, 1985; Caldwell *et al.*, 1988). Early observations noted disparity between the *in vitro* assessment of the *S/R* potency ratio versus the *in vivo* assessment of the *S/R* potency ratio for ibuprofen. For example, under *in vitro* conditions the *S/R* potency ratio of ibuprofen is 160, but *in vivo* this ratio reduces to about 1:1. These differences in potency ratios have since been reported for several, but not all, compounds in this class (Hutt and Caldwell, 1984). These observations regarding ibuprofen, coupled with the knowledge that both enantiomers were present in urine following administration of the *R*-isomer, suggested that *in vivo* inversion must be occurring (Nakamura *et al.*, 1981; Lee *et al.*, 1984). The mechanism of this inversion appears to be unidirectional (*R* to *S*) and is proposed to occur via coenzyme A thioester formation that is specific for the *R* isomer (Fig. 18).

When (*R*)-ibuprofen was administered to subjects, approximately 60% of the isomer was inverted to the *S* isomer with the half-life for the inversion being approximately 108 h in humans (Simmonds *et al.*, 1980; Lee *et al.*, 1984). The extent of the inversion can be affected by dose, route, disease and other drugs (Meffin *et al.*, 1986; Spahn *et al.*, 1987). The site for this inversion is uncertain, but similarity in plasma profiles between intravenous and oral dose administration suggest liver involvement. There is still much work to be done in this area. Until more is known about *in vivo* inversion, stereospecific assays for the active components are essential for accurate assessments of the concentration–effect relationship.

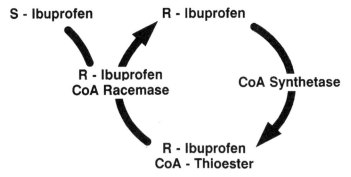

Fig. 18 Proposed mechanism for *in vivo* inversion.

5 Conclusion

Pharmacological and pharmacokinetic investigations over the past few decades have highlighted differences in the activity and disposition of enantiomeric pairs. Some of these differences can be used advantageously for the patient since the racemate may have multiple beneficial actions, or the unresolvable racemate may possess a truely unique mechanism of action and represent a significant therapeutic advancement, worthy of development despite the presence of an inactive 'impurity'. In contrast, enantiomeric differences may relate to toxicological aspects of the drug and dictate that development of a single isomer be pursued. In the future, drug development must include investigations aimed at understanding these enantioselective differences. Currently, regulatory guidelines do not prohibit the development of racemates. Regulatory authorities acknowledge that the decision to market a racemate or the isomer is complex and should include cost–benefit concerns (Kumkumian, 1988; Birkett, 1989; De Camp, 1989; Weissinger, 1989). However, these authorities also recognize that a decision about the safety and efficacy of a compound extends to understanding the action and disposition of each enantiomer. Therefore, these safety and efficacy decisions should come as a result of careful investigations into the pharmacology and pharmacokinetics of each isomer. With the recent technological advances, these investigative studies can and should be conducted to assure maximum efficacy with minimum risk for patients.

References

Anonymous, IUPAC (1970). Tentative rules for the nomenclature of organic chemistry, Section E. Fundamental stereochemistry. *J. Org. Chem.* **35**, 2849–2867.
Aps, C. and Reynolds, F. (1978). An intradermal study of the local anaesthetic and vascular effects of the isomers of bupivacaine. *Br. J. Clin. Pharmacol.* **6**, 63–68.
Ariens, E. J. (1984). Stereochemistry, a basis for sophisticated nonsense in pharmacokinetics and clinical pharmacology. *Eur. J. Clin. Pharmacol.* **26**, 663–668.
Baldwin, J. J. and Abrams, W. B. (1988). Stereochemically pure drugs: an industrial perspective. In *Drug Stereochemistry—Analytical Methods and Pharmacology* (ed. I. W. Wainer and D. E. Drayer), pp. 311–356. Marcel Dekker, New York.
Banfield, C., O'Reilly, R., Chan, E. and Rowland, M. (1983). Phenylbutazone–warfarin interaction in man: further stereochemical and metabolic consideration. *Br. J. Clin. Pharmacol.* **16**, 669–675.
Birkett, D. J. (1989). Racemates or enantiomers: regulatory approaches. *Clin. Exp. Pharmacol. Physiol.* **16**, 479–483.

Borgstrom, L., Nyberg, L., Jonsson, S., Lindberg, C. and Paulson, J. (1989). Pharmacokinetic evaluation in man of terbutaline given as separate enantiomers and as the racemate. *Br. J. Clin. Pharmacol.* **27**, 49–56.

Branch, R. A., Nies, A. S. and Shand, D. G. (1973). The disposition of propranolol. *Drug Metab. Dis.* **1**, 687–690.

Breckenridge, A., Orme, M., Wesseling, H., Lewis, R. J. and Gibbons, R. (1974). Pharmacokinetic and pharmacodynamics of the enantiomers of warfarin in man. *Clin. Pharmacol. Ther.* **15**, 424–430.

Brittain, R. T., Drew, G. M. and Levy, G. P. (1982). The α- and β-adrenoreceptor blocking potencies of labetolol and its individual stereoisomers in anaesthetized dogs and in isolated tissues. *Br. J. Pharmacol.*, **77**, 105–114.

Burnham, D., Gombar, C., Hyneck, M. L., Webb, D., Chretien, S., Wyle, F. and Friedman, C. (1989). Effects of low cimetidine dose on steady-state warfarin pharmacokinetics and prothrombin time. *Proceedings of the American College of Clinical Pharmacology*, Annual Meeting, Baltimore, MD.

Caccia, S., Ballabio, M. and De Ponte, P. (1979). Pharmacokinetics of fenfluramine enantiomers in man. *Eur. J. Drug Metab. Pharmacokin.* **4**, 129–132.

Cahn, R. S., Ingold, C. K. and Prelog, V. (1966). Specification of molecular chirality. *Angew. Chem. Int. Ed. Engl.,* **5**, 385–415.

Caldwell, J., Winter, S. M. and Hutt, A. J. (1988). The pharmacological and toxicological significance of the stereochemistry of drug disposition. *Xenobiotica* **18**, 59–70.

Campbell, R. W. F., Murray, A. and Julian, D. G. (1981). Ventricular arrhythmias in first 12 hours of acute myocardial infarction. *Br. Heart J.* **46**, 351–357.

Chandler, M. H. H., Scott, S. R. and Blouin, R. A. (1988). Age-associated stereoselective alterations in hexobarbital metabolism. *Clin. Pharmacol. Ther.* **43**, 436–441.

Cook, C. E., Seltzman, T. B., Tallent, C. R., Lorenzo, B. and Drayer, D. R. (1987). Pharmacokinetics of pentobarbital enantiomers as determined by enantioselective radioimmunoassay after administration of racemate to humans and rabbits. *J. Pharmacol. Exp. Ther.* **241**, 779–785.

Cotzias, G. C., Papavasiliou, P. S. and Gellene, R. (1969). Modification of Parkinsonism: chronic treatment with L-dopa. *N. Engl. J. Med.* **280**, 337–345.

Cox, P. J., Farmer, P. B., Jarman, M., Jones, M., Stec, W. J. and Kinas, R. (1976). Observations on the differential metabolism and biological activity of the optical isomers of cyclophosphamide. *Biochem. Pharmacol.* **25**, 993–996.

De Camp, W. H. (1989). The FDA perspective on the development of stereoisomers. *Chirality* **1**, 2–6.

Drayer, D. E. (1986). Pharmacodynamic and pharmacokinetic differences between drug enantiomers in humans: an overview. *Clin. Pharmacol. Ther.* **40**, 125–133.

Drayer, D. E. (1988a). The early history of stereochemistry: from the discovery of molecular asymmetry and the first resolution of a racemate by Pasteur to the asymmetrical carbon atom of van't Hoff and Le Bel. *In Drug Stereochemistry—Analytical Methods and Pharmacology* (eds I. W. Wainer and D. E. Drayer), pp. 3–29. Marcel Dekker, New York.

Drayer, D. E. (1988b). Pharmacokinetic differences between drug enantiomers in man. In *Drug Stereochemistry—Analytical Methods and Pharmacology* (eds I. W. Wainer and D. E. Drayer), pp. 209–225. Marcel Dekker, New York.

Echizen, H., Brecht, T., Niedergesass, S. Volgelgesang, B. and Eichelbaum, M. (1985). The effect of dextro-, levo-, and racemic verapamil on atrioventricular conduction in humans. *Am. Heart J.* **109**, 210–217.

Eichelbaum, M. (1984). Polymorphic drug oxidation in humans. *Fed. Proc.* **43**, 2298–2302.

Eichelbaum, M. (1988). Pharmacokinetic and pharmacodynamic consequences of stereoselective drug metabolism in man. *Biochem. Pharmacol.* **37**, 93–96.

Eichelbaum, M., Ende, M. Remberg, G., Schomerus, M. and Dengler, H. J. (1979). The metabolism of DL-[^{14}C]verapamil in man. *Drug Metab. Disp.* **7**, 145–147.

Eichelbaum, M., Mikus, G. and Vogelgesang, B. (1984). Pharmacokinetics of (+)-, (−)- and (±)-verapamil after intravenous administration. *Br. J. Clin. Pharmacol.* **17**, 453–458.

Fehske, K.J., Muller, W. E. and Wollert, U. (1981). The location of drug binding sites in human serum albumin. *Biochem. Pharmacol.* **30**, 687–692.

Freudenberg, K. (1966). Emil Fischer and his contributions to carbohydrate chemistry. In *Advances in Carbohydrate Chemistry, Vol. 21* (eds M. L. Wolfson and R. S. Tipson), pp. 1–38. Academic Press, London.

Giacomini, K. M., Nelson, W. L., Pershe, R. A., Valdevieso, L., Turner-Tamayasu, K. and Blaschke, T. F. (1986). *In vivo* interaction of the enantiomers of disopyramide in human subjects. *J. Pharmacokin. Biopharmacol.* **14**, 335–356.

Gillespie, L., Oates, J. A., Crout, J. R. and Sjoerdsma, H. (1962). Clinical and chemical studies with α-methyldopa in patients with hypertension. *Circulation* **25**, 281–291.

Hartling, O. J., Svendsen, T. L. and Trap-Jensen (1981). Systemic and forearm hemodynamic and metabolic fate of racemic propranolol or D-propranolol in healthy subjects. *Clin. Sci.* **60**, 675–679.

Hendel, J. and Brodthagen, H. (1984). Entero-hepatic cycling of methotrexate estimated by use of the D-isomer as a reference marker. *Eur. J. Clin. Pharmacol.* **26**, 103–107.

Hermans, J. J. R. and Thijssen, H. H. W. (1989). The *in vitro* ketone reduction of warfarin and analogues. Substrate stereoselectivity, product stereoselectivity and species differences. *Biochem. Pharmacol.* **38**, 3365–3370.

Hutt, A. J. and Caldwell, J. (1984). The importance of stereochemistry in the clinical pharmacokinetics of the 2-arylpropionic acid non-steroidal anti-inflammatory drugs. *Clin. Pharmacokinet.* **9**, 371–373.

Jenner, P. and Testa, B. (1973). The influence of sterochemical factors on drug disposition. *Drug Metabol. Rev.* **2**, 117–184.

Kidwell, G. A., Lima, J. J. Schaal, S. F. and Muir, W. M. (1989). Hemodynamic and electrophysiologic effects of disopramide enantiomers in a canine blood superfusion model. *J. Cardiovasc. Pharmacol.* **13**, 644–655.

Kroemer, H. K., Turgeon, J., Parker, R. A. and Roden, D. M. (1989a). Flecainide enantiomers: disposition in human subjects and electrophysiologic actions *in vitro*. *Clin. Pharmacol. Ther.* **46**, 584–590.

Kroemer, H. K., Funck-Brentano, C., Silberstein, D. J., Wood, A. J. J., Eichelbaum, M., Woosley, R. L. and Roden, D. M. (1989b). Stereoselective disposition and pharmacologic activity of propafenone enantiomers. *Circulation* **79**, 1068–1076.

Kumkumian, C. S. (1988). The use of stereochemically pure pharmaceuticals: a regulatory point of view. In *Drug Stereochemistry—Analytical Methods and Pharmacology* (eds I. W. Wainer and D. E. Drayer), pp. 299–310. Marcel Dekker, New York.

Le Corre, P., Gibassier, D., Sado, P. and Le Verge, R. (1988). Stereoselective metabolism and pharmacokinetics of disopyramide enantiomers in humans. *Drug. Metab. Disp.* **16**, 858–864.

Lee, E. J. D., Williams, K. M., Graham, G. G., Day, R. O. and Champion, G. D. (1984). Liquid chromatographic determination and the plasma concentration profile of optical isomers of ibuprofen in humans. *J. Pharmacol. Sci.* **73**, 1542–1544.

Lehmann, D. A. (1986). Stereoisomerism and drug action. *Trends Pharmacol. Sci.* **7**, 281–285.

Lennard, M. S., Tucker, G. T., Silas, J. H., Freestone, S., Ramsey, L. E. and Woods, H. F. (1983). Differential stereoselective metabolism of metoprolol in extensive and poor debrisoquine metabolizers. *Clin. Pharmacol. Ther.* **34**, 732–737.

Lima, J. J., Boudoulas, H. and Shields, B. J. (1985). Stereoselective pharmacokinetics of disopyramide enantiomers in man. *Drug. Metabol. Disp.* **13**, 572–577.

Lindner, W., Rath, M., Stoschitzky, K. and Semmelrock, H. J. (1989). Pharmacokinetic data of propranolol enantiomers in a comparative human study with (*S*)- and (*R,S*)-propranolol. *Chirality*, **1**, 10–13.

Mason, S. (1984). The left hand of nature. *New Sci.* **1393**, 10–14.

McErlane, K. M., Igwemezie, L. and Kerr, C. R. (1987). Stereoselective serum protein binding of mexiletine enantiomers in man. *Res. Comm. Chem. Pathol. Pharmacol.* **56**, 141–144.

McMenamy, R. H. and Oncley, J. L. (1958). The specific binding of L-tryptophan to serum albumin. *J. Biol. Chem.* **233**, 1436–1447.

Meffin, P. J., Sallestio, B. C., Purdie, Y. J. and Jones, M. E. (1986). Enantioselective disposition of 2-arylpropionic acid nonsteroidal anti-inflammatory drug. *J. Pharmacol Exp. Ther.* **238**, 280–287.

Muller, W. E. (1988). Stereoselective plasma protein binding of drugs. In *Drug Stereochemistry—Analytical Methods and Pharmacology* (eds I. W. Wainer and D. E. Drayer), pp. 227–244. Marcel Dekker, New York.

Nakamura, Y., Yamaguchi, T., Takajashi, S., Hashimoto, S., Iwatini, K. and Nagagawa, Y. (1981). Optical isomerization mechanism of *R*(−)-hydratropic acid derivates. *J. Pharmacobiodynamics* **4**, s1.

Notterman, D. A., Drayer, D. E., Metakis, L. and Reidenberg, M. M. (1986). Stereoselective renal tubular secretion of quinidine and quinine. *Clin. Pharmacol. Ther.* **40**, 511–517.

O'Reilly, R. A. (1974). Studies on the optical enantiomorphs of warfarin in man. *Clin. Pharmacol. Therp.* **16**, 348–354.

O'Reilly, R. A. (1980). Stereoselective interaction of trimethoprem–sulfamethoxazole with the separated enantiomorphs of racemic warfarin in man. *New Engl. J. Med.* **302**, 33–35.

Powell, J. R., Ambre, J. J. and Ruo, T. I. (1988). The efficacy and toxicity of drug stereoisomers. In *Drug Stereochemistry—Analytical Methods and Pharmacology* (eds I. W. Wainer and D. E. Drayer), pp. 245–270.

Relling, M. V. (1989). Polymorphic drug metabolism. *Clin. Pharm.* **8**, 852–863.

Romach, M., Piafsky, K. M. and Abel, J.G. (1981). Methadone binding to orosomucoid (alpha 1-acid glycoprotein): determinant of free fraction in plasma. *Clin. Pharmacol. Ther.* **29**, 211–217.

Schmidt, W. and Jahnchen, E. (1978). Species-dependent stereospecific serum protein binding of the oral antiagulant drug phenprocoumon. *Experientia* **34**, 1323–1325.

Schüttler, J., Stanski, D. R., White, P. F., Trevor, A. J., Horai, Y., Verotta, D. and Sheiner, L. B. (1987). Pharmacodynamic modeling of the EEG effects of ketamine and its enantiomers in man. *J. Pharmacokin. Biopharmacol.* **15**, 241–253.

Sedman, A. J., Bloedow, D. C. and Gal, J. (1982). Serum binding of tocainide and its enantiomers in human subjects. *Res. Comm. Chem. Pathol. Pharmacol.* **38**, 165–168.

Silber, B., Holford, N. H. G. and Riegelman, S. (1982). Stereoselective disposition and glucuronidation of propranolol in humans. *J. Pharmacol. Sci.* **71**, 699–704.

Simmonds, R. G., Woodage, T. J., Duff, S. M. and Green, J. N. (1980). Stereospecific inversion of (R)-$(-)$-benoxaprofen in rat and man. *Eur. J. Drug Metabol. Pharmacokin.* **5**, 169–172.

Simonyi, M. (1984). On chiral drug action. *Med. Res. Rev.* **4**, 359–413.

Smith, E. F., Kinter, L. B., Jugus, M., Eckardt, R. D. and Newton, J. F. (1989). Concentration-dependent stereoselective inhibition of the endotoxin-induced hemoconcentration in conscious rats with the peptidoleukotriene receptor antagonist SK&F 104353. *Eicosanoids* **2**, 101–107.

Spahn, H., Iwakawa, S. Benet, L. Z. and Lin, E. T. (1987). Influence of probenecid on the urinary excretion rates of the diastereomeric benoxaprofen glucuronides. *Eur. J. Drug. Metabol. Pharmacokinet.* **12**, 233–237.

Testa, B. (1989). Mechanism of chiral recognition in xenobiotic metabolism and drug-receptor interactions. *Chirality* **1**, 7–9.

Thibonnier, M., Holford, N. H. G., Upton, R. A., Blume, C. D. and Williams, R. L. (1984). Pharmacokinetic–pharmacodynamic analysis of unbound disopyramide directly measured in serial plasma samples in man. *J. Pharmacokinet. Bipharmacol.* **12**, 559–573.

Tobert, J. A., Cirillo, V. J., Hitzenberger, G., James, I., Pryor, J., Cook, T., Buntinx, A., Holmes, I. B. and Lutterbeck, P. M. (1981). Enhancement of uricosuric properties of indacrinone by manipulation of the enantiomer ratio. *Clin. Pharmacol. Ther.* **29**, 344–350.

Toon, S. and Trager, W. F. (1984). Pharmacokinetic implications of stereoselective change in plasma–protein binding: warfarin–sulfenpyrazone. *J. Pharmacol. Sci.* **73**, 1671–1673.

Toon, S., Low, L. K., Gibaldi, M., Trager, W. F., O'Reilly, R. A., Motley, C. H. and Goulart, D. A. (1986). The warfarin–sulfinpyrazone interaction: stereochemical considerations. *Clin. Pharmacol. Ther.* **39**, 15–24.

Toon, S., Hopkins, K. G., Garstang, F. M. and Rowland, M. (1987). Comparative effects of ranitidine and cimetidine on the pharmacokinetics and pharmacodynamics of warfarin in man. *Eur. J. Clin. Pharmacol.* **32**, 165–172.

Tucker, G. T. and Lennard, M. S. (1990). Enantiomer specific pharmacokinetics. *Pharmacol. Ther.* **45**, 309–329.

Vlasses, P. H., Irvin, Huber, P. B., Lee, R. B., Ferguson, R. K., Schrogie, J. J., Zacchei, A. G., Davies, R. O. and Abrams, W. B. (1981). Clinical pharmacology of the enantiomers and $(-)$-p-hydroxy-metabolites of indacrinone. *Clin. Pharmacol. Ther.* **29**, 798–807.

Wade, D. N., Mearrick, P. T. and Morris, J. L. (1973). Active transport of L-dopa in the intestine. *Nature* **242**, 463–465.

Wainer, I. W. and Marcotte, A. L. (1988). Stereochemical terms and concepts: an overview. In *Drug Stereochemistry—Analytical Methods and Pharmacology* (eds I. W. Wainer and D. E. Drayer), pp. 31–41. Marcel Dekker, New York.

Walle, T., Webb, J. G., Bagwell, E. E., Walle, U. K., Daniell, H. B. and Gaffney, T. E. (1988). Stereoselective delivery and actions of beta receptor antagonists. *Biochem. Pharmacol.* **37**, 115–124.

Wan, S. H., Matin, S. B. and Azarnoff, D. L. (1978). Kinetics, salivary excretion of amphetamine isomers, and effect of urinary pH. *Clin. Pharmacol. Ther.* **23**, 585–590.

Ward, S. A., Walle, T., Walle, U. K., Wilkinson, G. R. and Branch, R. A. (1989). Propranolol's metabolism is determined by both mephenytoin and debrisoquin hydroxylase activities. *Clin. Pharmacol. Ther.* **45**, 72–79.

Weissinger, J. (1989). Considerations in the development of stereoisomeric drugs: FDA viewpoint. *Drug Inf. J.* **23**, 663–667.

White, P. F., Ham, J., Way, W. L. and Trevor, A. J. (1980). Pharmacology of ketaminine isomers in surgical patients. *Anesthesiology* **52**, 231–239.

Wichelhaus, H., Knorr, L. and Duisberg, C. (1919). Emil Fischers verdienste um die Deutsche Chemische Gesellschaft. *Chem. Ber.* **52**, 129–168.

Wilkinson, G. R. and Shand, D. G. (1975). A physiological approach to hepatic drug clearance. *Clin. Pharmacol. Ther.* **18**, 377–390.

Williams, K. M. (1984). Kinetics of misonidazole enantiomers. *Clin. Pharmacol. Ther.* **36**, 817–823.

Williams, K. and Lee, E. (1985). Importance of drug enantiomers in clinical pharmacology. *Drugs.* **30**, 333–354.

Wingard, L. B., O'Reilly, R. A. and Levy, G. (1978). Pharmacokinetics of warfarin enantiomers; a search for intrasubject correlations. *Clin. Pharmacol. Ther.* **23**, 212–217.

Yacobi, A. and Levy, G. (1977). Protein binding of warfarin enantiomers in serum of humans and rats. *J. Pharmacokinet. Biopharmacol.* **5**, 123–131.

Yamada, H., Ichihashi, T., Hirano, K. and Kinoshita, H. (1981). Plasma protein binding and urinary excretion of *R* and *S* epimers of an arylmalonylamino-1-oxacephem. I: In humans. *J. Pharmacol. Sci.* **70**, 112–113.

2

Racemic Therapeutics—Problems all Along the Line

E. J. ARIENS
Groenewoudseweg 45, 6524 TP Nijmegen, The Netherlands

1 Introduction

The concept of stereochemistry and stereoselectivity in biological processes goes back to Pasteur and van't Hoff–Le Bel about 100 years ago. In their memoirs (Pasteur, 1901) Pasteur stated:

> Most natural organic products, the essential products of life are asymmetric and possess such asymmetry that they are not superposable on their images ... This establishes perhaps the only well marked line of dermarcation that can at present be drawn between the chemistry of dead matter and the chemistry of living matter.

Chirality, stereoselectivity and stereospecific production of chemicals are characteristics of nature. Many of the xenobiotics obtained by organic synthesis are also chiral. Contrary to natural products, synthetic chiral compounds are usually obtained as isomeric mixtures such as racemates. This situation rapidly changed with the development of stereospecific catalytic methods and the application of biotechnological methods which rely on the help of enzymes as catalysts. Stereospecific syntheses and/or separation of stereoisomers were, and to a certain extent still are, laborious tasks. As a consequence, most of the synthetic chiral agents applied as drugs are marketed as racemic mixtures or, in general, as mixtures of isomers, which illustrates that the line of demarcation between the chemistry of dead and living matter postulated by Pasteur still holds largely true for producers of drugs and pesticides (Fig. 1) (Ariens, 1990).

CHIRALITY IN DRUG DESIGN AND SYNTHESIS
ISBN 0-12-136670-7

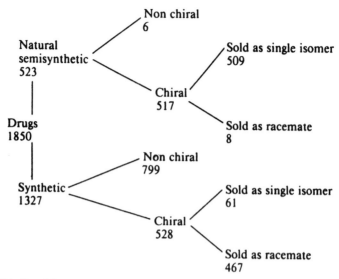

Fig. 1   Chirality of drugs: their application as single isomers or racemates. Products of natural origin are predominantly chiral and applied as single isomers found in nature. The few racemates originate from racemization of single-isomer natural products. Of the chiral synthetics, usually obtained as racemates, only 61 are applied as single isomers, 467, *ca.* 25% of the total number of drugs, is applied as racemic fixed ration mixtures. Derived from Kleeman and Engel (1982) and Bailey (1983–1986).

2   Implications of chirality in bioactive agents

Enantiomers, as indicated, usually differ greatly in their biological properties. This holds true for both dynamic (the desired and undesired actions) and kinetic properties, the latter particularly for the rate of enzymatic conversion, transport by carriers, protein binding and thus for distribution and elimination. Enantiomers must therefore be considered as essentially different chemical compounds. The distinction between 'active' and 'inactive' enantiomers is misleading. The enantiomer most potent for a particular, e.g. the desired, action is called the *eutomer* and the other one— often poorly active—is called the *distomer*. The distomer sometimes clearly contributes to undesired actions and can never be regarded as fully harmless. Isomers that do not contribute to the desired action are to be considered as undesired byproducts, or 'isomeric ballast', in drugs and pesticides.

Two important parameters have to be taken into consideration: the eudismic ratio and the eudismic proportion.

The *eudismic ratio* is the ratio of the activities or dynamics of the eutomer and distomer. The ratio usually differs for the components of the desired and undesired actions generated at different sites of action (receptors) (Lehmann *et al.*, 1976). The ratio is specific for a particular racemate in relation to a particular action and is only rarely equal to 1. The eudismic ratio tends to be large if the eutomer is highly potent, a phenomenon known as Pfeiffer's rule (Lehmann *et al.*, 1976; Ariens *et al.*, 1988a,b).

The *eudismic proportion* is the proportion of the concentrations of eutomer and distomer, [eut]/[dist], in, for instance, plasma. It is of particular significance in kinetics. In conversion of the enantiomers, this proportion will only exceptionally be equal to 1. For a racemate the eudismic proportion is 1 by definition. After absorption, among other things due to stereoselectivity in metabolic conversion, the eudismic proportion gradually changes until a steady state is reached for each of the isomers involved. Strictly speaking, there is no longer racemate in the body fluids. An exception is a rapid *in vivo* racemization. Whether the eutomer or the distomer is preferentially eliminated, or whether the eudismic proportion changes to values larger than or smaller than 1, can only be detected by means of chiral assays. The plasma concentration after application of a racemate, measured by non-chiral assays, only gives information on the *sum* of the eutomer and distomer and, since the eudismic proportion changes with time, is not related in a clear way to the response. The same holds true for pharmacokinetic constants such as the half-life of the 'racemate' which is in fact a fiction. The various pharmacokinetic constants, such as half-life, bioavailability and persistence, derived from 'racemate' concentrations based on non-chiral assays are comparable to parameters such as the age or body weight of a married couple. Suppose this is 125 years and 140 kg: what does it say about the age or body weight of the individual spouses? In the exceptional case that the eudismic ratio is 1, the eudismic proportion does not matter, but complications may still arise due to the stereoselectivity in the conversion to active metabolites.

3 Clinical pharmacology of racemic therapeutics

Neglect of stereoselectivity and, thereby, reliance on non-chiral assays in clinical pharmacology is more often the rule than the exception. Since about 25% of the therapeutics are racemates (Fig. 1) a large proportion of the studies on pharmacokinetics related to clinical evaluation of drugs is heavily biased (Ariens *et al.*, 1982, 1988b; Ariens and Wuis, 1987; Ariens, 1990). Usually the composite character, e.g. the racemic nature of bioactive products, is concealed in scientific publications and industrial information bulletins. This concealment begins the moment the product leaves the industrial laboratory. This is even more amazing since the many reviews on the chirality of drugs and pesticides, such as the series of articles on chirality in *TIPS*, of which Abbott (1986) is scientific editor, and Ariens *et al.*, 1982, 1988a, b; Ariens, 1984; Drayer, 1986; Ariens and Wuis, 1987; Wainer and Drayer, 1988; Jamali *et al.*, 1989; Smith, 1989, clearly illustrate stereo-selectivity in action and the broad spectrum of possibilities in this respect. In clinical pharmacology, particularly hospital pharmacy, there is still a kind of taboo on chirality. This goes so far that, usually on the basis of the fictitious plasma concentrations of the 'racemate' by means of computer-assisted curve fitting (based on mathematical equations derived and valid only for single compounds), impressive tables of pharmacokinetic constants of the racemate concerned are presented. Multicompartment systems for racemates are derived by computer-assisted fitting of postulated compart-ment systems to the multiphasic decline in the plasma concentration of the drug. Due to the great similarity in the physico-chemical characteristics of the enantiomers, their distributions based on passive transport will not differ. Processes such as protein binding, active transport and enzymatic conversion tend to be stereoselective such that the comparti-mental rate constants for the enantiomers differ. The eudismic proportions, i.e. the composition of the 'racemate', in the various compartments then differs. The number of phases in the decline of the plasma concentration increases with the number of compounds involved. Kinetics of racemates studied with non-chiral assays thus easily lead to impressive numbers of compartments. The more sophisticated the pharmacokinetic approach, for instance that based on 'systems dynamics', the more sophisticated is the nonsense generated by the neglect of stereoselectivity in the action of racemic mixtures (Rossum and Maes, 1985).

If computers could think, they would refuse to cooperate. The problem, however, is that the investigator himself is assumed to do some thinking. The data thus generated are erroneous and misleading, and, depending on the degree to which the clinician relies on it, even risky (Evans, 1988).

For a broad exemplification of the complications that may arise by the use of non-chiral methods in the study of mixtures of stereoisomers, see Ariens *et al.* (1982, 1988a, b), Ariens and Wuis (1987), Drayer (1986), Wainer and Drayer (1988), Ariens (1984), Jamali *et al.* (1989) and Smith (1989). Two examples are given here as an illustration. It is common knowledge that pharmacokinetic constants tend to differ for different routes of application and thus also for different delivery systems. This is especially true in comparisons of routes with different degrees of stereospecific presystemic elimination such as enteral, e.g. oral, vs. non-enteral, e.g. intravasal (intravenous, intraarterial, etc.), nasal, bronchial, vaginal or transdermal, application. A clear example is offered by the difference in the eudismic proportion in the plasma levels of verapamil after oral and intravenous administration to man. The eudismic ratio R/S for the negative dromotropic action on atrioventricular conduction is about 10. After oral application presystemic elimination is *ca.* 80% for the eutomer (R) and *ca.* 50% for the distomer (S) with a consequently relatively low systemic bioavailability (*ca.* 20%) for the eutomer as compared with *ca.* 50% for the distomer. The eudismic proportion in plasma is *ca.* 0.2 after oral and *ca.* 0.5 after intravenous administration. This implies that at equal 'racemate' plasma concentrations the eutomer concentration is low after oral and relatively high after intravenous administration (Vogelgesang *et al.*, 1984). For another calcium channel blocker, nivaldipine (a dihydropyridine derivative) the eudismic $(+)/(-)$ ratio for relaxation of the potassium induced contraction of dog coronary arteries is about 100 (Tokuma *et al.*, 1989). It too has a substantial presystemic elimination. Interestingly, for verapamil this elimination dominates for the eutomer while for nivaldipine this is the case for the distomer $(-)$. In man, C_{max} and AUC after oral administration the eudismic proportion in plasma is *ca.* 3. For the dog this is 3–5 but 1.5 after intravenous injection. For the male rat (oral) it is 0.6—here the elimination of the eutomer prevails—for the female it is 1. There is species, sex and route dependence in stereoselective disposition.

The reader may find out what investigation with non-chiral assays would have taught us here. The concealment of the composite character of racemates, etc., the neglect of stereospecificity in action and of chiral assays implies that important information remains hidden while useless and misleading data are generated. In a recent article on the pharmacokinetics of racemic terbutaline it is stated, among other things,

> For substances, like terbutaline, that are given as a racemate and whose enantiomers show differences in absorption and elimination it is of great experimental and clinical value to establish the enantiomer proportion after repeated dosing of the racemate. If enantiomers show differences in clearance this will not only effect the eudismic proportion at the steady state but also the time needed to reach steady conditions (Borgstrom *et al.*, 1989).

Chiral assays brought into the open remarkable implications of racemic mixtures in relation to genetic polymorphism (Meyer *et al.*, 1986), and species (El Mouelhi *et al.*, 1989), racial (Lennard *et al.*, 1989) and age (Chandler *et al.*, 1988) associated differences in pharmacokinetics. Caldwell *et al.* (1988) analysed the metabolic chiral inversion and dispositional enantioselectivity of the 2-arylpropionic acids, non-steroidal anti-inflammatory drugs (NSAIDs) and their biological consequences with highly elucidative results. Metabolic conversion of enantiomers at different rates to reactive intermediates means that positive results obtained with the microsome-dependent Ames test on racemates can be misleading. The distomer might be the culprit (Glatt and Oesch, 1988). In addition, racemic pro-drugs with different rates of conversion of the pro-eutomer and the pro-distomer may, if studied by non-chiral assay, lead to confusing results.

Two major problems arise:

(1) Avoidance of pollution of the literature on pharmacology and experimental therapeutics by preventing the neglect of the racemic nature of the drugs studied.
(2) Avoidance of medicinal pollution of patients by reduction to the scientifically feasible, technologically possible and economically acceptable limit of isomeric ballast in chiral therapeutics.

4 Ethical aspects of drug development, evaluation and use

In relation to the problems mentioned above there are two basic principles to be emphasized:

(1) 'Exposure of nature (including man) and its environment to xenobiotics (including drugs) is only justified if the desirable actions adequately compensate for the undesirable actions and the never fully excluded risks'. This implies, among other things, that one should 'Avoid isomeric ballast in therapeutics and the inherent medicinal pollution of patients'.
(2) 'In science the notion of the impossibility or inability to do things the proper way is no excuse to do them the wrong way'.

Protection of humans against the risks of exposure to xenobiotics, particularly to drugs, in todays chemistry-impregnated society received some attention in the 'World Medical Association Declaration of Helsinki'. Under 'Recommendations guiding medical doctors in biomedical research involving human subjects', it is stated under basic principles:

> 1.1 Biomedical research involving human subjects must conform to generally accepted scientific principles and should be based on adequately performed laboratory and animal experimentation and on a thorough knowledge of the scientific literature.
> 1.9 In any research on human beings each potential subject must be adequately informed about the aims, methods, anticipated benefits and potential hazards of the study, etc. [This implies 'informed consent'.]
> 1.8 Reports of experimentation not in accordance with the principles laid down in this declaration should not be accepted for publication.

There is something to be learned here by the ethical committees (the Institutional Review Boards, IRB) that supervise the evaluation of drugs on humans. Generation of invalid data in such studies must be considered unethical and thus not acceptable. In his book *Ethics and Regulation of Clinical Research*, Levine (1986) emphasizes in this relation that "research must be sufficiently well designed to achieve its purpose; otherwise it is not justified". The steady flow of heavily biased clinical studies on racemic therapeutics leaves no doubt about the deficiencies of many ethical committees and the 'misinformed' consent of patients. Addition to the committees of at least one investigator aware of the implications of chirality is required. Practice shows that at present the participation of hospital pharmacists in the ethical committees is no guarantee.

A simple and effective way to stop pollution of the literature with non-science generated in the study of racemic mixtures, etc., is the extension of the instructions to authors with an indication that:

> The composite character of drugs which are mixtures of stereoisomers must be brought to the attention of the reader. The prefix (RS)- or rac-, e.g. rac-propranolol, in the case of racemates and (Z/E)- or cis/trans- in the case of that type of isomers is obligatory. The implications of the composite and chiral nature of the drugs for the interpretation of the data measured and the conclusions drawn must be made explicit.

5 Non-information and disinformation in the field of chirality

As indicated above, in most scientific publications as well as industrial information bulletins dealing with racemic products the implications of the chiral composite nature of these products is neglected or even concealed. This as a matter of fact has its reasons and roots. In hardly any of the clinically orientated textbooks on pharmacology, pharmacokinetics or toxicology—including the highly recommended ones—are principles such as stereoselectivity, stereospecificity and stereochemistry paid attention to or even mentioned in the index. Pharmacokinetic parameters, particularly half-life and bioavailability, for racemic therapeutics derived from plasma concentrations measured with non-chiral assays, and thus largely senseless, are amply presented (Ariens et al., 1988b). The reader may consult the library to be convinced and astonished.

Goodman and Gilman (1985) present 65 pages (pp. 1668–1733) of pharmacokinetic constants for therapeutics, roughly a quarter of which are racemates. Almost without exception the constants are based on plasma levels determined with non-chiral assays. This means fiction anyway. The addition of the prefixes rac- or (RS)- to drug names in this case, as well as in most other textbooks, would only make the pharmacokinetic nonsense more sophisticated. The fictitious kinetic data should be eliminated; sufficient room would then be available for a discussion of stereoselectivity in action and its implications. The apparent stereophobia among teachers in the field should be combatted. Or do we have to wait for a new generation of educators?* These then hopefully will not leave their students with the false idea that something like 'plasma concentrations and pharmacokinetic parameters of racemates' really exists. What is real are plasma concentrations, etc., of the individual stereoisomers and their continuously changing eudismic proportion. For the many hundreds of therapeutic agents registered over the past 20 years, regulatory authorities have required pharmacokinetic data—including the hundreds of racemates among them. Such data with few exceptions were based on non-chiral assays and are thus practically worthless. The bill, many hundreds if not some billions of dollars, in the end was paid by the patients.

It is often difficult to locate proper information on chirality and the chiral properties of chemicals. As noted by Drayer (1987) and confirmed by the author the various reference books including the Merck index, 10th edn, pay no attention to the racemic nature of therapeutic racemates. A data source on, in particular, chiral bioactive products such as drugs, pesticides and toxic agents in general is badly needed.

6 Racemates as drug combinations

For fixed ratio combinations, for instance of an antihypertensive β-blocker and a saluretic, the authorities require full information on both components in the mixture as well as on the mixture as such. It would make sense to follow a similar approach in the case of mixtures of stereoisomers. Such information would make clear when—as often will be the case—the single eutomer or the racemic mixture is to be preferred. One should take into account that even in the exceptional case where there is some form of synergism between the stereoisomers, their proportion in the 1 : 1 racemate will only rarely be optimal. The proportion of an antihypertensive and a diuretic in a fixed ratio combination is not blindly chosen as 1 : 1 but is critically optimalized. For the racemic diuretic indacrinone the distomer with regard to the diuretic action antagonizes a side-effect, namely uric acid retention of the eutomer. The optimal eudismic proportion is found to be about 8 (Tobert et al., 1981). The question arises whether a well-balanced combination of a known non-chiral diuretic and a known non-chiral uricosuric is to be preferred. The idea that the pharmacokinetics of synergistic enantiomers in the racemate would be better synchronized than

---

* Happily, in British schools at least, the subject of chirality is already being introduced even at this level, and is certainly actively taught in all undergraduate chemistry courses: perhaps we can look forward to this subject receiving more attention in biomedical teaching soon—Editor.

for the case of a fixed ratio drug combination does not hold true. The enantiomers usually differ in pharmacokinetics.

In cases where the eudismic ratio for the therapeutic action is approximately 1, one has to take into account that this may not be the case for adverse effects that are not inherent to the mechanism of therapeutic action. Side-effects such as allergic reactions, mutagenic actions and embryotoxicity, but also e.g. intestinal side-effects of cardiovascular therapeutics, may be distributed over the enantiomers in a way different from the desired action. One should consider reevaluation in this respect in particular racemic therapeutics with a high incidence of side-effects such as Tocainide and Mexiletine, antiarrhythmics having a *ca.* 40% incidence of non-cardiac side-effects (Table 1) (Grech-Belanger *et al.*, 1986; Morganroth, 1987; Powel, 1988).

In cases where the eudismic ratio for the therapeutic action and for the side-effects is practically 1, or where as a result of a particular synergism between the enantiomers there is no isomeric ballast, complications may still arise from, for instance, stereoselective activation or toxification. Encainide is converted to active metabolites with a relatively long half-life which produce qualitatively different electrophysiological changes (Roden and Woosley, 1988).

Again, for the many types of complications that may arise from chirality in drug action and drug metabolism the reader is referred to the various reviews (Ariens *et al.* 1982, 1988a, b; Ariens, 1984; Drayer, 1986; Ariens and

Table 1 'New' antiarrhythmics

| | VPC patients efficacy[a] (%) | | Side-effect (%) | | | Potential for organ toxicity |
| | | | Proarrhythmia[f] | | | |
Drug	B or PL	MVA	VPC	MVA	Non-cardiac	
Tocainide[d]	40	15	2	3	40[b]	+++
Mexiletine[d]	40	15	2	3	40[b]	+
Encainide[e]	80	25	>1	10	10[c]	−

[a] VPC, ventricular premature complex; MVA, malignant ventricular arrhythmia; B or PL, benign or potentially lethal.
[b] Gastrointestinal and neurological.
[c] Blurred vision.
[d] Enantiomeric differences in metabolic conversion.
[e] Formation of active metabolites.
[f] Includes an estimate of serious and potentially life-threatening proarrhythmic effects only (Morganroth, 1987).

Table 2   The cascade of inadequacy in the generation of non-science in the study of racemic drugs

---

Pharmaceutical industry
Concealment of the racemic fixed-ratio character of products presented for research and evaluation.
Lack of stereoselective analytical methods required for proper investigation of racemic drugs.

Investigators, clinicians and/or hospital pharmacists
Proposals for research projects scientifically deficient due to the neglect of the racemic nature of the drug(s) to be studied.

Funding institutions
Poor judgement in the evaluation of and thus granting of funds for scientifically deficient research projects by the advisory experts and peers.

Ethics committees
Overlooking the fact that the generation of invalid data—in the evaluation of racemic therapeutics in studies on patients is unethical as is the implicit 'misinformed consent' obtained from the patient.

Investigators, clinicians and/or hospital pharmacists
Neglect of stereoselectivity in pharmacodynamics and pharmacokinetics in the study of racemic fixed-ratio mixtures.
Calculation of pharmacokinetic constants and derivation of multicompartment systems for such mixtures on basis of mostly non-existent plasma concentrations of the racemate with the use of equations valid only for single agents.
Presentation of dubious and strongly biased research reports and manuscripts for publication due to disregard of the racemic fixed-ratio nature of the therapeutic(s) studied.

Editorial boards and referees of scientific journals
Lack of the expertise required for proper evaluation of manuscripts dealing with studies on racemic drugs.

Prize-awarding agencies
Promotion of non-science by erroneous rewarding of astereognosis in the study of racemic agents.

IUPHAR, FIP and APhA[a]
Negligence in not taking adequate steps to stop or at least discourage pollution of scientific literature in the field of pharmacology and therapeutics due to neglect of stereoselectivity in the action of drugs.

Teachers and textbook writers
Neglect of stereochemistry in educational programmes, thus closing the vicious circle in the maintenance of a steady flow of astereognostic non-science in the field of pharmacology and therapeutics.

Regulatory authorities
Acceptance of invalid data based on non-chiral assays in the admission of racemic therapeutics, thus causing a large waste of money and research capacity and facilitating continuation of medicinal pollution of patients via isomeric ballast in their medicines.

---

[a] IUPHAR, International Union of Pharmacology; FIP, Fédération Internationale Pharmaceutique; APhA, American Pharmaceutical Association.

Wuis, 1987; Wainer and Drayer, 1988; Jamali *et al.*, 1989; Smith, 1989). Implications of the neglect of stereoselectivity in the pharmacology and experimental therapeutics of racemates is summarized in Table 2. The literature is rich in examples like the many studies on, for instance, β-adrenergic agents, adrenoreceptor blockers, combined β- and α-adreno-receptor blockers, calcium channel blockers, non-steroidal antiphlogistic agents, etc. Soons *et al.* (1989) give an example particularly suitable for instruction since it matches Table 2 quite closely. It even was awarded the 'Pharmatec prize' for its outstanding scientific qualities! This under the auspices of the Féderation Internationale Pharmaceutique (FIP).

For the investigation and evaluation of racemic therapeutics chiral assays are inevitable already for proper pre-clinical study. Industry definitely should supply clinical investigators involved in the evaluation of their racemic therapeutics in patients with the necessary stereoselective analytical tools. They should at least avoid generation of misleading data and under no circumstances should they conceal the composite nature of their products.

7 Perspectives

The climate is changing. Japan, in a leading position, in 1987 adopted requirements for racemic products. Full pharmacology and toxicology is required for each of the enantiomers and for the racemate. As a matter of fact, for the latter only kinetic data based on chiral assays should and probably will be accepted. The European Economic Community (EEC) in *The Rules Governing Medicinal Products in the European Community*, Vol. II, 1989, extended the section on stereoisomerism. It states:

> Possible problems relating to stereoisomerism, which should be discussed in the appropriate Expert Report and cross referenced, should include: the batch to batch consistency of the ratio of stereoisomers in the various batches used—the toxicological issues—the pharmacological aspects (including evidence on which stereoisomers have the desired pharmacological properties)—pharmacokinetics including information on the relative metabolism of the stereoisomers—extrapolation of the pre-clinical data (paying particular attention to possible problems relating to species differences in handling of the stereoisomers)—the significant clinical issues.

This at least opens the possibility to require essential information on each of the enantiomers or stereoisomers in general as well as on the racemate or in general composite chiral products. Chiral assays will, strictly taken, be inevitable. Further it is stated that

> Where a mixture of stereoisomers has previously been marketed and it is now proposed to market a product containing only one isomer, full data on this isomer should be provided. The US authorities (FDA) still have the matter in consideration.

This change in policy will at least strongly reduce if not eliminate the flow of heavily biased articles in the scientific literature as far as new products are concerned. Table 2 will still be applicable to most investigations and publications on the hundreds of racemic therapeutics already on the market, unless the editorial boards of the scientific journals come to the conclusion reached now by the regulatory authorities and decide to stop the pollution of scientific literature. The participants in the cascade presented in Table 2 have an output large enough to warrant a new journal. 'Current Nonsense in Pharmacology and Experimental Therapy'. There is an alternative solution. The definition of 'Isomeric ballast' as the isomer(s) in the mixture that does not contribute to the desired action, taking into account that no chemical (isomer) is absolutely free of risks, combined with the principle that 'exposure of nature (including man) and its environment to xenobiotics (including drugs) is only justified if the desirable actions adequately compensate for the undesirable actions and the never fully excluded risks' implies: 'avoid isomeric ballast in therapeutics and the inherent medicinal pollution of patients'. A further consequence of this is that therapeutics polluted by isomeric ballast should be withdrawn from the market as soon as ballast-free preparations are available at an acceptable price. Often only a small fraction of the price paid in the pharmacy is related to that for the drug substance in the product. The approach indicated should apply to generics as well as to brand products. The resulting incentive for the innovative industry and the rapid development of chiral techniques in chemistry can help us to reduce the pollution of patients.

The recognition of these problems had to wait for 100 years after Pasteur generated the basic insights. It should not take another 100 years to eliminate polluting isomeric ballast from therapeutics, although the perspectives in this respect are not very encouraging.

8 Summary

Racemic therapeutics are in fact fixed ratio mixtures of stereoisomers, biologically to be regarded as different compounds. Usually only one of the isomers fully contributes to the therapeutic action whereas the other often is to be classified as a medicinal pollutant. Due to differences in the turnover, in pharmacokinetics the proportion of the enantiomers (1 : 1 in the racemate) continuously changes in plasma. The implications of the neglect of stereoselectivity at the various levels in the investigation of racemic drugs are elucidated, discussed and summarized in the 'cascade of inadequacy' (Table 2).

The fact that clinicians and regulatory authorities have been content for decennia with invalid pharmacokinetic data on *ca.* 25% of the therapeutics (the racemates) in use, makes the benefit of and need for kinetics in general questionable. Biopharmacists, in particular hospital pharmacists, might be invited to review in a critical way their contribution over the past 10 years to pharmacokinetics of racemic therapeutics, a major topic in their field of research.

Chemical pollution of the *milieu interne* of patients by the isomeric ballast present in about 25% of the drugs already on the market will go on for many decennia. For new chiral drugs the choice between using the racemate or the single compound will hopefully be based on a critical evaluation of the chiral characteristics both therapeutically and toxicologically. Whether pollution of the scientific literature based on non-chiral pharmacokinetic studies of racemic drugs will continue is largely in the hands of the editorial boards. Whether violation of fundamental rights of patients as formulated in the Helsinki conventions will continue largely depends on the ethical attitude of clinical investigators and their pharmaceutical and industrial informants.

References

Abbott, A. (1986). Series on Chirality TIPS. 7, 20–24, 60–65, 112–115, 155–158, 200–205, 227–230, 281–301.

Ariens, E. J. (1984). Stereochemistry, a basis for sophisticated nonsense in pharmacokinetics and clinical pharmacology. *Eur. J. Clin. Pharmacol.* 26, 663–668.

Ariens, E. J. (1990). Stereoselectivity in pharmacodynamics and pharmacokinetics. *Schweiz. med. Wschr.* 120, 131–134.

Ariens, E. J. and Wuis, E. W. (1987). Bias in pharmacokinetics and clinical pharmacology. *Clin. Pharmacol. Ther.* 42, 361–363.

Ariens, E. J., Soudijn, W. and Timmermans, P. B. M. W. M. (1982). *Stereochemistry and Biological Activity of Drugs*, pp. 1–19. Oxford: Blackwell Scientific Publications.

Ariens, E. J., Rensen, J. J. S. and Welling, W. (1988a). *Stereoselectivity of Pesticides—Biological and Chemical Problems.* Elsevier, Amsterdam.

Ariens, E. J., Wuis, E. W. and Veringa, E. J. (1988b). Stereoselectivity of bioactive xenobiotics. A pre-Pasteur attitude in medicinal chemistry, pharmacokinetics and clinical pharmacology. *Biochem. Pharmacol.* 37, 9–18.

Bailey, D. M. (ed.) (1983–1986). *Annual Reports in Medicinal Chemistry*, Vols 19–21. Academic Press, London.

Borgstrom, L., Chang Xiao, L. and Walhagen, A. (1989). Pharmacokinetics of the enantiomers of terbutaline after repeated oral dosing with racemic terbutaline. *Chirality* 1, 174–177.

Caldwell, J., Hutt, A. J. and Fournel-Gigleux, S. (1988). The metabolic chiral inversion and dispositional enantioselectivity of the 2-arylpropionic acids and their biological consequences. *Biochem. Pharmacol.* 37, 105–114.

Chandler, M. H. H., Scott, S. R. and Blouin, R. A. (1988). Age-associated stereoselective alterations in hexobarbital metabolism. *Clin. Pharmacol. Ther.* 43, 436–441.

Drayer, D. E. (1986). Pharmacodynamic and pharmacokinetic differences between drug enantiomers in humans: an overview. *Clin. Pharmacol. Ther.* **40**, 125–133.

Drayer, D. E. (1987). On the use of drugs administered as racemates. *Clin. Pharmacol. Ther.* **42**, 364.

El Mouelhi, M., Ruelius, H. W., Fenselau, C. and Dulik, D. M. (1987). Species-dependent enantioselective glucuronidation of three 2-arylpropionic acids. *Drug Metab. Dispos.* **15**, 767–772.

Evans, A. M. (1988). Stereoselective drug disposition: potential for misinterpretation of drug disposition data. *Br. J. Clin. Pharmacol.* **26**, 771–780.

Glatt, H. and Oesch, F. (1988). Mutagenicity of cysteine and penicillamine and its enantiomeric selectivity. *Biochem. Pharmacol.* **34**, 3725–3728.

Goodman and Gilman (1985). 7th edn.

Grech-Belanger, O., Turgeon, J. and Gilbert, M. (1986). Stereoselective disposition of mexiletine in man. *Br. J. Clin. Pharmacol.* **21**, 481–487.

Jamali, F., Mehvar, R. and Pasutto, F. M. (1989). Enantioselective aspects of drug action and disposition. Therapeutic Pitfalls. *J. Pharm. Sci.* **78**, 695–715.

Kleeman, A. and Engel, J. (1982). *Pharmazeutische Wirkstoffe.* Thieme Verlag, Stüttgart.

Lehmann, F. P. A., Rodrigues De Miranda, J. F. and Ariens, E. J. (1976). Stereoselectivity and affinity in molecular pharmacology. In *Progress Research* (ed. E. Jucker, Vol. 20, pp. 101–142, Birkhauser Verlag, Basel.

Lennard, M. S., Tucker, G. T., Woods, H. F., Silas, J. H. and Iyun, A. O. (1989). Stereoselective metabolism of metoprolol in Caucasians and Nigerians—relationship to debrisoquine oxidation phenotype. *Br. J. Clin. Pharmacol.* **27**, 613–616.

Levine, R. J. (1986). *Ethics and Regulation of Clinical Research*, 2nd edn, pp. 393–429. Urban & Schwarzenberg Baltimore.

Meyer, U. A., Gut, J., Kronbach, I., Skoda, C., Meier, U. T. and Catin, T. (1986). The molecular mechanisms of two common polymorphisms of drug oxidation—evidence for functional changes in cytochrome P-450 isoenzymes catalysing bufuralol and mephenytoin oxidation. *Xenobiotica* **16**, 449–464.

Morganroth, J. (1987). New antiarrhythmic agents: mexiletine, tocainide, flecainide, encainide and amiodarone. *Rational Drug Ther. Am. Soc. Pharmacol. Exp. Therap.*, **21**, 1–5.

Pasteur, L. (1901). On the asymmetry of naturally occurring organic compounds, the foundations of stereochemistry. In *Memoirs by Pasteur, Van t'Hoff, Le Bel and Wislicenus* (ed. G. M. Richardson), pp. 1–33.

Powel, J. R. (1988). The efficacy and toxicity of drug stereoisomers. In *Drug Stereochemistry* (ed. I. W. Wainer and D. E. Drayer), p. 245. Marcel Dekker, New York.

Roden, D. M. and Woosley, R. L. (1988). Clinical pharmacokinetics of encainide. *Clin. Pharmacokin.* **14**, 141–147.

Rossum, J. M. and Maes, R. A. A. (1985). *Pharmacokinetics: Classic and Modern*, pp. 1–162. VCH Verlagsgesellschaft mbH, Weinheim.

Soons, P. A., De Boer, A. G., Van Brummelen, P. and Breimer, D. D. (1989). Oral absorption profile of nitrendipine in healthy subjects: a kinetic and dynamic study. *Br. J. Clin. Pharmacol.* **27**, 179–189.

Smith, D. F. (1989). The stereoselectivity of drug action. *Pharmacol. Toxicol.* **65**, 321–331.

Tobert, J. A., Cirillo, V. J., Hitzenberger, G., James, I., Pryor, J., Cook, T., Buntinx, A., Holmes, I. B. and Lutterbeck, P. M. (1981). Enhancement of uricosuric properties of indacrinone by manipulation of the enantiomer ratio. *Clin. Pharmacol. Ther.* **29**, 344–350.

Tokuma, Y., Fujiwara, T., Niwa, T., Hashimoto, T. and Noguchi, H. (1989). Stereoselective disposition of nivaldipine, a new dihydropyridine calcium antagonist, in the rat and dog. *Res. Comm. Chem. Pathol. Pharmacol.* **63**, 249–262.

Vogelgesang, B., Echizen, H., Schmidt, E. and Eichelbaum, M. (1984). Stereoselective first-pass metabolism of highly cleared drugs: studies of the bioavailability of L- and D-verapamil examined with a stable isotope technique. *Br. J. Clin. Pharmacol.* **18**, 733–740.

Wainer, I. W. and Drayer, D. E. (1988). *Drug Stereochemistry, Analytical Methods and Pharmacology.* Marcel Dekker, New York.

3

Chirality, Drug Metabolism and Action

DONALD S. DAVIES

Department of Clinical Pharmacology, Royal Postgraduate Medical School, London W12 0NN, UK

1 Introduction

Molecules which possess a chiral centre exist in two forms (enantiomers) which are indistinguishable in terms of most of their chemical and physical properties. However, when chiral compounds are placed in a chiral environment differences between enantiomers become evident.

Biological systems are largely constructed from chiral molecules such as L amino acids or D sugars. In this highly chiral environment it is not surprising that some drugs, which possess an asymmetric centre or centres exhibit a high degree of stereoselectivity in their interactions with biological macromolecules. Stereoselectivity in drug action at specific receptors, with ion channels or enzymes, is well-known (Timmermans, 1983). However, stereoselective drug action is by no means the rule. Antiarrhythmic drugs such as flecainide appear not to exhibit stereoselectivity in action on sodium channels in the heart or isolated Purkinje fibres. Enantiomers may exhibit similar, opposing or different actions, sometimes at the same receptor. For example, the antihypertensive agent labetol is both an α- and β-adrenoceptor antagonist. The drug possesses two chiral centres and is used as a mixture of four diastereoisomers. The R,R form provides most of the β-blocking activity whilst the S,R diastereoisomer is an α-receptor antagonist. The S,S and R,S forms do not contribute significantly to the pharmacology of the drug (Brittain *et al.*, 1982).

In recent years stereoselectivity in drug disposition and metabolism have emerged as important variables in the action or toxicity of some drugs (Caldwell *et al.*, 1988a) and complicating the interpretation of plasma concentration data in relation to therapeutic effect.

CHIRALITY IN DRUG DESIGN AND SYNTHESIS
ISBN 0-12-136670-7

2   Stereochemistry and drug disposition

Drug disposition in which the drug molecule interacts specifically with a chiral biological macromolecule may exhibit stereoselectivity. However, a number of the events involved in the disposition of drugs in an organism do not involve specific interactions.

2.1   Drug absorption

The vast majority of drugs are absorbed from the intestine, the airways or through the skin by passive diffusion of the unionized form of the drug across lipid membranes. The diffusion is controlled by the degree of ionization of the drug (determined by the pK_a) at the site of absorption and the lipid solubility of the unionized form, two parameters which do not show stereoselectivity. A small number of drugs are actively transported across the intestinal wall and, since this involves a specific interaction with a chiral macromolecule, stereoselectivity in absorption may be observed. Two drugs which exhibit this phenomenon are methotrexate (Hendel and Brodthagen, 1984) and dopa (Wade et al., 1973); the L enantiomers of these drugs are actively absorbed but the D forms cross the intestine by passive diffusion.

2.2   Drug distribution

As with drug absorption, most drugs penetrate organs or cross the blood–brain barrier by passive diffusion, a process not influenced by the stereochemical nature of the molecule. However, for a very small number of drugs, distribution involves active processes and specific interactions with chiral macromolecules. The S enantiomer of propranolol is selectively bound in the heart (Bai et al., 1983), whilst the R isomers of 2-arylpropionic acids such as ibuprofen are selectively incorporated into adipose tissue (Williams et al., 1986).

2.3   Protein binding

The majority of drugs are reversibly bound to proteins in plasma and it is generally assumed that drug action is related to the unbound concentration in plasma water. For highly bound ($>95\%$) drugs minor differences in the plasma protein binding of enantiomers may have a significant effect on the enantiomeric composition of the drug in plasma water and hence on drug action. Acidic drugs which bind to albumin exhibit stereoselectivity as do basic drugs binding to α_1-acid glycoprotein (Muller, 1988). Stereoselective displacement of (R)-warfarin from albumin by sulfinpyrazone is part of the complex interaction between these two drugs (see below) and leads to increased clearance of the R isomer (Toon et al., 1986).

2.4   Renal excretion

Renal clearance is a major route of elimination for a number of drugs and thus stereoselectivity in the process may have important effects on the intensity and duration of drug action. Glomerular filtration is not stereoselective but only free drug in plasma water is filtered. Stereoselective protein binding, leading to a difference in the enantiomeric composition of drug in plasma water will result in isomers exhibiting differences in renal clearance by glomerular filtration.

Drugs which are cleared by active secretion in the renal tubules may exhibit marked stereoselective elimination. The renal clearance of plasma quinidine is four times greater than quinine, its diastereoisomer. The renal clearance of quinidine which is free in plasma water is six-fold greater than that of creatinine, whilst that of quinine is similar to that of creatinine indicating that the quinidine, unlike its isomer, is a substrate for tubular secretory processes (Notterman et al., 1986).

2.5   Drug metabolism

Stereoselectivity is commonly encountered in the metabolism of drugs by phase I and phase II reactions (Caldwell et al., 1988a). The rate and/or route of metabolism may be stereoselective, or one enantiomer may undergo chiral inversion as is seen with 2-arylpropionic acids. Differences in rates of metabolism to the same product are not usually very great. For example, aromatic hydroxylation of propranolol is three times as rapid for the R as for the S isomer (Walle et al., 1988). However, the enantiomers of mephenytoin are oxidized at vastly different rates and by different routes. The S enantiomer is 4-hydroxylated and the R form is N-demethylated. In extensive metabolizers the half-life of the S form is 2 h, whilst that of the R enantiomer is 76 h (Wedlund et al., 1985).

The calcium channel blocker, verapamil, has a low systemic bio-availability due to extensive presystemic metabolism. Stereoselectivity in the extent of presystemic metabolism results in a five-fold greater concentration of the R isomer in plasma following oral doses (Vogelgesang et al., 1984). Since the S enantiomer is ten times as potent as the R form, stereoselective presystemic metabolism complicates the interpretation of plasma concentration–effect curves.

Chiral inversion is a rare metabolic pathway but is of considerable importance in the action and elimination of non-steroidal anti-inflammatory 2-arylpropionic acids (reviewed by Caldwell *et al.* (1988b) and Caldwell (1990)). Most 2-arylpropionic acids are used as racemates but anti-inflammatory activity resides in the *S* isomer. The inactive *R* forms undergo chiral inversion, the extent being dependent upon substrate and species. As a consequence, the relative anti-inflammatory potencies measured *in vitro* are often not observed *in vivo*. Thus the *S* to *R* potency of 160 measured *in vitro* for ibuprofen is considerably attenuated *in vivo* (two-fold) because of the efficient unidirectional chiral inversion of *R* to *S*. Chiral inversion has been found in man with ibuprofen (Kaiser *et al.*, 1976), benoxaprofen (Bopp *et al.*, 1979), cicloprofen (Hutt and Caldwell, 1983), fenprofen (Rubin *et al.*, 1985) and thioxaprofene (Diekmann, 1979). The mechanism of the *R–S* inversion probably involves the formation of a coenzyme-A thioester of the drug followed by racemization and hydrolysis to release the drug. Since only *R* isomers form the coenzyme-A thioester the chiral inversion is unidirectional from *R* to *S*.

3 Stereoselective metabolism and drug action

It is evident that the processes of drug disposition and elimination, particularly metabolism, do exhibit stereoselectivity but does this have a significant effect on drug action or toxicity? The answer appears to be 'not frequently' and even when it does it may not greatly influence the way a drug is used.

As described above, the calcium channel blocking drug verapamil is subject to extensive presystemic metabolism when given orally and this results in a ratio of inactive *R* to active *S* isomer in plasma of 5:1. As a consequence (Table 1) for a *given* plasma concentration, verapamil appears to be three times as potent after intravenous as after oral dosing (Echizen *et al.*, 1985). In contrast, β-receptor blockade is greater for a given plasma concentration of propranolol after oral rather than intravenous doses (Table 1; Coltart and Shand, 1970). These authors attributed the observation to the presence in plasma of the β-blocking metabolite, 4-hydroxypropranolol, after oral dosing. However, a recent study (Lindner *et al.*, 1989) suggests that greater systemic bioavailability of the β-blocking *S* enantiomer is probably responsible for the discrepancy in the concentration–response curves following oral or intravenous dosing. Verapamil and propranolol provide intriguing pharmacokinetic problems but the stereoselective effects on drug kinetics do not present clinical

Table 1 Plasma concentration effect relationship after oral or intravenous administration

		Plasma concentration $(ng\,ml^{-1})$		
Drug	Effect	Intravenous	Oral	Ratio IV: oral
(R,S)-Verapamil	PR prolongation[a]	40	120	3
(R,S)-Propranolol	Inhibition of exercise[b] tachycardia	38	11	0.3

[a] 20% PR prolongation.
[b] 50% Inhibition of exercise tachycardia.

problems as drug action not plasma concentration is used to monitor therapy.

Drug–drug interactions may be stereoselective and can present complex kinetic problems. The effects of sulfinpyrazone on the metabolism of warfarin is such a case (Toon *et al.*, 1986). Sulfinpyrazone enhances the pharmacodynamic (hypoprothrombinemia) effect of racemic warfarin but does not decrease its total body clearance. However, it does decrease the clearance of the more active S form by inhibiting its oxidation. Sulfinpyrazone is a less potent inhibitor of the metabolism of R warfarin. However, since sulfinpyrazone selectively displaces the R form from binding sites on plasma proteins (see above) it increases its free concentration in plasma water, thereby attenuating the effect of enzyme inhibition on the clearance of the R form. The net result is a heightened pharmacologic effect with little or no change in the kinetics of racemic warfarin (Table 2).

Drug toxicity is often unrelated to pharmacologic effect but may be mediated through the generation of chemically reactive metabolites. Stereoselective production of toxic metabolites has not been demonstrated but the observations that optic-neuritis caused by pencillamine is probably

Table 2 Effects of sulfinpyrazone on warfarin

It enhances the pharmacodynamic effect of racemic warfarin.

It does not decrease the clearance of racemic warfarin.

It decreases the clearance of the more active S form by inhibiting its oxidation.

It has a less inhibitory effect on the metabolism of the R form.

It stereoselectively displaces the R form from protein binding, thereby increasing the free concentration and attenuating the effect of enzyme inhibition on the clearance of the R form.

through the L isomer whilst D-dopa may be responsible for the granulocytopenia initiated by that drug, suggests that further work on enantiomer-specific toxicity is warranted. However, the small number of examples suggests that this is unlikely to be a major problem.

4 Conclusions

There are no general guidelines for the development of drugs with chiral centres. A case-by-case approach must be used to evaluate safety and efficacy. The evaluation is made easier when it is known how isomers differ in their pharmacologic effects, kinetics, metabolism and toxicity profile. Other important parameters are the shape of the dose–response curve and the therapeutic index. Numerous examples of stereoselective differences in the pharmacokinetics and metabolism of drugs have been described and these complicate the interpretation of plasma concentration–effect data. However, drug therapy is very rarely dictated by plasma concentrations. Clinically significant stereoselective effects are far fewer in number. Nevertheless it would be prudent, technology and cost permitting, to use single enantiomers wherever possible.

References

Bai, S. A., Walle, U. K., Wilson, M. J. and Walle, T. (1983). Stereo-selective binding of the (−) enantiomer of propranolol to plasma and extravascular binding sites in the dog. *Drug Metab. Dispos.* **11**, 394–395.

Bopp, R. J., Nash, J. F., Ridolfo, A. S. and Shepard, E. R. (1979). Stereo-selective inversion of (*R*)-(−)-benoxaprofen to the (*S*)-(+)-enantiomer in humans. *Drug Metab. Dispos.* **7**, 356–359.

Brittain, R. T., Drew, G. M. and Levy, G. P. (1982). The alpha- and beta-adrenoceptor blocking potencies of labetalol and its individual stereoisomers. *Br. J. Pharmacol.* **77**, 105–114.

Caldwell, J., Winter, S. M. and Hutt, A. J. (1988a). The pharmacological and toxicological significance of the stereochemistry of drug disposition. *Xenobiotica* **18**, 59–70.

Caldwell, J., Hutt, A. J. and Fournel-Gigleux, S. (1988b). The metabolic chiral inversions and dispositional enantio-selectivity of the 2-aryl propionic acids and their biological consequences. *Biochem. Pharmacol.* **37**, 105–114.

Caldwell, J. (1990). Metabolic and kinetic criteria in the development of chiral drugs. In *Basic Science in Toxicology* (eds G. N. Volans, J. Sim, F. M. Sullivan and P. Turner), pp. 79–90.

Coltart, D. J. and Shand, D. G. (1970). Plasma propranolol levels in the quantitative assessment of β-adrenergic blockade in man. *Br. Med. J.* **3**, 731–734.

Diekmann, H., Garbe, A., Steiner, K., Buhring, K. U., Faro, H. P. and Nowak, H. (1979). Disposition of thixaprofene: kinetics of the stereoisomers. *Naunyn Scmiedeberg's Arch. Pharmacol.* **307**, (Suppl.) R3.

Echizen, H., Vogelgesang, B. and Eichelbaum, M. (1985). Effects of *d,l*-verapamil on atrioventricular conduction in relation to its stereo-selective first-pass metabolism. *Clin. Pharmacol. Ther.* **37**, 71–76.

Hendel, J. and Brodthagen, H. (1984). Entero-hepatic cycling of methotrexate estimated by use of the D-isomer as a reference marker. *Eur. J. Clin. Pharmacol.* **26**, 103–107.

Hutt, A. J. and Caldwell, J. (1983). The metabolic chiral inversion of 2-arylpropionic acids — a novel route with pharmacological consequences. *J. Pharm. Pharmacol.* **35**, 693–704.

Kaiser, D. G., Vangiessen, G. J., Reischer, R. J. and Wechter, W. J. (1976). Isomeric inversion of ibuprofen (*R*)-enantiomer in humans. *J. Pharm. Sci.* **65**, 269–273.

Lindner, W., Rath, M., Ftofchitzky, K., and Femmelrock, H. J. (1989). Pharmacokinetic data on Propranolol enantiomers in a comparative human study with (*S*)- and (*R,S*)-Propranolol. *Chirality* **1**, 10–13.

Muller, W. E. (1988). Stereo-selective plasma protein binding of drugs. In *Drug Stereochemistry* (eds I. W. Wainer and D. E. Drayer), pp. 227–244. Marcel Dekker, New York.

Notterman, D. A., Drayer, D. E., Metakis, L. and Reidenberg, M. M. (1986). Stereo-selective renal tubular secretion of quinidine and quinine. *Clin. Pharmacol. Ther.* **40**, 511–517.

Rubin, A., Knadler, M. P., Ho, P. P. K., Bechtol, L. D. and Wolen, R. L. (1985). Stereoselective inversion of (*R*)-fenoprofen to (*S*)-fenoprofen in humans. *J. Pharm. Sci.* **74**, 82–84.

Timmermans, P. B. M. W. M. (1983). Stereo-selectivity in various drug fields. In: Stereochemistry and Biological Activity of Drugs (eds E. J. Ariens, W. Soudijn and P. B. M. W. M. Timmermans), pp. 161–180, Blackwell, Oxford.

Toon, S., Low, L. K., Gibaldi, M., Trager, W. F., O'Reilly, R. A. and Motley, C. H. (1986). The warfarin–sulfinpyrazone interaction: stereochemical considerations. *Clin. Pharmacol. Ther.* **39**, 15–24.

Vogelgesang, B., Echizen, H., Schmidt, E. and Eichelbaum, M. (1984). Stereoselective first-pass metabolism of highly cleared drugs: studies of the bioavailability of *l*- and *d*-verapamil examined with a stable isotope technique. *Br. J. Clin. Pharmacol.* **18**, 733–740.

Wade, D. N., Mearrick, P. T. and Morris, J. L. (1973). Active transport of L-dopa in the intestine. *Nature* **242**, 463–465.

Walle, T., Webb, J. G., Bagwell, E. E., Walle, U. K., Daniell, H. B. and Gaffney, T. E. (1988). Stereoselective delivery and actions of beta-receptor antagonists. *Biochem. Pharmacol.* **37**, 115–124.

Wedlund, P. J., Aslanian, W. S., Jacqz, E., McAllister, C. B., Branch, R. A. and Wilkinson, G. R. (1985). Phenotypic differences in mephenytoin pharmacokinetics in normal subjects. *J. Pharmacol. Exp. Ther.* **234**, 662–669.

Williams, K., Day, R., Knihinicki, R. and Duffield, A. (1986). The stereo-selective uptake of ibuprofen enantiomers into adipose tissue. *Biochem. Pharmacol.* **35**, 3403–3405.

4

From Enzyme Mimics to Molecular Self-Assembly Processes

J. FRASER STODDART

Department of Chemistry, The University, Sheffield S3 7HF, UK

1 Introduction

The last two decades have seen an enormous drive on the part of chemists to design and synthesize asymmetric catalysts (Sharpless, 1986; Brown and Davies, 1989) to allow them to control and determine the handedness of chiral products emanating from chemical reactions. Although many of the early and successful homogeneous catalysts have been constructed around organometallic and metallo-organic compounds, the importance of purely organic catalysts (Bosnich, 1986) has not been ignored.

In this chapter, the development of enzyme mimics and analogues (Stoddart, 1980, 1984, 1987a, b, c) is traced from those systems inspired by one of nature's gifts — the cyclodextrins (Stoddart, 1989) — through to some of the many wholly synthetic examples which have been realized in the wake of the accidental discovery of the crown ethers by Pedersen (1967, 1971) in the 1960s. It will be suggested that a second generation of such man-made compounds, which are larger in terms of molecular weight and ultimately even more sophisticated structurally speaking than the members of the first generation, will emerge from a new synthetic strategy that relies on the self-assembly, molecule-by-molecule, of supramolecular and polymolecular structures (Lehn, 1988).

2 A gift from nature

It is almost a century since the crystalline compounds we now recognize as cyclodextrins (CDs) were isolated from culture media of *Bacillus macerans*

CHIRALITY IN DRUG DESIGN AND SYNTHESIS
ISBN 0-12-136670-7

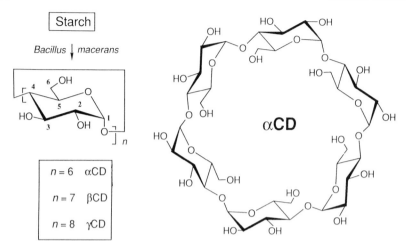

Fig. 1 The microbiological source of the CDs and the structure of αCD revealing its averaged C_6 molecular symmetry.

grown on starch. The CDs (Fig. 1) are cyclic oligosaccharides, commonly containing six, seven or eight α1,4-linked D-glucopyranose residues: we shall refer to them as αCD, βCD, and γCD, respectively. Their gross structures and shapes, shown in Fig. 2, reveal them to be rigid doughnut-shaped molecules of sufficient sizes to accommodate other smaller molecules inside them. An interesting example (Stoddart and Zarzycki, 1988; Alston *et al.*, 1989) is portrayed in Fig. 3 in the form of an X-ray crystal structure of the 1 : 1 adduct formed between αCD and the anti-tumour drug carboplatin.

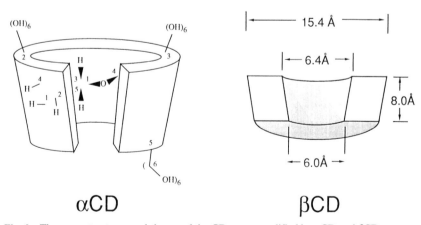

Fig. 2 The gross structures and shapes of the CDs as exemplified by αCD and βCD.

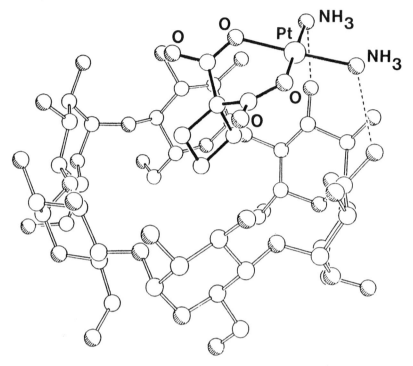

Fig. 3 A ball-and-stick representation of the solid-state structure of the 1 : 1 adduct formed between αCD and carboplatin. Note that the cyclobutane ring of the platinum complex penetrates into the cavity of the CD with additional stabilization coming from hydrogen bonds between the ammine ligands on the metal and secondary hydroxyl groups on the CD.

Therefore, these molecules are all-purpose molecular containers for organic, inorganic, organometallic, and metallo-organic compounds that may be neutral, cationic, anionic, or even radicals. As a result, they are used (Duchêne, 1987) in separation science, in cosmetics and toiletries, and also in the pharmaceutical, agrochemical, and food industries. Specifically, because of their innocuous starch-like properties and their promiscuous behaviour in forming inclusion compounds with many different pharmaceuticals (Szejtli, 1982, 1988), they are highly attractive compounds for development as drug-delivery systems. They also behave as molecular reaction vessels displaying both covalent (*e.g.* cyclic phosphate ester hydrolysis) and non-covalent (*e.g.* regioselective electrophilic aromatic substitution) catalysis (Komiyama and Bender, 1984; Bender, 1987; Komiyama, 1989).

Above all, Cramer (1982) was the person who recognized, appreciated, and demonstrated, between 1951 and 1966, the inclusion-complex forming characteristics of CDs, including

(1) their abilities, as highly symmetrical but chiral compounds, to discriminate in their complexation of enantiomers both as ground state (illustrated by the resolution of racemic modifications) and as transition state (expressed in the kinetic resolution of racemic modifications) phenomena; and
(2) their propensities to catalyse reactions on bound substrates.

As one of the pioneers of molecular recognition, he had to fight as a young man for his ideas and beliefs. Nowadays, Cramer (1987) relates the strength of opposition he met in 1948 as a young scientist when he first proposed 'the idea that a molecule even in solution can envelop another molecule' and, more specifically, 'the conjecture that cyclodextrins form inclusion compounds even in solution'. He reflected almost 40 years later: 'When I presented my results for the first time at a meeting in Lindau, Lake Konstanz, I met fierce opposition from some parts of the establishment. One of my older (and very important) colleagues even stated publicly and bluntly in the discussion that he would try to remove a young man with such crazy ideas from the academic scene. But there was also a good number of supporters, so I finally made it.'

As a class of naturally occurring *chiral* receptor molecules, the CDs are somewhat atypical (Jones *et al.*, 1969) in having high axial symmetries, *e.g.* although αCD, displayed in Fig. 1, contains 30 chiral centres, it belongs to point group C_6. It is fascinating indeed that these receptors with high axial symmetries bind with such an extremely broad range of substrates, *i.e.* substrate specificity is very poor indeed. Although we are conditioned into believing and accepting that the majority of biologically important receptor sites are asymmetric—that is, they are associated with molecules that belong to point group C_1—it is well to reflect upon the likely consequences of substrate binding to biologically active receptor sites that are symmetric or even pseudo-symmetric. In common with CDs, such receptor sites would be expected to be very much less discriminating toward substrate molecules, particularly those that are either achiral, and so have reflection symmetry, or chiral, but also have axial symmetry, *e.g.* they belong to point groups C_2, C_3, *etc.* Some reflection on this fundamental dichotomy between chirality and symmetry in a biological context might be more than justified. It might be quite revealing.

The remarkable developments in the use of CDs as enzyme models and analogues, particularly the more recent examples (Breslow, 1983, 1984,

1988; Tabushi, 1984; Thiem *et al.*, 1988) that have been designed to exhibit covalent catalysis, have depended on the production of chemically modified CDs (Croft and Bartsch, 1983). Most of these derivatives are constitutionally unsymmetrical and, as a result, have no molecular symmetry, except for the identity element. This means that every glucopyranose residue, substituted or otherwise, is 'different' and so it becomes possible (Spencer *et al.*, 1987), using very high field ^{1}H and ^{13}C two-dimensional NMR spectroscopic techniques, to 'map out' the complete structure of an asymmetric CD derivative. In principle, given the vastly increased number of NMR spectroscopic probes, molecular recognition at such a CD receptor site should be more easy to define and to describe.

Although there are a limited number of chemical modifications the chemist can inflict upon the CDs themselves and still retain their all-important water solubility characteristics, there have been some promising synthetic advances of a fundamental type during the last few years. A recent example is illustrated in Fig. 4. From a readily available derivative of αCD, it is possible (Ellwood and Stoddart, 1990) to convert all the glucopyranose units into 3,6-anhydro-D-glucose residues, so affording per-3,6-anhydro-αCD, with, once again, averaged C_6 molecular symmetry. This fascinating αCD derivative in which the conformations of *all* the pyranose rings have been interconverted ($^4C_1 \rightarrow \ ^1C_4$) is, believe it or not, still soluble in water as

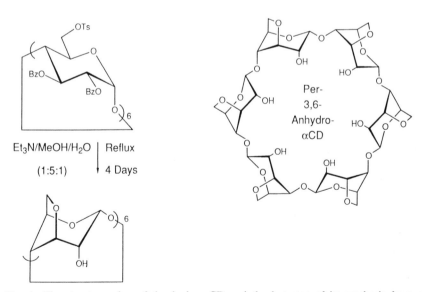

Fig. 4 The structure of per-3,6-anhydro-αCD and the last step of its synthesis from a derivative of αCD.

well as in organic solvents such as dichloromethane. The fact that αCD—
and indeed βCD—can be turned 'outside in' rather easily opens up another
family of molecular receptors around which to design and create new
enzyme mimics. Also, the fact that CD glucotransferases can be encouraged
(Cottaz and Driguez, 1989) to convert substituted disaccharide derivatives
into chemically modified αCD derivatives with C_3 symmetry, without
having to resort to extensive protecting group chemistry, suggests that
enzymes are going to play an increasing role in the synthesis of cyclic oligosaccharides. Then, following the first total synthesis (Takahashi and Ogawa,
1987) of αCD, the stepwise production (Mori *et al.*, 1989) of the '*manno*-
isomer' of αCD suggests that a range of torus-shaped molecular receptors,
based on monosaccharide residues other than glucose as the pyranose sugar,
are now, in principle at least, within the reach of highly skilled synthetic
chemists.

Despite all this considerable activity, however, nature's receptors, even
chemically modified ones and other variations on the naturally occurring
structural theme, are not going to be accepted by everyone in search of
enzyme mimics as enough by themselves. And, after all, why should the
synthetic chemist not launch out into the world of unnatural products?
Chemists have the knowledge and expertise to become independent of
biological systems if they choose and nobody is going to be able to stand in
the way of those who wish to develop the art and science of making wholly
synthetic enzyme mimics—that behave as either chiral reagents or chiral
catalysts—from taking up this challenge.

3   Needs of enzyme mimics

The commonly recognized features of enzymes need not necessarily all be
shared by artificial enzymes. Indeed, enzyme mimics can have many
advantages—including much greater stabilities to reaction conditions—
over enzymes. They can also be modified structurally to satisfy a given set of
requirements (Lehn, 1979). They must display at least some of the following
properties:

(i)   specific substrate binding;
(ii) rapid association of the substrate;
(iii) rapid dissociation of the product;
(iv) selective reaction of the bound substrate;
(v)   regeneration of the active site following the reaction; and
(vi) high turnover numbers of the reaction.

While some (iv–vi) of these properties are essential, others (i–iii) are optional. In fact, broad substrate specificity can be an advantage and catalytic efficiency does not need to be high, provided reaction selectivity is maintained.

The requirements listed above are, of course, for substrate complexes with enzyme mimics. Equally well, one can consider the formation of reagent complexes with enzyme mimics in which the reagent assumes the characteristics of a kind of artificial coenzyme with the enzyme mimic behaving like a chiral auxiliary, hopefully in a catalytic fashion. This kind of enzyme mimic is very simple in its conception and so is particularly attractive in practical terms.

4 Serendipity yet again

It was during the 1960s that Pedersen (1967, 1971) made his accidental discovery (Fig. 5) of dibenzo-18-crown-6 (DB18C6) whilst he was trying to make a quinquedentate ligand starting from a sample of the tetra-hydropyranyl 'ether' of catechol that still contained some 10% of the diphenol present as an impurity. It was these so-called crown ethers, which led to the blossoming of host–guest (Cram, 1988) and supramolecular (Lehn, 1988) chemistry, that gave a long overdue fillip to the design and synthesis of wholly synthetic enzyme models and analogues.

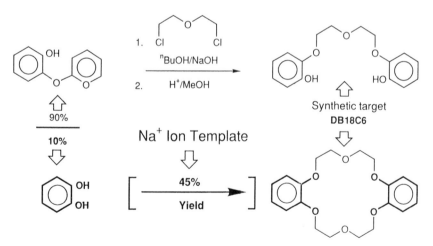

Fig. 5 The accidental discovery of dibenzo-18-crown-6 (DB18C6) by Pedersen (1971) who commented '*My excitement which had been rising during this investigation, now reached its peak and ideas swarmed into my brain. I applied the epithet "crown" to the first member of this class of macrocyclic polyethers because its molecular model looked like one and, with it, cations could be crowned and uncrowned without physical damage to either, just as the heads of royalty*'.

Substrate complex

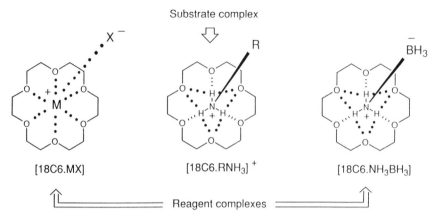

[18C6.MX]   [18C6.RNH₃]⁺   [18C6.NH₃BH₃]

══════════════════ Reagent complexes ══════════════════

Fig. 6   Examples of substrate and reagent complexes involving 18-crown-6 (18C6). In all three complexes, the macrocyclic ring adopts a conformation where the 12 C–O bonds have *anti* geometries and the six C–C bonds have *gauche* geometries with alternating clockwise and anticlockwise helicities. This overall geometry confers local D_{3d} symmetry (*cf.* the chair conformation of cyclohexane) on the macrocycle. In the [18C6·MX] complex, if M⁺ is a K⁺ ion, then it will be located at the centre of the macrocyclic ring, entering into pole–dipole interaction (●●●●) with the six oxygen atoms and a pole–pole interaction (●●●●) with X⁻ to afford an ion pair. In both the [18C6·RNH₃⁺] and [18C6·NH₃BH₃] complexes, the NH₃⁺ centre is hydrogen bonded (ıııı) to the nearer triangle of oxygen atoms in a face-to-face manner. The more distant triangle of oxygen atoms provide additional pole–dipole stabilization (●●●●), shown as occurring to the hydrogen atoms where most of the formal positive charge on the NH₃⁺ is probably concentrated.

In any enzyme mimic, a source of non-covalent bonding—or temporary covalent bonding—must be established between it and the substrate and/or the reagent. Crown ethers, such as 18-crown-6 (18C6) provide (Fig. 6) ideal binding sites for both metal (M⁺) and primary alkyl ammonium (RNH₃⁺) ions (Pedersen, 1967, 1971; Cram and Cram, 1974, 1978; Lehn, 1978; Stoddart, 1979, 1987a; Sutherland, 1986). Since electrostatic interactions, including hydrogen bonds, are involved, highly structured complexes are formed both in the solid state and in solution, particularly when the solvent is an apolar organic one. The [18C6·MX] complex and the [18C6·NH₃BH₃] adduct (Colquhoun *et al.*, 1984) are both examples of reagent complexes, whereas the [18C6·RNH₃]⁺ complex is an example of a substrate complex (Fig. 6).

The 18-crown-6 constitution affords a primary binding site for substrates, including α-amino acid ester salts. Functionality can be introduced to provide secondary binding sites and/or catalytic groups. Chirality can also be incorporated usually such that the homotopicity of the two faces of the macrocyclic polyether is preserved, *i.e.* axial symmetry is often a feature of chiral 18C6 derivatives. In this way, only one complex with 1:1 stoichiometry can be formed. This is an important consideration in the design of chiral macrocyclic receptors, be they crown ethers or otherwise. Numerous examples of chiral crown ethers employed successfully in asymmetric synthesis and catalysis, including (a) acyl transfer reactions, (b) Michael addition reactions, (c) oxidative decarboxylations, and (d) hydride transfer reactions, have been discussed elsewhere (Stoddart, 1980, 1984, 1987a, b, c).

5 A chiral crown ether as a reagent

The (R,R,R,R) and (S,S,S,S) enantiomers (Fig. 7) of 2,3,11,12-tetraphenyl-18-crown-6 have been employed (Allwood *et al.*, 1984) successfully as chiral auxiliaries in *stoichiometric* amounts to form NH_3BH_3 adducts, capable of effecting enantioselective reductions of prochiral aromatic ketones [PhCOR where R = Me, Et, Pr^i, Bu^t] to the corresponding S and R aromatic secondary alcohols. The chiral TP18C6 derivatives can be synthesized (Crosby *et al.*, 1989) in one step in large quantities (*ca.* 10 g) from the now readily available chiral hydrobenzoins (Jacobsen *et al.*, 1988; Wai *et al.*, 1989; McKee *et al.*, 1990).

The solid-state structure (Fig. 8) of $[(R,R,R,R)$-TP18C6·$NH_3BH_3]$ reveals that the macrocyclic polyether ring adopts the familiar all-*gauche* conformation with local D_{3d} symmetry. Since two vicinal phenyl groups are oriented axially and the other two equatorially on the macrocycle, the symmetry of the receptor as a whole is reduced to C_2. The NH_3BH_3 molecule is hydrogen bonded through its NH_3^+ centre to the three facing

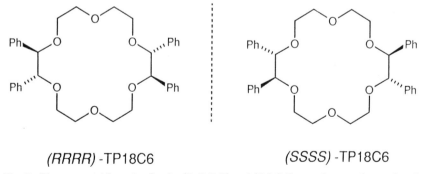

(RRRR) -TP18C6   *(SSSS)* -TP18C6

Fig. 7   The structural formulae for the (R,R,R,R) and (S,S,S,S) enantiomers of tetraphenyl-18-crown-6 (TP18C6). Note that, on account of their D_2 symmetries, the two faces of the macrocycles, in each case, are homotopic, *i.e.* only one adduct is formed with NH_3BH_3.

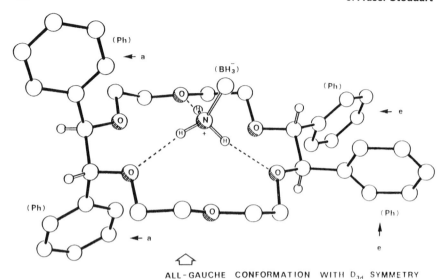

ALL-GAUCHE CONFORMATION WITH D_{3d} SYMMETRY

Fig. 8 A ball-and-stick representation of the solid-state structure of the $[(R,R,R,R)$-TP18C6·NH$_3$BH$_3$] adduct, showing the hydrogen bonding (----) of the NH$_3^+$ centre to the nearer triangle of oxygen atoms and the relative dispositions of the axial (a) and equatorial (e) phenyl groups with respect to the all-*gauche* conformation with local D_{3d} symmetry for the macrocyclic ring itself.

alternate oxygen atoms of the macrocycle, affording a binary face-to-face adduct.

Table 1 records the outcome of a competitive reduction of a mixture of the four prochiral aromatic ketones with stoichiometric amounts of $[(S,S,S,S)$-TP18C6·NH$_3$BH$_3$] in toluene containing some BF$_3$ as a Lewis acid catalyst in the temperature range -75°C, warming up to -40°C over

Table 1 The competitive reduction of four prochiral aromatic ketones (PhCOR) with $[(S,S,S,S)$-TP18C6·NH$_3$BH$_3$] in toluene at -78°C, warming up to -40°C over 85 min

PhCOR	Mol %	Conversion (%)	Enantiomeric excess (%)
PhCOMe	28	90	24 (R)
PhCOEt	27	76	38 (R)
PhCOPr^i	18	12	42 (R)
PhCOBu^t	27	68	67 (R)

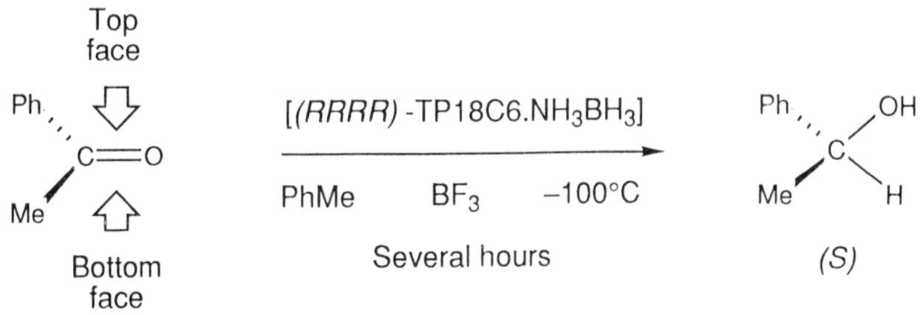

Top
face

Ph
⟍
⟍
‸
C=O

Me
⟋

Bottom
face

[(RRRR)-TP18C6.NH₃BH₃]
$$\xrightarrow{\hspace{3cm}}$$
PhMe   BF₃   −100°C

Several hours

Ph   OH
⟍   ⟋
C
⟍
Me   H

(S)

Fig. 9 The [(R,R,R,R)-TP18C6·NH₃BH₃] adduct acting as a chiral reagent in the conversion of acetophenone into predominantly (S)-1-phenylethanol. Under the stated reaction conditions, hydride attack is occurring 19 times out of 20 to the bottom face of the ketone.

85 min. Enantiomeric excesses of the R alcohols range from 24 to 67% in going down the series from PhCOMe to PhCOBu^t, and, somewhat surprisingly, one ketone, PhCOPr^i, was much less reactive than the other three ketones. The reason for the substrate specificities indicated by the percentage conversions in Table 1 is unclear. Temperature is, of course, important in determining the extent of the enantioselectivity. Enantiomeric excesses of >90% have been obtained (Fig. 9) by carrying out the reaction on PhCOMe for several hours at −100°C. Detailed investigations of the reaction conditions have established that toluene is the preferred solvent, given the low-temperature requirement. For example, much lower enantiomeric excesses were obtained in dichloromethane. Also, replacement of the phenyl groups in TP18C6 by other aryl groups, such as α-naphthyl, β-naphthyl, or anisyl (Allwood et al., 1988), had a detrimental effect upon the enantioselectivities.

Although a number of crystalline adducts between chiral crown ethers incorporating asymmetric carbohydrate units and NH₃BH₃ have also been characterized (Shahriari-Zavareh et al., 1985) by X-ray crystallography, none of them reduce the range of prochiral aromatic ketones listed in Table 1 with enantiomeric excesses greater than 13%. This observation might reflect the fact that these chiral crown ethers have diastereotopic faces and so can form two 'different' adducts with NH₃BH₃. It is wiser to appeal to axial symmetry (as in TP18C6) and so avoid this complicating factor.

In the [TP18C6·NH₃BH₃] adducts, although the NH₃BH₃ behaves like a coenzyme (cf. NADH) and the chiral TP18C6, in its binding of NH₃BH₃, shows some of the characteristics of an enzyme, the system is only stoichiometric and the chiral auxiliary has to be recovered by chromatography after the reaction and recycled.

6   The same chiral crown ether as a catalyst

The formation of cyanohydrin derivatives of aromatic aldehydes is catalysed (Chênevert *et al.*, 1983) by 18C6 in a reaction where only 10 mol% of the catalyst is required. When benzaldehyde was subjected (Stoddart, 1987c) to asymmetric phase transfer cyanohydrin formation (Fig. 10) with [(*R,R,R,R*)-TP18C6·KCN] in toluene at −78°C, warming up to 0°C during 150 min and using benzoyl chloride as a trapping reagent, the enantiomeric excess of the benzoylated cyanohydrin, obtained in 62% chemical yield, was 40% in favour of the *R* product. The nature of the active catalyst is suggested by the solid state structure (Fig. 11) of the 1 : 1 complex formed between Ca(NO₃)₂ and (*S,S,S,S*)-TP18C6 (Crosby *et al.*, 1989). The Ca²⁺ ion is located in the centre of the macrocycle and is ion paired to NO₃⁻ ions on both faces of the macrocycle. If, in the [(*R,R,R,R*)-TP18C6·KCN] complex, the K⁺ ion is also located in the middle of the 18C6 ring, then it is not unlikely that the CN⁻ ion is ion paired through its nitrogen atom to the electrostatically bound K⁺ ion, leaving the weakly anchored anion suitably disposed to express its nucleophilicity to the prochiral substrate through its exposed carbon end. In this manner, KCN also behaves a little like a coenzyme and, as before in the case of NH₃BH₃, the (*R,R,R,R*)-TP18C6 can be reclaimed and recycled.

This type of chiral phase-transfer catalyst, where the substrate only becomes temporarily and weakly associated with it, offers an attractive area for further research. However, the chiral phase-transfer catalysts would benefit from being even more highly structured, provided they can be elaborated from inexpensive starting materials without too much difficulty. One way in which this challenge could be met is discussed below.

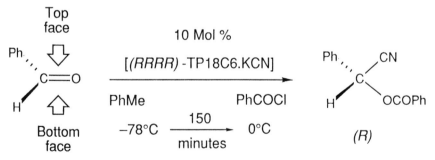

Fig. 10   The [(*R,R,R,R*)-TP18C6·KCN] complex acting as a chiral catalyst in the conversion of benzaldehyde into predominantly the *R* isomer of the benzoylated cyanohydrin derivative. Under the stated reaction conditions, cyanide attack occurs seven times out of ten to the top face of the aldehyde.

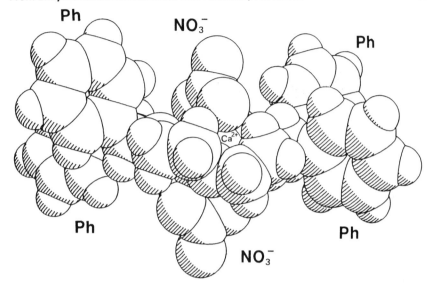

Fig. 11   The space-filling representation of $[(S,S,S,S)\text{-TP18C6}\cdot\text{Ca(NO}_3)_2]$ in the solid state. Note how the NO_3^- anions are ion paired to the encircled Ca^{2+} ion above and below the macrocyclic ring which does not—for once—adopt the all-*gauche* conformation with local D_{3d} symmetry, possibly on account of the relatively small size of the Ca^{2+} ion compared with the 'hole' size of 18C6 and the steric bulk of the axially disposed NO_3^- ions.

7   Coordination through the second sphere

Our fascination (Colquhoun *et al.*, 1986; Stoddart, 1988) with the concept of second-sphere coordination (Werner, 1913) was to introduce us, quite by accident, to the ideas of molecular self-assembly. It transpires (Colquhoun *et al.*, 1985a) that the large and flexible dibenzo-30-crown-10 (DB30C10) wraps itself (Fig. 12) around the dicationic $[\text{Pt(bipy)(NH}_3)_2]^{2+}$ metal complex such that the positive charge is solvated by the polyether chains while the π-electron deficient bipyridyl (bipy) ligand enters into charge transfer (CT) and other dispersive interactions with the π-electron rich catechol rings of DB30C10 stacked at the ideal distance of 3.5 Å. In aceto-nitrile solution, the free energy of binding, calculated from the K_a value of 191 000 M^{-1}, amounts to a remarkably high 30.1 kJ mol^{-1} at room temperature when the counterions are soft hexafluorophosphates.

Next, the obvious constitutional similarities between $[\text{Pt(bipy)(NH}_3)_2]^{2+}$ and $[\text{DQT}]^{2+}$, the Diquat dication, which constitutes one of the two well-known bipyridinium herbicides (Summers, 1980), led to the demonstration (Colquhoun *et al.*, 1985b) that DB30C10 also complexes in a similar

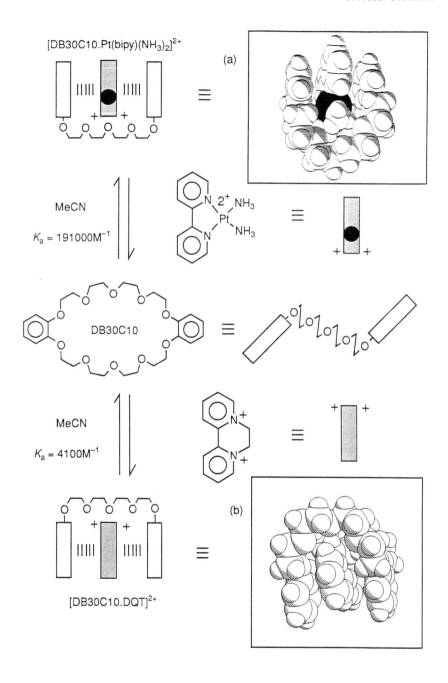

$[DB30C10 \cdot Pt(bipy)(NH_3)_2]^{2+}$

(a)

MeCN

$K_a = 191000 M^{-1}$

$2+$

NH_3

Pt

NH_3

DB30C10

MeCN

$K_a = 4100 M^{-1}$

$[DB30C10 \cdot DQT]^{2+}$

(b)

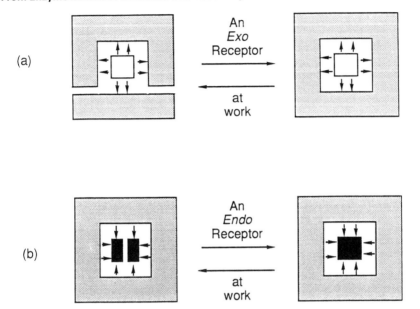

Fig. 13   Template-directed synthesis—a self-fulfilling phenomenon?

supramolecular fashion (Fig. 12) to the $[DQT]^{2+}$ dication, although this time the π-stacking distance between parallel donor and acceptor rings is reduced to 3.4 Å. Despite this even tighter fit, there is a considerably smaller free energy of complexation of 20.6 kJ mol^{-1}, reflecting the K_a value of 4100 M^{-1} obtained in acetonitrile at room temperature when, once again, the counterions are soft hexafluorophosphates.

The manner in which DB30C10 organizes itself spontaneously around the $[Pt(bipy)(NH_3)_2]^{2+}$ and $[DQT]^{2+}$ dications is reminiscent of the templating action (Pedersen, 1971) of Na$^+$ ions during the high yielding (45%) synthesis (Fig. 5) of DB18C6. In principle, we have now reached the stage in molecular self-assembly processes where we can use molecular recognition (Fig. 13) in an *exo* sense to template the efficient construction of molecular

---

Fig. 12 The spontaneous self-assembly of dibenzo-30-crown-10 around the (a) $[Pt(bipy)(NH_3)_2]^{2+}$ and (b) $[DQT]^{2+}$ dications in acetonitrile solutions. Note the definition and use of chemical cartoons to aid in the display of supramolecular structures. The long dashes (ıııı) indicate the existence of stabilising dispersive forces in CT interactions associated with π-donor/ π-acceptor stacking interactions. In both case (a) and case (b) there is inset a space-filling representation of the solid-state structures of the 1 : 1 complexes.

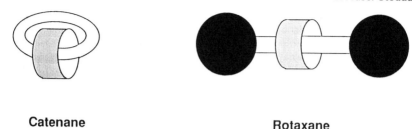

Catenane   **Rotaxane**

Fig. 14 Schematic representations of a catenane and a rotaxane.

assemblies. The question remains to be answered—can we use these molecular assemblies in an *endo* context as the next generation of enzyme mimics? To answer this question, we need to learn how to build large molecules and molecular assemblies molecule-by-molecule in addition to the familiar atom-by-atom and group-by-group approach involving the time-consuming and often not so efficient functional group manipulations and transformations that rely upon the delicate and intricate use of protecting groups. Biological systems are rich in precedents of self-assembly.

8 Planned molecular self-assembly

The kind of self-assembly processes employed in biological systems might be easier to establish within chemical systems—at least in the beginning—if the relatively small molecules contained an element of mechanical entanglement in addition to the non-covalent bonding that also has to be an integral part of molecular components making up such assemblies. The nature of the mechanical entanglement could ultimately involve inter-twining as in the spontaneous assembly of double or triple helices, or it could involve, more logically to start with, interlocking, as in the formation of catenanes and rotaxanes (Schill, 1971; Dietrich-Buchecker and Sauvage, 1987), of appropriate molecular components. And so the possibility (Fig. 14) that catenanes and rotaxanes might serve as prototypes for the construction of large, ordered, and structured molecular assemblies is worthy of consideration.

9 From host–guest chemistry to molecular assemblies

When a guest is complexed by a host (Fig. 15(a)), the 1 : 1 complex is usually in equilibrium in solution with the molecular components. A number of

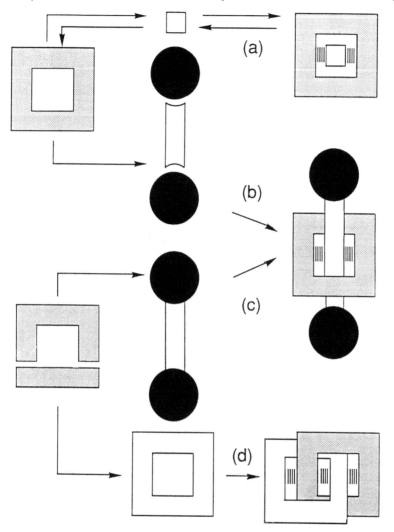

Fig. 15 Representations, using chemical cartoons of (a) 1 : 1 complex formation and some of the means of production of (b and c) rotaxanes and (d) catenanes.

different examples have already been discussed, (see Figs 6 and 12). By contrast, formation of a rotaxane by either a threading (Fig. 15(b)) or a clipping (Fig. 15(c)) process will be irreversible. And so will the formation of a catenane by a clipping process (Fig. 15(d)).

The Paraquat dication, which constitutes the other well-known bipyridinium herbicide (Summers, 1980), is complexed (Allwood *et al.*,

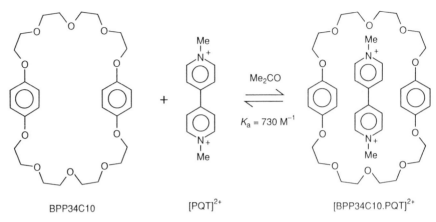

BPP34C10   [PQT]$^{2+}$ [BPP34C10.PQT]$^{2+}$

Fig. 16   The formation of the 1 : 1 complex between BPP34C10 and [PQT]$^{2+}$ dications.

1987; Ashton *et al.*, 1987; Slawin *et al.*, 1987) by bisparaphenylene-34-crown-10 (BPP34C10), a constitutional isomer of DB30C10. The [PQT]$^{2+}$ dication forms (Fig. 16) a 1 : 1 complex with BPP34C10. In acetone, the stability constant (K_a = 730 M^{-1}) associated with the formation of this complex at room temperature, when the counterions are soft hexafluorophosphates, corresponds to a free energy of complexation of 16.3 kJ mol^{-1}. Stabilization arises from:

(1) electrostatic attractions, including (C–H$\cdots$O) hydrogen bonding between the positively charged guest and the crown ether oxygen atoms present in the host, and
(2) dispersive forces, including CT interactions between the π-electron accepting bipyridinium moiety of the guest and the π-electron donating hydroquinol rings of the host.

As in the case (Fig. 12) of the [DB30C10·DQT]$^{2+}$ complex, the CT interactions give rise to a deep orange colour for the [BPP34C10·PQT]$^{2+}$ complex in both the solution and solid states. The X-ray crystal structure (Fig. 17) of the [BPP34C10·PQT]$^{2+}$ complex reveals a pseudo-rotaxane-like character to the molecular assembly with a distance of 3.7 Å between the mean planes of the π-donors and the π-acceptor.

Having shown (Fig. 18(a)) that [PQT]$^{2+}$ dications are complexed by BPP34C10, the next question to be addressed was—could a neutral molecule with a π-electron rich aromatic ring, like 1,4-dimethoxybenzene (1/4 DMB), be complexed by a tetracationic macrocycle of the appropriate

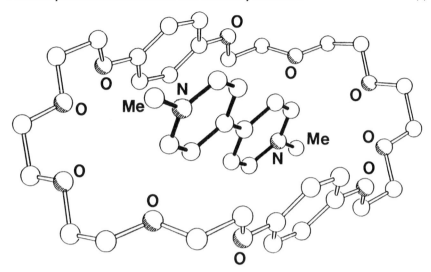

Fig. 17   A ball-and-stick representation of the solid state structure of the [BPP34C10·PQT]$^{2+}$ complex.

dimensions, wherein two [PQT]$^{2+}$ dicationic units are held approximately 7 Å apart in a rigid face-to-face manner. The answer, shown in Fig. 18(b), was the tetracationic macrocycle [BISPQT]$^{4+}$ containing two bipyridinium rings joined 'top' and 'bottom' by two p-xylylenyl residues.

The compound [BISPQT][PF$_6$]$_4$ was synthesized (Odell *et al.*, 1988) with considerable difficulty, presumably in view of the macrocyclic ring strain, and shown (Ashton *et al.*, 1988) to form a 1 : 1 complex with 1/4 DMB in acetonitrile (Fig. 19). The relatively small K_a value of 16 M^{-1}, obtained at room temperature, corresponds to a free energy of complexation of 6.9 kJ mol^{-1}, arising from mainly dispersive forces involving the two π-electron deficient rings in the host and the π-electron-rich guest.

The X-ray crystal structure (Fig. 20) of the 1 : 1 complex formed between the tetracationic macrocycle [BISPQT]$^{4+}$ and 1/4 DMB shows that the guest is inserted pseudo-rotaxane-like through the centre of the host. In addition to π-stacking interactions, there are also weak, but nonetheless stabilizing edge-to-face interactions (Ashton *et al.*, 1988) involving the aromatic hydrogen atoms on 1/4 DMB and the π-systems of the orthogonally-aligned p-phenylene units in the tetracationic macrocycle [BISPQT]$^{4+}$. This kind of electrostatic interaction is found (Gould *et al.*, 1985; Burley and Petsko, 1986) in widely diverse situations such as the solid-state structures of benzene and naphthalene on the one hand and in the crystal structures of

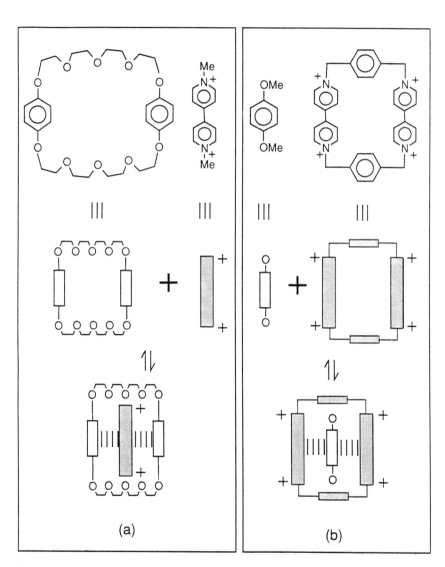

Fig. 18 A schematic representation, using chemical cartoons, of the design feature used in evaluating 1 : 1 complex formation (a) between BPP34C10 and the $[PQT]^{2+}$ dication and (b) between 1/4 DMB and the tetracationic macrocycle $[BISPQT]^{4+}$.

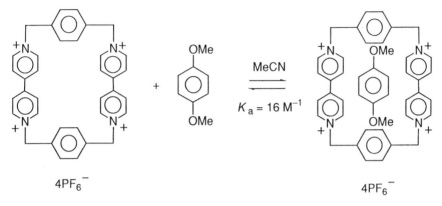

Fig. 19 The formation of the 1 : 1 complex between the tetracationic macrocycle [BISPQT]$^{4+}$ and 1/4 DMB.

proteins, rich in amino acids carrying aromatic-containing side chains, on the other hand.

The observations that BPP34C10 complexes with the [PQT]$^{2+}$ dication and that the tetracationic macrocycle [BISPQT]$^{4+}$ complexes with 1/4 DMB, when considered alongside the occurrence of the continuous alternating donor-acceptor stack formed (Ortholand *et al.*, 1989) when 1,5-dinaphtho-44-crown-12 crystallizes with two molar equivalents of

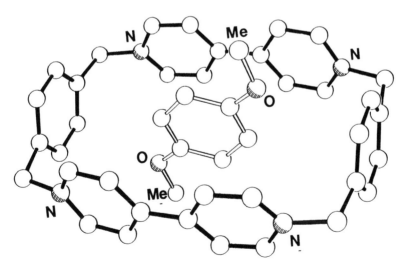

Fig. 20 Ball-and-stick representation of the solid-state structure of the 1 : 1 complex formed between the tetracationic macrocycle [BISPQT]$^{4+}$ and 1/4 DMB.

74

Fraser Stoddart

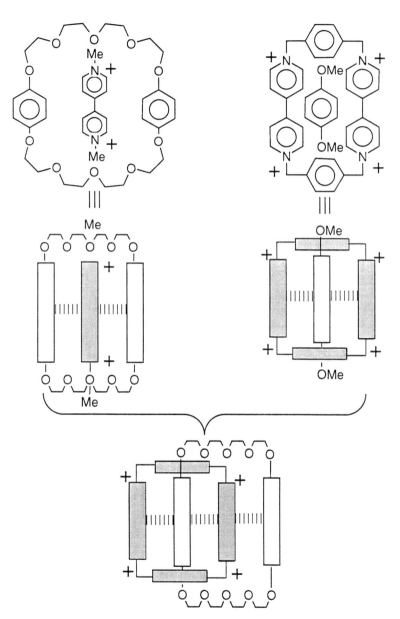

Fig. 21 A schematic representation, using chemical cartoons, of the design concept behind the realization of the [2]catenane.

the [PQT]$^{2+}$ dication, suggested (Ashton *et al.*, 1989) the possibility of combining these two supramolecular features simultaneously into the design (Fig. 21) of a [2]catenane.

10 Structure-directed synthesis

When the reaction between the bis(pyridinium) bis(hexafluorophosphate), shown in the scheme in Fig. 22, and 1,4-bis(bromomethyl)benzene, is carried out (Ashton *et al.*, 1989) in acetonitrile at room temperature in the presence of three molar equivalents of BPP34C10, the [2]catenane is formed in a remarkably high 70% yield as a crystalline tetrakis(hexafluoro-phosphate), following purification and counterion exchange. Indeed, it is very much easier to construct this molecular assembly than it is to make one of the components, namely the tetracationic macrocycle, by itself. This highly encouraging observation holds out considerable promise for the future development of this kind of template-directed synthetic chemistry.

The solid-state structure (Fig. 23) of the [2]catenane provides a convincing demonstration of just how highly ordered are the components that comprise this intriguing molecular assembly. The interplanar separations between the associated bipyridinium moieties and hydroquinol rings are *ca.* 3.5 Å in all cases. The structure is stabilized by both π-stacking and edge-to-face interactions involving the appropriate aromatic rings. Dynamic ^{1}H NMR spectroscopy established (Ashton *et al.*, 1989) that the [2]catenane is also highly ordered in solution, *i.e.* the order, which templates their formation and is evident in the solid state, 'lives on' in the [2]catenane molecules when the compound is dissolved in polar solvents. This means that we can envisage ultimately storing and transferring information in molecules of this type. With the introduction of chirality—not an impossible task, let it be

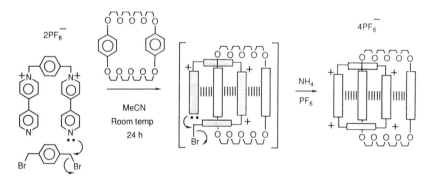

Fig. 22 Making the [2]catenane to order.

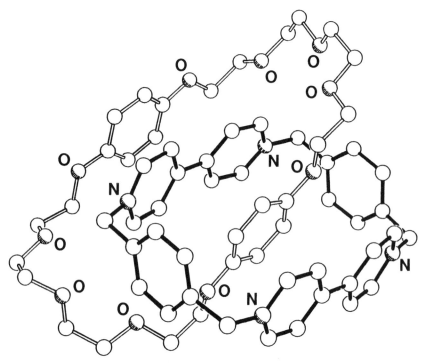

Fig. 23 Ball-and-stick representation of the solid-state structure of the [2]catenane.

said—molecular assemblies of this type could form the basis for the development of a new generation of enzyme mimics.

What is particularly exciting is that the [2]catenane actually templates its own formation. The first nucleophilic substitution between the bis(pyridinium) dication and the dibromide will produce a trication which, in view of the similarity of the bipyridinium moiety to a $[PQT]^{2+}$ dication, should thread its way through the centre of the macrocyclic ring of BPP34C10. The second nucleophilic substitution is then a highly ordered event, *i.e.* entropically, it is not a bad reaction. There may also be present some enhancement of reactivity in the final intramolecular cyclization as a consequence of the increased nucleophilicity of the nitrogen as part of a developing bipyridinium moiety which lies alongside a π-electron-rich hydroquinol ring. Whatever the details of the mechanism, the reaction is amazingly efficient.

The [2]catenane is the first member of a new series of [n]catenanes and [n]rotaxanes we have been able to construct using a modular approach to chemical synthesis (Anelli *et al.*, in preparation). Without exception, it is very much easier to make the catenanes—and also the rotaxanes—themselves than it is to prepare some of the molecular components of these assemblies. These new chemical compounds are products of non-covalent self-assembly, followed by covalent bond formation. They are examples of what we have called (Kohnke *et al.*, 1989) structure-directed synthesis—a hypothesis which we have summarized as follows: *there are inherently simple ways of making apparently complex unnatural products from appropriate substrates without the need for reagent control or catalysis.*

11 The future

In 1990, as we look towards the next century (Fig. 24) a lot is surely going to happen at the molecular level in chemistry! Unnatural product synthesis will grow in importance relative to natural product synthesis. Not only will this change in emphasis lead—as it has done in the past—to new drugs, but it will also uncover novel chiral catalysts that could not have been contemplated a few years ago.

Chemical synthesis is a highly creative medium. It is now clear from the activities in a number of laboratories around the world that synthetic chemistry is set to undergo a conceptual revolution. As the main targets for chemical synthesis move from being natural to unnatural products, the emphasis in chemistry will be less and less on discovery and more and more on invention.

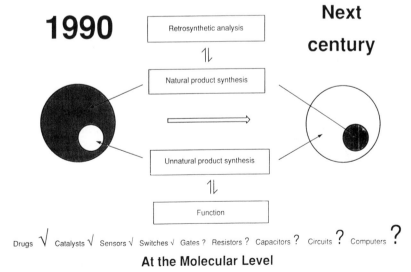

Fig. 24 The changing face of chemistry.

Acknowledgements

I thank my many talented coworkers and research collaborators, whose names appear along with my own among the following list of references for their individual contributions to the story told in this short article. The research has been generously supported by the Science and Engineering and Agricultural and Food, Research Councils in the UK as well as by a number of the major British Chemical companies and overseas governments. We are all grateful to our sponsors.

References

Allwood, B. L., Shahriari-Zavareh, H., Stoddart, J. F. and Williams, D. J. (1984). Enantioselective reductions of aromatic ketones with ammonia-borane complexes of chiral tetraphenyl-18-crown-6 derivatives. *J. Chem. Soc., Chem. Commun.* 1461–1464.

Allwood, B. L., Spencer, N., Shahriari-Zavareh, H., Stoddart, J. F. and Williams, D. J. (1987). Complexation of paraquat by a bisparaphenylene-34-crown-10 derivative. *J. Chem. Soc., Chem. Commun.* 1064–1066.

Allwood, B. L., Crosby, J., Pears, D. A., Shahriari-Zavareh, H., Slawin, A. M. Z., Stoddart, J. F. and Williams, D. J. (1988). The 1 : 1 adduct between the *trans-transoid-trans* isomer of 2,3,11,12-tetra-anisyl-18-crown-6 with the (*RRRR*)-configuration and borane ammonia, BH_3NH_3. *Acta Crystallogr., Sect. C.* **44**, 1118–1121.

Alston, D. R., Ashton, P. R., Lilley, T. H., Stoddart, J. F., Zarzycki, R., Slawin, A. M. Z. and Williams, D. J. (1989). Second sphere coordination of carboplatin and rhodium complexes by cyclodextrins. *Carbohydr. Res.* **192**, 259–281.

Anelli, P. L., Ashton, P. R., Ballardini, R., Balzani, V., Gandolfi, M. T., Goodnow, T. T., Kaifer, A. E., Pietraszkiewicz, M., Prodi, M., Reddington, M. V., Slawin, A. M. Z., Spencer, N., Stoddart, J. F., Vicent, C. and Williams, D. J. manuscript in preparation.

Ashton, P. R., Slawin, A. M. Z., Spencer, N., Stoddart, J. F. and Williams, D. J. (1987). Complex formation between bisparaphenylene-($3n + 4$)-crown-n ethers and the paraquat and diquat dications. *J. Chem. Soc., Chem. Commun.* 1066–1069.

Ashton, P. R., Odell, B., Reddington, M. V., Slawin, A. M. Z., Stoddart, J. F. and Williams, D. J. (1988). Isostructural, alternately-charged receptor stacks. The inclusion complexes of hydroquinone and catechol dimethyl ethers with cyclobis(paraquat-*p*-phenylene). *Angew. Chem. Int. Ed. Engl.* **27**, 1550–1553.

Ashton, P. R., Goodnow, T. T., Kaifer, A. E., Reddington, M. V., Slawin, A. M. Z., Spencer, N., Stoddart, J. F., Vicent, C. and Williams, D. J. (1989). A [2]catenane made to order. *Angew. Chem. Int. Ed. Engl.* **28**, 1396–1399.

Bender, M. L. (1987). Enzyme models—cyclodextrins (cycloamyloses). In *Enzyme Mechanisms* (eds M. I. Page and A. Williams), pp. 56–66. Royal Society of Chemistry, London.

Bosnich, B. (ed.) (1986). *Asymmetric Catalysis*, p. 154. Martinus Nijhoff, Dordrecht.

Breslow, R. (1983). Artificial enzymes. *Chem. Br.* **19**, 126–131.

Breslow, R. (1984). Enzyme models related to inclusion compounds. In *Inclusion Compounds* (eds J. L. Atwood, J. E. D. Davies and D. D. MacNicol), Vol. 3, pp. 473–508. Academic Press, London.

Breslow, R. (1988). Molecules that mimic enzymes. *New Sci.* **1621**, 44–47.

Brown, J. M. and Davies, S. G. (1989). Chemical asymmetric synthesis. *Nature* **342**, 631–636.

Burley, S. K. and Petsko, G. A. (1986). Dimerization energetics of benzene and aromatic amino acid side chains. *J. Am. Chem. Soc.* **108**, 7995–8001.

Chênevert, R., Plante, R. and Voyer, N. (1983). Crown ether catalysis in the synthesis of cyanohydrin derivatives. *Synth. Commun.* **13**, 403–409.

Colquhoun, H. M., Jones, G., Maud, J. M. and Stoddart; J. F. (1984). Crystal and supramolecular structures of $BF_3NH_3 \cdot 18$-crown-6 and $BH_3NH_3 \cdot 18$-crown-6. *J. Chem. Soc., Dalton Trans.* 63–66.

Colquhoun, H. M., Doughty, S. M., Maud, J. M., Stoddart, J. F., Williams, D. J. and Wolstenholme, J. B. (1985a). Second sphere coordination of $[Pt(bipy)(NH_3)_2]^{2+}$ by dibenzo-crown ethers. *Isr. J. Chem.* **25**, 15–26.

Colquhoun, H. M., Goodings, E. P., Maud, J. M., Stoddart, J. F., Wolstenholme, J. B. and Williams, D. J. (1985b). The complexation of the diquat dication by dibenzo-3n-crown-n ethers. *J. Chem. Soc., Perkin Trans. 2*, 607–624.

Colquhoun, H. M., Stoddart, J. F. and Williams, D. J. (1986). Second-sphere coordination—a novel rôle for molecular receptors. *Angew. Chem. Int. Ed. Engl.* **25**, 487–507.

Cottaz, S. and Driguez, H. (1989). First regiospecific synthesis of $6^A,6^C,6^E$-tri-O-methylcyclomaltohexaose. *J. Chem. Soc. Chem. Commun.* 1088–1089.

Cram, D. J. (1988). The design of molecular host, guests, and their complexes. (Nobel Lecture). *Science* **240**, 760–767.

Cram, D. J. and Cram, J. M. (1974). Host–guest chemistry. *Science* **183**, 803–809.

Cram, D. J. and Cram, J. M. (1978). Design of complexes between synthetic hosts and organic guests. *Acc. Chem. Res.* **11**, 5–14.

Cramer, F. (1982). Cyclodextrin—a paradigmatic model. In *Proc. First Int. Symp. Cyclodextrins, Budapest, 1981* (ed. J. Szejtli), pp. 3–24. Reidel, Dordrecht.

Cramer, F. (1987). Introduction. In *Cyclodextrins and their Industrial Uses* (ed. D. Duchêne), pp. 11–20. Editions de Santé, Paris.

Croft, A. P. and Bartsch, R. A. (1983). Synthesis of chemically modified cyclodextrins. *Tetrahedron* **39**, 1417–1474.

Crosby, J., Fakley, M. E., Gemmell, C., Martin, K., Quick, A., Slawin, A. M. Z., Shahriari-Zavareh, H., Stoddart, J. F. and Williams, D. J. (1989). An efficient procedure for the synthesis and isolation of (+)-(2R,3R,11R,12R)- and (−)-(2S,3S,11S,12S)-tetraphenyl-18-crown-6. *Tetrahedron Lett.* **30**, 3849–3852.

Dietrich-Buchecker, C. O. and Sauvage, J.-P. (1987). Interlocking of molecular threads: from the statistical approach to the templated synthesis of catenands. *Chem. Rev.* **87**, 795–808.

Duchêne, D. (ed.) (1987). *Cyclodextrins and their Industrial Uses*. Editions de Santé, Paris.

Ellwood, P. and Stoddart, J. F. (1990). Synthesis and characterisation of per-3,6-anhydrocyclodextrins. In *Proc. Fifth Int. Symp. Cyclodextrins, Paris, 1990* (ed. D. Duchêne), in press. Editions de Santé, Paris.

Gould, R. O., Gray, A. M., Taylor, P. and Walkinshaw, D. (1985). Crystal environments and geometries of leucine, isoleucine, valine and phenylalanine provide estimates of minimum nonbonded contact and preferred van der Waals interaction distances. *J. Am. Chem. Soc.* **107**, 5921–5927.

Jacobsen, E. N., Markó, I., Mungall, W. S., Schröder, G. and Sharpless, K. B. (1988). Asymmetric dihydroxylation via ligand-accelerated catalysis. *J. Am. Chem. Soc.* **110**, 1968–1970.

Jones, J. K. N., Stoddart, J. F. and Szarek, W. A. (1969). Large heterocyclic rings from carbohydrate precursors. *Can. J. Chem.* **47**, 3213–3215.

Kohnke, F. H., Mathias, J. P. and Stoddart, J. F. (1989). Structure-directed synthesis of new organic materials. *Angew. Chem. Adv. Mater.* **101**, 1129–1135.

Komiyama, M. (1989). α-Cyclodextrin-catalyzed regioselective P–O(2′) cleavages of 2′,3′-cyclic monophosphates of ribonucleosides. *J. Am. Chem. Soc.* **111**, 3046–3050.

Komiyama, M. and Bender, M. L. (1984). Cyclodextrins as enzyme models. In *The Chemistry of Enzyme Action* (ed. M. I. Page), pp. 505–527. Elsevier, Amsterdam.

Lehn, J.-M. (1978). Cryptates. The chemistry of macropolycyclic inclusion complexes. *Acc. Chem. Res.* **11**, 49–57.

Lehn, J.-M. (1979). Macrocyclic receptor molecules: aspects of chemical reactivity, investigations into molecular catalysis and transport processes. *Pure Appl. Chem.* **51**, 979–997.

Lehn, J.-M. (1988). Supramolecular chemistry — scope and perspectives. Molecules, supermolecules, and molecular devices. (Nobel Lecture). *Angew. Chem. Int. Ed. Engl.* **27**, 89–112.

McKee, B. H., Gilheany, D. G. and Sharpless, K. B. (1990). *R,R*-1,2-Diphenyl-1,2-ethanediol (stilbene diol). *Org. Synth.* (submitted).

Mori, M., Ito, Y. and Ogawa, T. (1989). A highly efficient and stereoselective cycloglycosylation. Synthesis of cyclo {→4)-[α-Man-(1→4)]5-α-Man-(1→}, a manno isomer of α-cyclodextrin. *Tetrahedron Lett.* **30**, 1273–1276.

Odell, B., Reddington, M. V., Slawin, A. M. Z., Spencer, N., Stoddart, J. F. and Williams, D. J. (1988). Cyclobis(paraquat-*p*-phenylene). A tetracationic multipurpose receptor. *Agnew. Chem. Int. Ed. Engl.* **27**, 1547–1550.

Ortholand, J.-Y., Slawin, A. M. Z., Spencer, N., Stoddart, J. F. and Williams, D. J. (1989). A polymolecular donor–acceptor stack made of paraquat and a 1,5-dihydroxynaphthalene-derived crown ether. *Angew. Chem. Int. Ed. Engl.* **28**, 1394–1395.

Pedersen, C. J. (1967). Cyclic polyethers and their complexes with metal salts. *J. Am. Chem. Soc.* **89**, 7017–7036.

Pedersen, C. J. (1971). Macrocyclic polyethers for complexing metals. *Aldrichim. Acta* **4**, 1–4.

Schill, G. (1971). *Catenanes, Rotaxanes, and Knots.* Academic Press, New York.

Shahriari-Zavareh, H., Stoddart, J. F., Williams, M. K., Allwood, B. L. and Williams, D. J. (1985). The supramolecular structure and reactivities of some complexes of chiral crown ethers with borane–ammonia. *J. Incl. Phenom.* **3**, 355–377.

Sharpless, K. B. (1986). The discovery of asymmetric epoxidation. *Chem. Br.* **22**, 38–44.

Slawin, A. M. Z., Spencer, N., Stoddart, J. F. and Williams, D. J. (1987). The dependence of the solid state structures of bisparaphenylene-(3*n* + 4)-crown-*n* ethers upon macrocyclic ring size. *J. Chem. Soc., Chem. Commun.* 1070–1072.

Spencer, C. M., Stoddart, J. F. and Zarzycki, R. (1987). The structural mapping of an unsymmetrical chemically-modified cyclodextrin by high field nuclear magnetic resonance spectroscopy. *J. Chem. Soc., Perkin Trans.* **2**, 1323–1336.

Stoddart, J. F. (1979). From carbohydrates to enzyme analogues. *Chem. Soc. Rev.* **8**, 85–142.

Stoddart, J. F. (1980). The design and development of enzyme analogues. In *Enzymic and Non-Enzymic Catalysis* (eds P. Dunnill, A. Wiseman and N. Blackbrough), pp. 84–110. Ellis-Horwood, Chichester.

Stoddart, J. F. (1984). Crown ethers are enzyme models. In *The Chemistry of Enzyme Action* (ed. M. I. Page), pp. 529–561. Elsevier, Amsterdam.

Stoddart, J. F. (1987a). Chiral crown ethers. In *Topics in Stereochemistry* (eds E. L. Eliel and S. H. Wilen), Vol. 17, pp. 207–288. Wiley, New York.

Stoddart, J. F. (1987b). Enzyme models—crown ethers. In *Enzyme Mechanisms* (eds M. I. Page and A. Williams), pp. 35–55. Royal Society of Chemistry, London.

Stoddart, J. F. (1987c). The extramolecular chemical approach to enzyme analogues. *Biochem. Soc. Trans.* **15**, 1188–1191.

Stoddart, J. F. (1988). Conception and birth of new receptor chemistry from dibenzo-18-crown-6. *Pure Appl. Chem.* **60**, 467–472.

Stoddart, J. F. (1989). A century of cyclodextrins. *Carbohydr. Res.* **192**, xi–xv.

Stoddart, J. F. and Zarzycki, R. (1988). Cyclodextrins as second-sphere ligands for transition metal complexes. *Rec. Trav. Chim. Pays-Bas* **107**, 515–528.

Summers, L. A. (1980). *The Bipyridinium Herbicides*. Academic Press, London.

Sutherland, I. O. (1986). Molecular recognition by synthetic receptors. *Chem. Soc. Rev.* **15**, 63–91.

Szejtli, J. (1982). *Cyclodextrins and their Inclusion Complexes*. Akadémiai Kiadó, Budapest.

Szejtli, J. (1988). *Cyclodextrin Technology*. Kluwer, Dordrecht.

Tabushi, I. (1984). Design and synthesis of artificial enzymes. *Tetrahedron* **40**, 269–292.

Takahashi, Y. and Ogawa, T. (1987). Total synthesis of cyclomaltohexaose. *Carbohydr. Res.* **164**, 277–296.

Thiem, H.-J., Brandl, M. and Breslow, R. (1988). Molecular modelling calculations on the acylation of β-cyclodextrin by ferrocenylacrylate esters. *J. Am. Chem. Soc.* **110**, 8612–8616.

Wai, J. S. M., Marko, I., Svendsen, J. S., Finn, M. G., Jacobsen, E. N. and Sharpless, K. B. (1989). A mechanistic insight leads to a greatly improved osmium-catalyzed asymmetric dihydroxylation process. *J. Am. Chem. Soc.* **111**, 1123–1125.

Werner, A. (1913). *Neure Anschauungen auf dem Gebiete der anorganische Chemie*, 3rd edn. Vieweg, Braunscheig.

5

Modelling of Drug–Receptor Interactions: Stereoselectivity of 5-Hydroxytryptamine and Dopamine Receptors in the Brain

ULI HACKSELL, ANETTE M. JOHANSSON,
ANDERS KARLÉN, KRISTINA LUTHMAN
and CHARLOTTA MELLIN
Department of Organic Pharmaceutical Chemistry,
Uppsala Biomedical Centre, Uppsala University,
S-751 23 Uppsala, Sweden

1 Introduction

Neurotransmitters such as dopamine (DA) and serotonin (5-HT) (Fig. 1) are achiral and fairly flexible molecules that act on a variety of biological targets. DA stimulates D_1-receptors and pre- and post-synaptic D_2-receptors (Seeman *et al.*, 1986) and 5-HT interacts with at least seven subtypes of 5-HT-receptors (Hartig, 1989). In addition, these neurotransmitters are nonselective, that is, they interact also with other neurotransmitter receptors and drugs with such pharmacological profiles would probably not be useful as therapeutic agents. The nonselective actions of the neurotransmitters are not surprising when considering that many of their receptors belong to the G-protein coupled receptor superfamily (Dixon, *et al.*, 1988). There are considerable amino acid homologies between receptors in this class. In particular, the seven putative transmembrane regions, which appear to be common to all G-protein bound receptors and which may be responsible for ligand binding, have very similar

CHIRALITY IN DRUG DESIGN AND SYNTHESIS
ISBN 0-12-136670-7

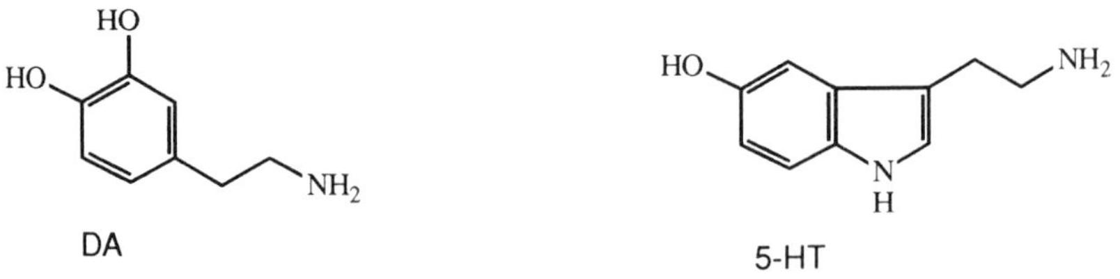

Fig. 1   The structure of dopamine (DA) and serotonin (5-HT).

amino acid sequences. Furthermore, the various receptors appear to transmit the chemical message from the neurotransmitter by similar mechanisms.

It is a well-established strategy among medicinal chemists to introduce structural modifications in neurotransmitters in order to obtain drugs with the desired pharmacological selectivity. Such modifications may also introduce chirality and, almost always, the neurotransmitter receptors discriminate between the resulting enantiomers. This can be illustrated with a phenyl-piperidine derivative, 3-PPP, which was synthesized as a conformationally restricted analogue of DA (Hacksell *et al.*, 1981, Hjorth *et al.*, 1981). 3-PPP interacts in a stereoselective fashion with DA-receptors (Hjorth *et al.*, 1983; Wikström *et al.*, 1984). The *R* enantiomer is a moderately potent agonist with a pharmacological profile similar to that of DA, that is, it acts as an agonist both at pre- and post-synaptic D_2-receptors. In contrast, the *S* antipode (Fig. 2) behaves as an agonist at presynaptic receptors and as an antagonist at postsynaptic receptors in most assays.

Recently, two D_2-receptor isoforms have been identified (Monsma *et al.*, 1989, Giros *et al.*, 1989). These two isoforms differ in the third cytoplasmic loop, a region which probably is responsible for the coupling to G-proteins. The two receptor isoforms may correspond to pre- and post-synaptic D_2-receptors and the apparent possibility that their coupling to/interaction with G-proteins may be different would provide an attractive rationale for the

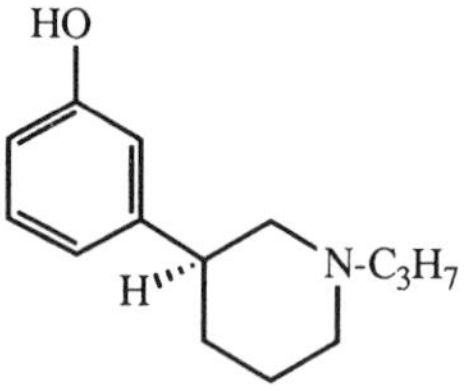

(*S*)-3-PPP

Fig. 2   The structure of (*S*)-3-PPP, a phenylpiperidine derivative.

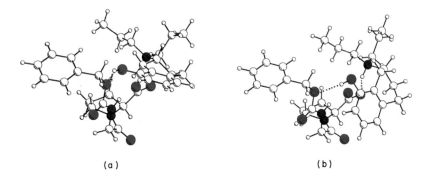

(a)   (b)

Plate 1 Starting geometry (*a*) and energy minimized (MMX) conformation (*b*) of a complex between (*R*)–8–OH DPAT and L–ZGP. Oxygen atoms are red, nitrogen atoms are blue and hydrogen bonds are indicated by dotted lines. In the starting geometry, 8–OH DPAT adopts a half-chair conformation with a pseudo-equatorial dipropylammonium group. During the minimization, the tetralin conformation changes into a boat. In contrast, the conformation of L–ZGP does not change appreciably.

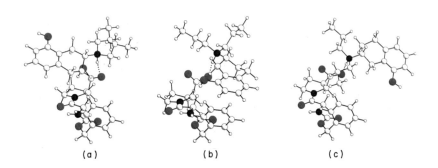

(a)   (b)   (c)

Plate 2 Three energy-minimized (MMX) complex conformations obtained by different dockings of identical conformations of (*R*)–8–OH DPAT and L–ZGP. Complexes (*b*) and (*c*) are 2.9 and 4.0 kcal mol⁻¹ more stable than complex (*a*). In fact, conformation (*a*) is one of the least stable complexes identified by docking these conformations of L–ZGP and (*R*)–8–OH DPAT. Oxygen atoms are red, nitrogen atoms are blue and hydrogen bonds are indicated by dotted lines.

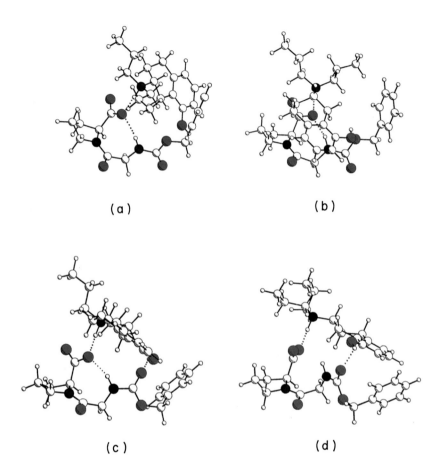

(a)

(b)

(c)

(d)

Plate 3 Minimum-energy conformations of complexes between L–ZGP and (R)– and (S)–8–OH DPAT ((a) and (c), respectively). Also shown are the best diastereomeric complexes found starting with the same conformations of L–ZGP and (S)– and (R)–8–OH DPAT ((b) and (d), respectively). Oxygen atoms are red, nitrogen atoms are blue and hydrogen bonds are indicated by dotted lines.

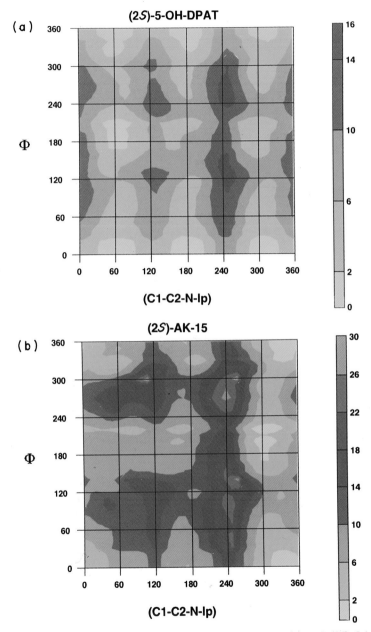

Plate 4 Conformational energy maps of (2S)–5–OH DPAT (*a*) and (2S)–5–hydroxy–1, 1–dimethyl–2–(dipropylamino) tetralin ((2S)–AK–15) (*b*). Φ is the tetralin inversion angle (see Karlén *et al*. (1986) for definition) and τ (C1, C2, N, lone pair) describes the rotation about the C2–N bond. Colour coding of energies (kcal mol⁻¹) is given to the right. The maps were generated by use of the one-bond torsional angle driver in the MM2–85 program.

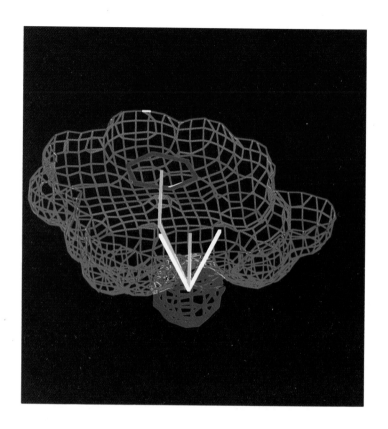

Plate 5 Partial 5–HT$_{1A}$–receptor excluded volume and agonist pharmacophore. The latter consists of an aromatic pharmacophore element (red) and a nitrogen–dummy atom vector (white lines define the outer limits of permitted vector orientations). The oxygen at the receptor which binds to the agonists is shown in red. The yellow lines correspond to descriptors that define the model further. For clarity, the receptor-excluded volume has been sliced in a plane parallel to and 1 Å above the plane of the aromatic pharmacophore element.

observation that presynaptic DA-receptors generally are more sensitive to agonist stimulation than those located postsynaptically. Thus, both enantiomers of 3-PPP may be partial agonists and the apparent antagonistic action of (S)-3-PPP on postsynaptic D_2-receptors would be due to a smaller efficacy than that of the antipode.

The above discussion provides a good example of how results from molecular biology may help to rationalize pharmacological results. However, even though the amino acid sequences of the D_2-receptors are known, the precise three-dimensional structure of the ligand binding site is unknown and we have no knowledge about the precise mechanism for the information transmission; for example, how is the interaction of DA with its receptor transmitted to the G-proteins and subsequently to an effector such as adenylyl cyclase? Thus, even though the knowledge of amino acid sequences of receptors has increased our pharmacological understanding, it does not help us to understand why (S)-3-PPP is less efficacious than (R)-3-PPP.

2 Interactions between L-ZGP and 8-OH DPAT

At present the three-dimensional structures of receptors in the G-protein bound receptor superfamily appear to be elusive. However, even if the precise three-dimensional structures were known, it would be difficult to use the information for rational drug design. The difficulty in studying the details of the receptor–ligand interaction may be illustrated by the following example. We are currently trying to establish factors which produce separation of enantiomers of various racemic aminoalcohols on achiral LC-columns when L-ZGP (benzyloxycarbonyl protected glycylproline) is added as a chiral counter ion (Pettersson and Josefsson, 1986). Initially, we have attempted to study the interaction between L-ZGP and 8-OH DPAT (Fig. 3), a racemic amino phenol which is separated into the enantiomers on several solid phases (Karlsson *et al.*, 1988).

According to molecular-mechanics (MMX) calculations, L-ZGP is able to adopt numerous (around 250) conformations with relative steric energies

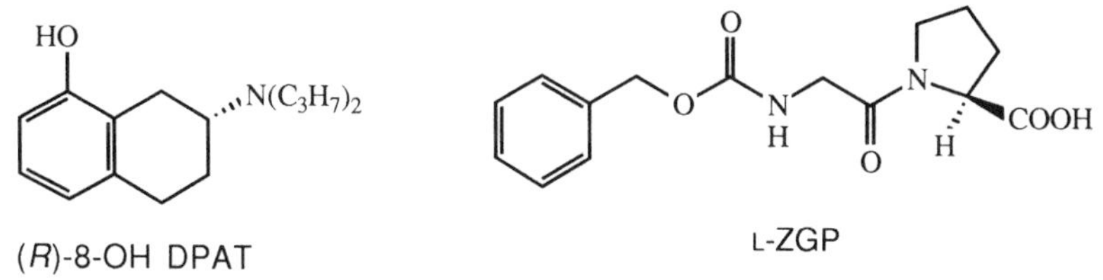

(R)-8-OH DPAT   L-ZGP

Fig. 3   The structure of (R)-8-OH DPAT and L-ZGP.

below 3 kcal mol^{-1} (Luthman and Hacksell, 1990). Ionized ZGP prefers to adopt conformations with a *cis* arrangement around the glycine–proline amide bond, whereas the protonated form shows a preference for a *trans* arrangement. The difference in main conformational characteristics is due to electrostatic repulsions between the carboxylate and the amide carbonyl oxygen in the *trans* but not the *cis* conformations of deprotonated ZGP. It is also noteworthy that many conformations with a *cis* oriented carbamate group appear to be favoured energetically. Also 8-OH DPAT possesses a fair degree of conformational flexibility (Arvidsson *et al.*, 1988). MMP2 calculations demonstrate that about 40 conformations of 8-OH DPAT have relative steric energies below 3 kcal mol^{-1}. The main conformational characteristics indicated from the calculations are supported by results obtained from NMR spectroscopy.

Dockings between 8-OH DPAT and L-ZGP were performed as flexible fittings using the MMX force field. In flexible dockings, the atoms in both molecules are allowed to move during the minimization. In contrast, in the simpler, less informative, and more frequently used rigid dockings, the geometries of the docked conformations are fixed. The result of a flexible docking of (*R*)-8-OH DPAT and L-ZGP is shown in Plate 1. As a result of the minimization, the conformation of (*R*)-8-OH DPAT changed from a half-chair to a boat.

The dominating interaction between the molecules in the energy-minimized complexes is a reinforced electrostatic interaction between the carboxylate group and the protonated nitrogen. Many complexes are further stabilized by inter- or intra-molecular hydrogen bonds and by attractive aromatic interactions. Interestingly, the minimum-energy conformation of L-ZGP is absent in complexes having a relative steric energy below 4 kcal mol^{-1}.

Based on the number of energetically allowed conformations one would need about 40×250 fittings to test all pairwise combinations of accessible conformations of L-ZGP and one of the enantiomers of 8-OH DPAT. However, in reality, the problem is much more complicated since there are a large number of local minima possible for each combination of ions. The numerous possibilities are illustrated by dockings of a half-chair conformation of (*R*)-8-OH DPAT with a *cis*(amide), *trans*(carbamate) conformation of L-ZGP (Plate 2). About 20 different minimized complex conformations were obtained depending on the relative orientation of the two molecules at the start of the docking. Two complex conformations with perpendicular relative orientations [(a) and (c)] and one conformation in which the molecules are aligned (b) are shown in Plate 2.

The minimum-energy conformation of the (*R*)-8-OH DPAT–L-ZGP complex is shown in Plate 3(a). In this complex, L-ZGP adopts a *cis*(amide), *trans*(carbamate) conformation. The complex is stabilized by a reinforced electrostatic interaction and, in addition, by an intramolecular hydrogen bond between the carbamate N–H and the carboxylate group. The diastereomeric complex obtained when docking the same conformations of (S)-8-OH DPAT and L-ZGP (Plate 3(b)) retains the intramolecular hydrogen bond and is only 0.4 kcal mol^{-1} less stable. The relative orientations of the 8-OH DPAT enantiomers in the two diastereomeric complexes are, however, very different. The most stable complex obtained with (S)-8-OH DPAT (Plate 3(c)) is also shown. In this complex, L-ZGP adopts a cis(amide), cis(carbamate) conformation which is stabilized by the same intramolecular hydrogen bond and the complex receives extra stabilization from an intermolecular hydrogen bond between the carbamate carbonyl and the phenol group. In fact, complex (c) is about 1.5 kcal mol^{-1} more stable than (a). Again, when the other enantiomer [(R)-8-OH DPAT] is docked with the same L-ZGP conformation [cis(amide), cis(carbamate)], the resulting complex [Plate 3(d)] is less stable (by about 7 kcal mol^{-1}) and the relative orientations of the two molecules are completely different. The major reason for the higher energy of the latter complex is the loss of the intramolecular hydrogen bond in L-ZGP.

3 Modelling of drug–receptor interactions

The problem of accurately searching the conformational space of small molecules has been addressed repeatedly (Howard and Kollman, 1988; Saunders et al., 1990). The above results indicate that the conformational multiple-minimum problem becomes much larger in studies of two molecules interacting with each other. Thus, the difficulties one would face if attempting to use information on receptor structure for making quantitative predictions about drug–receptor interactions are huge. Most likely, the very complicated information which may be offered by the three-dimensional structure of the receptor protein would be useful mainly for qualitative assessments. Instead, simple models will probably provide the most useful information. Such models may be derived from physico-chemical and pharmacological properties of series of receptor ligands and are referred to as indirect models since the structure of the target is unknown (Cohen et al., 1990).

One frequently used strategy for construction of simple indirect models is the active analogue approach (AAA) (Sufrin et al., 1981). The basic idea in the AAA is that each active analogue in a series must be able to present the biological target with a pharmacophore, that is a number of important functionalities in proper relative spatial positions. This pharmacophore is defined and then used as a template for the fitting (superposition) of various analogues. The combined van der Waals volume of the active analogues

88   U. Hacksell *et al.*

defines a receptor excluded volume. Furthermore, and by definition, inactive analogues must either lack pharmacophore groups, be unable to adjust to the pharmacophore for other reasons or they must produce excess volume which is part of the receptor essential volume. This latter volume may be defined as the common excess volume of inactive analogues which can adjust (or fit) to the pharmacophore.

We have been studying interactions between 2-aminotetralins and serotonin and dopamine receptors for several years. One theme has consisted of introducing methyl groups in various positions in the tetralin moiety. The resulting derivatives have been resolved into the enantiomers to enable studies of pharmacological stereoselectivities. As shown below, such information may be valuable when defining a pharmacophore for a biological response.

4 DA D₂-receptor agonists and antagonists

When applying the AAA to a series of analogues it is of great help to have access to test data of some fairly rigid and potent analogues. Fortunately, data were available on two potent DA D₂-receptor agonists with restricted mobility when we wanted to deduce an indirect model for DA D₂-receptor agonists (Johansson *et al.*, 1986). These compounds, (*R*)-apomorphine (APO) and the octahydrobenzo[f]quinoline derivative 1 (Wikström *et al.*, 1985) (Fig. 4) were subjected to conformational analysis by MMP2 calculations in order to define geometries of conformations with relative steric energies below 3 kcal mol⁻¹. Previous structure–activity relationship studies had indicated that a D₂ pharmacophore should consist of a phenolic hydroxyl group, an aromatic ring and a protonated nitrogen (Cannon, 1985; Miller *et al.*, 1988). Thus pairwise fittings of these structural elements were performed on each of the identified conformations. Only the superposition of the minimum-energy conformations of the two compounds produced a

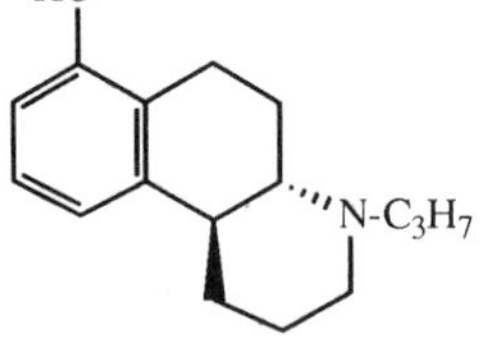

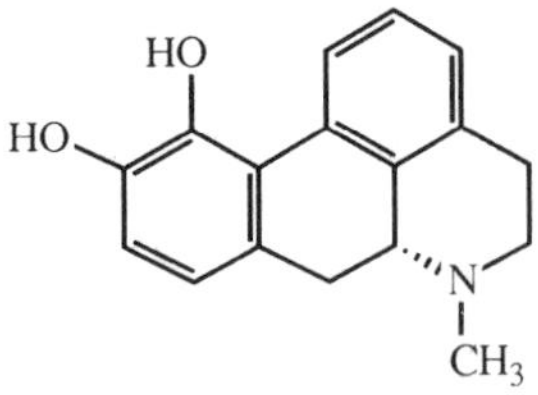

Fig. 4 The structure of the octahydrobenzo[*f*]quinoline derivative **1** and (*R*)-APO.

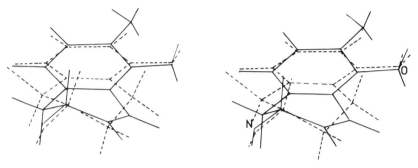

Fig. 5 Stereoscopic representation of a computer-generated best fit of (R)-apomorphine (solid lines) and (4aS,10bS)-7-hydroxy-4-propyl-1,2,3,4,4a,5,6,10b-octahydrobenzo[f]-quinoline (**1**) (dashed lines) in their minimum-energy (MMP2) conformations. For clarity, only the 2-aminotetralin fragments are shown. The relative positions of the coinciding hydroxyl groups, aromatic rings, nitrogens, and the nitrogen lone pairs of electrons ($N–H^+$) define the DA D_2-receptor agonist pharmacophore.

good fit. No other conformations gave a good overlap between the selected pharmacophore groups. Thus, the fit of the minimum-energy conformations was used to define a putative DA D_2-receptor agonist pharmacophore (Fig. 5). It is likely that a compound which has to pay a large energy penalty to adopt a biologically active conformation will show a modest activity (Karlén et al., 1989). Therefore, it was particularly satisfying that the only good fit was obtained with the minimum-energy conformations.

Having arrived at a pharmacophore hypothesis, we set out to test it by use of the series of optically pure 2-aminotetralin derivatives shown in Table 1. These compounds are particularly interesting because they exhibit pronounced conformational differences (Plate 4): For example, the rotational mobility about the C–N bond differs considerably. It is evident from NMR spectroscopy and molecular-mechanics calculations that the methyl substituted analogues prefer to adopt only one staggered rotamer of the dipropylammonium group whereas 5-OH DPAT adopts all three staggered conformations (Johansson et al., 1986, 1987a; Karlén et al., 1986, Hacksell et al., 1990). Also, the preferred location of the substituents on the cyclohexene ring may differ. In the *trans* derivative AJ-116, MMP2 calculations and NMR data indicate that half-chair conformations with dipseudo-axial and dipseudo-equatorial substituents are equally stable. In contrast, in the *cis* analogue UH-242 only half-chair conformations with an equatorially located nitrogen substituent are energetically relevant.

It is interesting to note that analogues which are potent D_2-receptor agonists readily adopt pharmacophore conformations and that agonists of

Table 1 Dopaminergic potency and relative steric energy of the pharmacophore conformation of some 2-aminotetralins

Compound	Dopaminergic agonist potency	Relative steric energy of the pharmacophore conformation (kcal mol^{-1})
(*S*)-5-OH-DPAT	Very potent	0.5
(1*R*,2*S*)-UH-242	Potent	0
(1*S*,2*S*)-AJ-116	Weakly potent	2.4
(*S*)-AK-15	Weakly potent	>2.5
(2*R*,3*S*)-AJ-166	Very potent	0
(2*R*,3*R*)-AJ-164	Weakly potent	>2.5

low potency prefer to adopt other conformations (Table 1). Thus, the ease of adopting pharmacophore conformations appears to be correlated with the dopaminergic agonist potency. This strengthens the pharmacophore hypothesis. One may argue that (1R,2S)-UH-242 ought to possess higher potency than observed. However, it is quite possible that the reduced potency may be due to the steric bulk of the pseudo-axial methyl group which may interfere with an optimal receptor interaction. One possibility might be that the methyl group does not permit the protonated nitrogen to interact optimally with a negatively charged amino acid residue at the receptor.

The pharmacology of the tricyclic analogues 1 and 2 (Fig. 6) (Wikström *et al.*, 1985) provides further support for the pharmacophore hypothesis. Thus, whereas (1S,2S)-AJ-116 is a weakly potent agonist, the corresponding tricyclic *trans* derivative 1, which resides almost entirely in a pharmacophore conformation, is a potent agonist. In addition, the inactive tricyclic *cis* derivative 2 is not able to adopt pharmacophore conformations, whereas the tetralin analogue (1R,2S)-UH-242, which is a fairly potent agonist, preferentially adopts a pharmacophore conformation.

Since the hypothetical D_2-receptor agonist pharmacophore appears to be correct, it was used as a template for potent agonists. Thus, (R)-APO 1, (S)-5-OH DPAT and (2R,3S)-AJ-166 were fitted to the pharmacophore and their van der Waals volumes were combined to generate a partial DA D_2-receptor excluded volume (Johansson *et al.*, 1987a). The resulting model may be of predictive value—compounds which can adopt energetically accessible pharmacophore conformations without producing van der Waals volume outside that of the receptor excluded volume should be able to activate DA D_2-receptors.

The interaction of 5-OH DPAT with the D_2-receptor is highly stereoselective. This is consistent with the pharmacophore model because (R)-5-OH DPAT cannot adopt an energetically favourable pharmacophore conformation due to severe van der Waals repulsions between C2–H and N^+–H. In fact, (R)-5-OH DPAT does not appear to be an agonist at all but

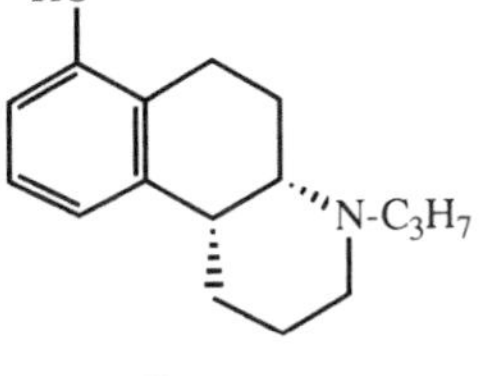

2

Fig. 6 The structure of the tricyclic analogue **2**.

92   U. Hacksell *et al.*

behaves as a weak antagonist (Karlsson *et al.*, 1990). Several reports have
appeared in which (*R*)-5-OH DPAT has shown weak agonist properties.
However, in these studies, the enantiomeric purity has not been
unambiguously established. We have developed a new resolution method
which gives an enantiomeric excess of (*R*)-5-OH DPAT of more than 99.7%
ee. (*S*)-5-OH DPAT (0.05 mmol kg^{-1}) produces a significant decrease in
limbic and striatal DOPA levels when given to rats treated with a DOPA
decarboxylase inhibitor. This action is expected from a stimulation of
presynaptic DA D$_2$-receptors. In contrast, treatment with (*R*)-5-OH DPAT
at 100- and 1000-fold higher doses, produces a significant increase in rat
striatal DOPA levels but does not affect the limbic DA-synthesis rate. The
reason for the absence of effects in the limbic brain areas is not understood, but the result obtained in the striatal brain portions demonstrates
that (*R*)-5-OH DPAT acts as a weakly potent DA-receptor antagonist.

Several other 2-aminotetralins and related chiral derivatives consist of
one enantiomer with potent dopaminergic agonist properties and one
enantiomer which behaves as an antagonist. A series of *cis*-Cl-methyl
substituted derivatives of 5-OH DPAT provides one such example. The
1*R*,2*S* enantiomer of UH-242 (Table 1) is a D$_2$-receptor agonist, whereas the
antipode behaves as an antagonist (Johansson *et al.*, 1985, 1987b; Svensson
et al., 1986b). In fact, (1*S*, 2*R*)-UH-242 has served as the lead compound for
a series of structurally related antagonists with interesting pharmacological
profiles (Svensson *et al.*, 1986a). The antagonist potency of (1*S*,2*R*)-UH-242
is increased by methylation of the phenol functionality (Johansson *et al.*,
1987b). In contrast, *O*-methylation of (*S*)-5-OH DPAT produces a
derivative in which the affinity for D$_2$-receptors is decreased more than 100-
fold. In fact, when pharmacological data from a series of agonists and
antagonists derived from UH-242 were studied in detail, it became apparent
that lipophilicity was important for antagonist activity of the 1*S*,2*R*
derivatives (Grol *et al.*, 1990). In contrast, agonist potency was not
correlated with lipophilicity in the 1*R*,2*S* enantiomers. These results are
consistent with a tentative model in which the agonists have three important
intermolecular interactions with the receptor, whereas the antagonists only
have two (Fig. 7). According to this model, the agonists, but not the
antagonists, would be able to donate a hydrogen bond from the phenolic
hydroxyl group to the receptor.

5   5-HT$_{1A}$-receptor agonists and antagonists

When the hydroxy substituent of 5-OH DPAT is moved to the C8-position,
the dopaminergic activity is lost. Instead, a potent 5-HT$_{1A}$-receptor agonist,
8-OH DPAT, is formed (Arvidsson *et al.*, 1981; Hjorth *et al.*, 1982). In

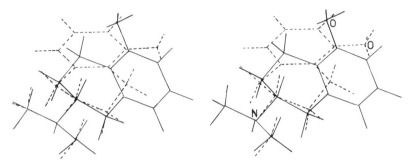

Fig. 7 Stereoscopic view of a computer-generated fit of 5-hydroxy-2-(dimethylamino)tetralin moieties of (S)- and (R)-5-OH DPAT (dashed and solid lines, respectively). This fit indicates that only the hydroxyl group of (S)-5-OH DPAT is able to donate a hydrogen bond to the DA D_2-receptor and that both enantiomers probably are anchored to the receptor by a similar reinforced electrostatic bond.

contrast to 5-OH DPAT, which interacts in a stereospecific fashion with DA D_2-receptors, the interaction between 8-OH DPAT and the 5-HT_{1A}-receptors is only weakly stereoselective—in most assays for 5-HT_{1A}-receptor agonist activity, the R enantiomer is about twice as potent as the antipode (Arvidsson et al., 1981; Björk et al., 1989). Both enantiomers appear to have a pronounced selectivity for 5-HT_{1A}-receptor sites, for example, the affinity for D_2-receptors is about 500 times lower than that for 5-HT_{1A}-receptors. The difference in pharmacological stereoselectivity between the 5- and 8-substituted analogues indicates that they have different modes of interaction with their respective receptors. This is emphasized further by the different effects of introducing methyl substituents in the two series. trans-C1-Methyl substitution decreases activity in both series, but much more in the 8-OH DPAT series since the resulting derivative (ALK-4; see Fig. 10) appears to be devoid of activity (Arvidsson et al., 1987). This may be related to a severe peri interaction between the 8-hydroxy substituent and a pseudo-equatorial C1-methyl substituent which forces the molecule to adopt a conformation with the C1 and C2 substituents in pseudo-axial positions. In fact, NMR spectroscopy supports this idea since the coupling constant between C1–H and C2–H is very small (2.2 Hz), which is typical for a diequatorial coupling. Introduction of a cis-C1-methyl substituent in 8-OH DPAT, to give ALK-3 (Fig. 8) increases stereoselectivity dramatically—from two-fold to more than 1000-fold (Arvidsson et al., 1987; Hjorth et al., 1989). It may be noted that the cis-C1-methyl substituent considerably decreases the conformational mobility. Thus, only eight conformations with relative steric energies below

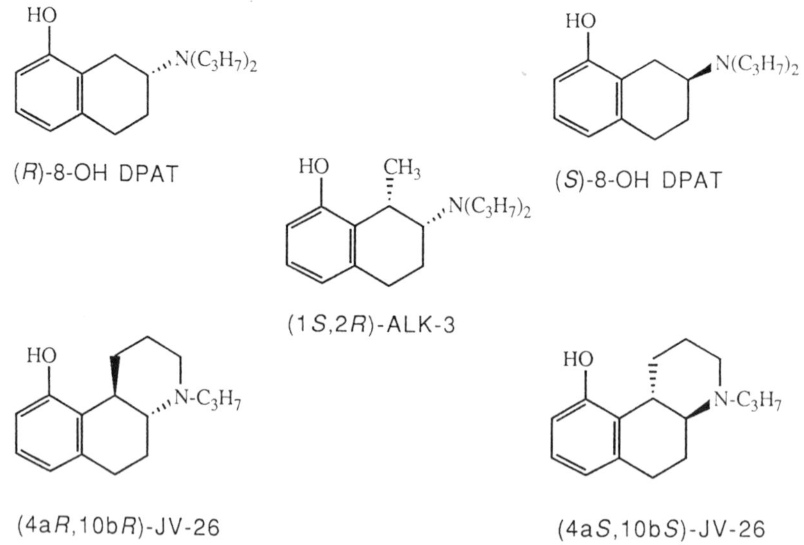

(R)-8-OH DPAT

(1S,2R)-ALK-3

(S)-8-OH DPAT

(4aR,10bR)-JV-26

(4aS,10bS)-JV-26

Fig. 8   Structures of some potent 5-HT$_{1A}$-receptor agonists.

3 kcal mol^{-1} were identified by MMP2 calculations. This may be compared with 8-OH DPAT which adopts about 40 energetically favourable conformations. Thus, ALK-3 is a valuable compound for modelling purposes. Even more valuable for modelling, however, are the enantiomers of JV-26 (Fig. 8), which are tricyclic *trans* derivatives of 8-OH DPAT (Mellin *et al.*, 1990). Both JV-26 enantiomers are potent agonists and possess very little conformational mobility. Therefore, these derivatives provide important clues for deducing an indirect model for 5-HT$_{1A}$-receptor agonists. The introduction of C3-methyl substituents in 8-OH DPAT decreases potency but increases stereoselectivity (Mellin *et al.*, 1988; Björk *et al.*, 1987). It is noteworthy that the two enantiomers which possess agonist potency have opposite configurations at the nitrogen bearing carbon (Fig. 9).

By use of a modification of the AAA, it was possible to arrive at a model for 5-HT$_{1A}$-receptor agonists which rationalizes, in a qualitative sense, the observed activities of the compounds shown in Figs 8–10 (Mellin *et al.*, 1990): various pharmacophore hypotheses were tested but the only pharmacophore which was consistent with the data set consists of an aromatic ring and a dummy atom connected to the positively charged nitrogen. The latter pharmacophore group is supposed to mimic a reinforced electrostatic bond between the protonated nitrogen and a carboxylate anion at the receptor. In the pharmacophore model, allowed

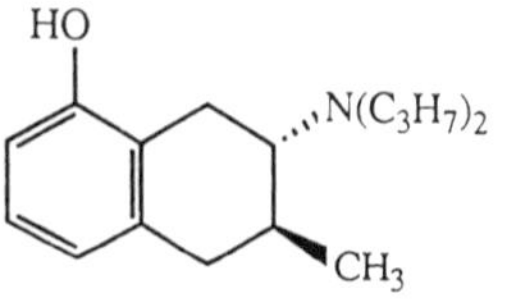

(2S,3S)-CM-12

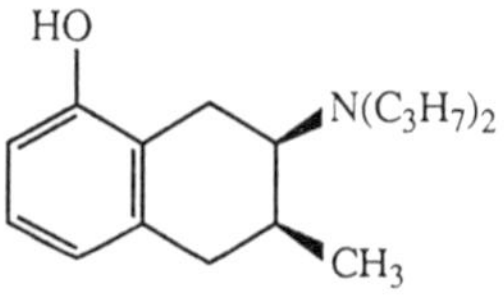

(2R,3S)-CM-11

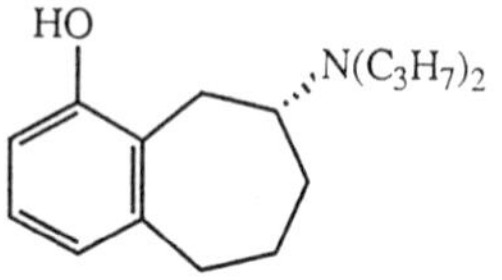

(R)-LY-14

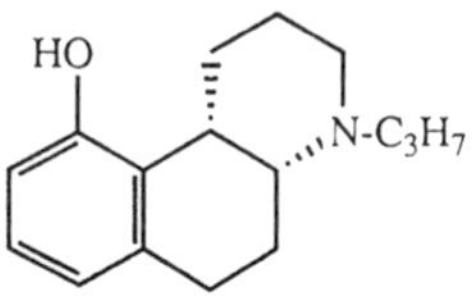

(4aR,10bS)-OHBQ

Fig. 9 Structures of some moderately potent 5-HT$_{1A}$-receptor agonists.

orientations of the nitrogen–dummy atom vectors are restricted as shown in Plate 5. Potent agonists were fitted to the pharmacophore and their van der Waals volumes were added to generate a 5-HT$_{1A}$-receptor-excluded volume. None of the moderately potent agonists (Fig. 9) or inactive compounds (Fig. 10) were able to fit the pharmacophore without producing excess volume. It was also possible to extend the model and include the moderately potent agonists, since this extended model was able to differentiate between agonists and inactives. Thus, by use of the AAA it was possible to generate a model which differentiates between potent and moderately potent 5-HT$_{1A}$-receptor agonists and compounds without apparent efficacy. The model appears to have some generality and it should be of predictive value. However, it is highly simplified since it does not take into account the electronic properties of the aromatic ring. Consequently, the model in its present form is not able to rationalize one of our most exciting findings which deals with 8-OH DPAT derivatives substituted with a 5-fluoro substituent.

In contrast to racemic 8-OH DPAT, which behaves as a very potent 5-HT$_{1A}$-receptor agonist *in vivo*, the racemic 5-fluoro substituted derivative, UH 301, appeared to be completely devoid of serotonergic activity when tested in rats. However, (±)-UH 301 was able to displace [^{3}H]8-OH DPAT from 5-HT$_{1A}$-receptors *in vitro*. Therefore, we decided to prepare and study pharmacologically the pure enantiomers (Hillver *et al.*, 1990): (R)-UH 301, has a pharmacological profile similar to that of 8-OH DPAT, but is slightly

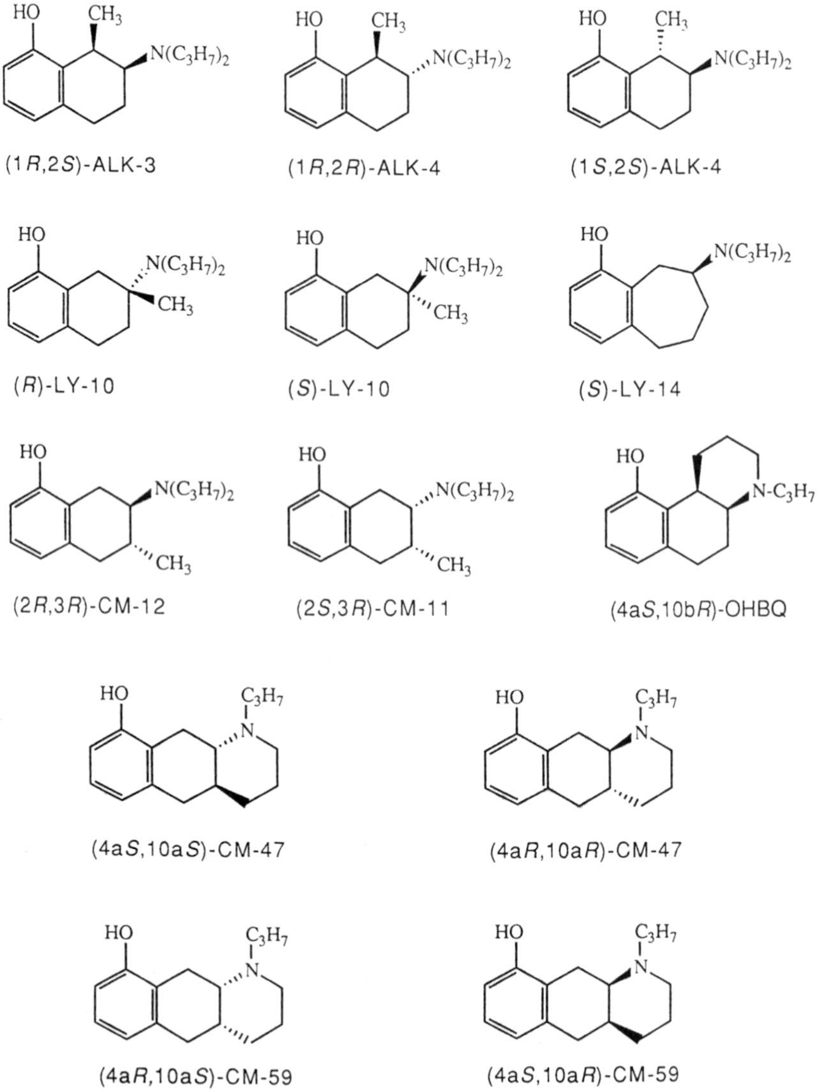

Fig. 10 Structures of some compounds which are structurally related to the 5-HT$_{1A}$-receptor agonists but lack ability to stimulate 5-HT$_{1A}$-receptors.

less potent. In contrast, (S)-UH 301 (Fig. 11) is able to bind to 5-HT$_{1A}$-receptors but has no ability to elicit a response, that is, it lacks efficacy. Thus, introduction of a 5-fluoro substituent in (S)-8-OH DPAT appears to diminish affinity and abolish efficacy. In fact, (R)-UH 301 is an effective

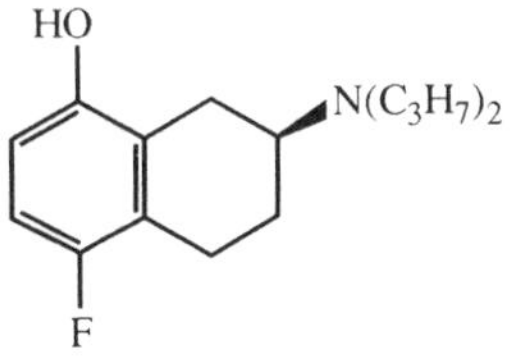

(S)-UH-301

Fig. 11   The structure of (S)-UH-301.

antagonist of 8-OH DPAT induced $5-HT_{1A}$-receptor stimulation in all assays studied so far. This indicates the exciting possibility that the simple model described above may be extended to describe the efficacy of $5-HT_{1A}$-receptor agonists in terms of electronic properties of the aromatic ring and its substituent(s). Since partial $5-HT_{1A}$-receptor agonists appear to be of value as anxiolytic agents (Traber and Glaser, 1987), the possibility to design compounds with a spectrum of pharmacological profiles by modification of stereochemistry and aromatic substituents seems particularly promising.

Acknowledgements

The research presented herein was supported by grants from the Swedish Natural Science Council, the Swedish National Board for Technical Development, and 'Centrala Försöksdjursnämnden'. The excellent contributions from our coworkers, whose names are cited in the references, are gratefully acknowledged.

References

Arvidsson, L.-E., Hacksell, U., Svensson, U., Nilsson, J. L. G., Hjorth, S., Carlsson, A., Sanchez, D., Lindberg, P. and Wikström, H. (1981). 8-Hydroxy-(2-di-n-propylamino)tetralin, a new centrally acting 5-HT-receptor agonist. *J. Med. Chem.* **24**, 921–923.

Arvidsson, L.-E., Johansson, A. M., Hacksell, U., Nilsson, J. L. G., Svensson, K., Hjorth, S., Magnusson, T., Carlsson, A., Andersson, B. and Wikström, H. (1987). (+)-*cis*-8-Hydroxy-1-methyl-2-(di-n-propylamino)tetralin: a potent and highly stereoselective 5-hydroxytryptamine receptor agonist. *J. Med. Chem.* **30**, 2105–2109.

Arvidsson, L.-E., Karlén, A., Norinder, U., Kenne, L., Sundell, S. and Hacksell, U. (1988). Structural factors of importance for 5-hydroxytryptaminergic activity. Conformational preferences and electrostatic potentials of 8-hydroxy-2-(di-n-propylamino)tetralin (8-OH DPAT) and some related agents. *J. Med. Chem.* **31**, 212–221.

Björk, L., Mellin, C., Hacksell, U. and Andén, N.-E. (1987) Effects of the C3-methylated derivatives of 8-hydroxy-2-(di-n-propylamino)tetralin (8-OH-DPAT) on central 5-hydroxytryptaminergic receptors. *Eur. J. Pharmacol.* **143**, 55–63.

Björk, L., Backlund Höök, B., Nelson, D. L., Andén, N.-E. and Hacksell, U. (1989). Resolved *N,N*-dialkylated 2-amino-8-hydroxytetralins: stereoselective interactions with 5-HT$_{1A}$ receptors in the brain. *J. Med. Chem.* **32**, 779–783.

Cannon, J. G. (1985). Dopamine agonists: Structure–activity relationships. *Prog. Drug Res.* **29**, 303–414.

Cohen, N. C., Blaney, J. M., Humblet, C., Gund, P. and Barry, D. C. (1990). Molecular modelling software and methods for medicinal chemistry. *J. Med. Chem.* **33**, 883–894.

Dixon, R. A., Strader, C. D. and Sigal, I. S. (1988). Structure and function of G-protein coupled receptors. *Ann. Rep. Med. Chem.* **23**, 221–233.

Giros, B., Sokoloff, P., Martres, M.-P., Riou, J.-P., Emorine, L. J. and Schwartz, J.-C. (1989). Alternative splicing directs the expression of two D$_2$ dopamine receptor isoforms. *Nature* **342**, 923–926.

Grol, C. J., Nordvall, G., Johansson, A. M. and Hacksell, U. (1990). 5-Oxygenated *N*-alkyl-2-amino-1-methyltetralins. Effects of structure and stereochemistry on dopamine D$_2$-receptor affinity (in manuscript).

Hacksell, U., Arvidsson, L.-E., Svensson, U., Nilsson, J. L. G., Sanchez, D., Wikström, H., Lindberg, P., Hjorth, S. and Carlsson, A. (1981). 3-Phenyl-piperidines. Central dopamine-autoreceptor stimulating activity. *J. Med. Chem.* **24**, 1475–1482.

Hacksell, U., Johansson, A. M., Karlén, A., Svensson, K. and Grol, C. J. (1990). Stereochemical parameters of importance for dopamine D$_2$-receptor activation. In *Chirality and Biological Activity* (eds B. Holmstedt, H. Frank and B. Testa), pp. 247–266. Alan R. Liss, New York.

Hartig, P. (1989). Molecular biology of 5-HT receptors. *Trends Pharmacol. Sci.* **10**, 64–69.

Hillver, S.-E., Björk, L., Li, Y.-L., Svensson, B., Ross, S., Andén, N.-E. and Hacksell, U. (1990). (*S*)-5-Fluoro-8-hydroxy-2-(dipropylamino)tetralin: a putative 5-HT$_{1A}$-receptor agonist. *J. Med. Chem.* **33**, 1541–1544.

Hjorth, S., Carlsson, A., Wikström, H., Lindberg, P., Sanchez, D., Hacksell, U., Arvidsson, L.-E., Svensson, U. and Nilsson, J. L. G. (1981). 3-PPP, A new centrally acting DA-receptor agonist with selectivity for autoreceptors. *Life Sci.* **28**, 1225–1238.

Hjorth, S., Carlsson, A., Lindberg, P., Sanchez, D., Wikström, H., Arvidsson, L.-E., Hacksell, U. and Nilsson, J. L. G. (1982). 8-Hydroxy-2-(di-n-propyl-amino)tetralin, 8-OH-DPAT, a potent and selective simplified ergot congener with central 5-HT-receptor stimulating activity. *J. Neural Transm.* **55**, 169–188.

Hjorth, S., Carlsson, A., Clark, D., Svensson, K., Wikström, H., Sanchez, D., Lindberg, P., Hacksell, U., Arvidsson, L.-E., Johansson, A. and Nilsson, J. L. G. (1983). Central dopamine receptor agonist and antagonist actions of the enantiomers of 3-PPP. *Psychopharmacology* **81**, 89–99.

Hjorth, S., Sharp, T. and Hacksell, U. (1989). Partial postsynaptic 5-HT$_{1A}$ agonist properties of the novel stereoselective 8-OH-DPAT analogue (+)-*cis*-8-hydroxy-1-methyl-2-(di-n-propylamino)tetralin, (+)-ALK-3. *Eur. J. Pharmacol.* **170**, 269–274.

Howard, A. E. and Kollman, P. A. (1988). An analysis of current methodologies for conformational searching of complex molecules. *J. Med. Chem.* **31**, 1669–1675.

Johansson, A. M., Arvidsson, L.-E., Hacksell, U., Nilsson, J. L. G., Svensson, K., Hjorth, S., Clark, D., Carlsson, A., Sanchez, D., Andersson, B. and Wikström, H. (1985). Novel dopamine receptor agonists and antagonists with preferential action on autoreceptors. *J. Med. Chem.* **28**, 1049–1053.

Johansson, A. M., Karlén, A., Grol, C. J., Sundell, S., Kenne, L. and Hacksell, U. (1986). Dopaminergic 2-aminotetralins: affinities for dopamine D_2-receptors, molecular structures and conformational preferences. *Mol. Pharmacol.* **30**, 258–269.

Johansson, A. M., Nilsson, J. L. G., Karlén, A., Hacksell, U., Svensson, K., Carlsson, A., Kenne, L. and Sundell, S. (1987a). C3-Methylated 5-hydroxy-2-(dipropylamino)tetralins: conformational and steric parameters of importance for central dopamine receptor activation. *J. Med. Chem.* **30**, 1135–1144.

Johansson, A. M., Arvidsson, L.-E., Hacksell, U., Nilsson, J. L. G., Svensson, K. and Carlsson, A. (1987b). Resolved *cis*- and *trans*-2-amino-5-methoxy-1-methyltetralins: central dopamine receptor agonists and antagonists. *J. Med. Chem.* **30**, 602–611.

Karlén, A., Johansson, A. M., Kenne, L., Arvidsson, L.-E. and Hacksell, U. (1986). Conformational analysis of the dopamine-receptor agonist 5-hydroxy-2-(dipropylamino)tetralin and its C(2)-methyl substituted derivative. *J. Med. Chem.* **29**, 917–924.

Karlén, A., Helander, A., Kenne, L. and Hacksell, U. (1989). Topography and conformational preferences of 6,7,8,9-tetrahydro-1-hydroxy-*N,N*-dipropyl-5*H*-benzocyclohepten-6-ylamine. A rationale for the dopaminergic inactivity. *J. Med. Chem.* **32**, 765–774.

Karlsson, A., Pettersson, C., Sundell, S., Arvidsson, L.-E. and Hacksell, U. (1988). Improved preparation, chromatographic separation and X-ray crystallographic determination of the absolute configuration of the enantiomers of 8-hydroxy-2-(dipropylamino)tetralin (8-OH DPAT). *Acta Chem. Scand., Ser. B.* **42**, 231–236.

Karlsson, A., Björk, L., Pettersson, C., Andén, N.-E. and Hacksell, U. (1990). (*R*)- and (*S*)-5-hydroxy-2-(dipropylamino)tetralin (5-OH DPAT): assessment of optical purities and dopaminergic activities. *Chirality* **2**, 90–95.

Luthman, K. and Hacksell, U. (1990). Conformational analysis of benzyloxy-carbonylglycyl-L-proline—MMX-calculations and NMR-spectroscopy (in manuscript).

Mellin, C., Björk, L., Karlén, A., Johansson, A. M., Sundell, S., Kenne, L., Nelson, D. L., Andén, N.-E. and Hacksell, U. (1988). Central dopaminergic and 5-hydroxytryptaminergic effects of C3-methylated derivatives of 8-hydroxy-2-(di-n-propylamino)tetralin. *J. Med. Chem.* **31**, 1130–1140.

Mellin, C., Vallgårda, J., Nelson, D. L., Björk, L., Hong, Y., Andén, N.-E., Csöregh, I., Arvidsson, L.-E. and Hacksell, U. (1990). A 3-D model for 5-HT_{1A}-receptor agonists based on stereoselective methyl substituted and conformationally restricted analogues of 8-hydroxy-2-(dipropylamino)tetralin. *J. Med. Chem.* (in press).

Miller, D. D., Harrold, M., Wallace, R. A., Wallace, L. J. and Uretsky, N. J. (1988). Dopaminergic drugs in the cationic form interact with D_2 dopamine receptors. *Trends Phamacol. Sci.* **9**, 282–284.

Monsma, F. J., Jr., McVittie, L. D., Gerfen, C. R., Mahan, L. C. and Sibley, D. R. (1989). Multiple D_2 dopamine receptors produced by alternative RNA splicing. *Nature* **342**, 926–929.

Pettersson, C. and Josefsson, M. (1986). Chiral separation of aminoalcohols by ion-pair chromatography. *Chromatographia* **21**, 321–326.

Saunders, M., Houk, K. N., Wu, Y.-D., Still, W. C., Lipton, M., Chang, G. and Guida, W. C. (1990). Conformations of cycloheptadecane. A comparison of methods for conformational searching. *J. Am. Chem. Soc.* **112**, 1419–1427.

Seeman, P., Grigoriadis, D. E. and Niznik, H. B. (1986). Selectivity of agonists and antagonists at D_2 dopamine receptors compared to D_1 and S_2 receptors. *Drug Dev. Res.* **9**, 63–69.

Sufrin, J. R., Dunn, D. A. and Marshall, G. R. (1981). Steric mapping of the L-methionine binding site of ATP: L-methionine (*S*)-adenosyltransferase. *Mol. Pharmacol.* **19**, 307–313.

Svensson, K., Carlsson, A., Johansson, A. M., Arvidsson, L.-E. and Nilsson, J. L. G. (1986a). A homologous series of *N*-alkylated *cis*-(+)-(1*S*,2*R*)-5-methoxy-1-methyl-2-aminotetralins: central dopamine-receptor antagonists showing profiles ranging from classical antagonism to selectivity for auto-receptors. *J. Neural Transm.* **65**, 29–38.

Svensson, K., Hjorth, S., Clark, D., Carlsson, A., Wikström, H., Andersson, B., Sanchez, D., Johansson, A. M., Arvidsson, L.-E., Hacksell, U. and Nilsson, J. L. G. (1986b). (+)-UH 232 and (+)-UH 242: novel stereoselective dopamine receptor antagonists with preferential action on autoreceptors. *J. Neural Transm.* **65**, 1–27.

Traber, J. and Glaser, T. (1987). 5-HT_{1A}-Related anxiolytics. *Trends Pharmacol. Sci.* **8**, 432–437.

Wikström, H., Sanchez, D., Lindberg, P., Hacksell, U., Arvidsson, L.-E., Johansson, A. M., Thorberg, S.-O., Nilsson, J. L. G., Svensson, K., Hjorth, S., Clark, D. and Carlsson, A. (1984). Resolved 3-(3-hydroxyphenyl)-*N*-n-propyl-piperidine and its analogues: central dopamine receptor activity. *J. Med. Chem.* **27**, 1030–1036.

Wikström, H., Andersson, B., Sanchez, D., Lindberg, P., Arvidsson, L.-E., Johansson, A. M., Nilsson, J. L. G., Svensson, K., Hjorth, S. and Carlsson, A. (1985). Resolved monophenolic 2-aminotetralins and 1,2,3,4,4a,5,6,10b-octahydrobenzo[*f*]quinolines: structural and stereochemical considerations for centrally acting pre- and postsynaptic dopamine-receptor agonists. *J. Med. Chem.* **28**, 215–225.

6

Molecular Basis of the Activity of Antibiotics of the Vancomycin Group: Guides for Peptide–Peptide Binding

DUDLEY H. WILLIAMS, ANDREW J. DOIG,
JONATHAN P. L. COX, IAN A. NICHOLLS
and MARK GARDNER

Cambridge Centre for Molecular Recognition,
University Chemical Laboratory,
Lensfield Road, Cambridge, UK

1 Introduction

Antiobiotics of the vancomycin group have assumed increasing clinical importance during the last 15 years, in part because of the increasing prevalence of *Staphylococcus aureus* bacteria which are resistant to methicillin (Wise *et al.*, 1978). In addition, vancomycin itself has found extensive use in the treatment of post-operative diarrhoea, caused by *Clostridium difficile* in the gut. The antiobiotic is then given orally, and has been found to be very efficient in curing a dangerous condition.

As the importance of the antibiotics in this group has increased, pharmaceutical companies in many parts of the world have initiated efforts to find new members. As a result, the group now consists of a large number of structures, all of which are heptapeptides. For a vancomycin group antibiotic produced by any one actinomycete, there are often a number of variants, frequently differing in the nature of the attached sugars or fatty acid groups. The total number of structural variants which have been reported is in the region of 100; these variants can be encompassed by the

CHIRALITY IN DRUG DESIGN AND SYNTHESIS
ISBN 0-12-136670-7

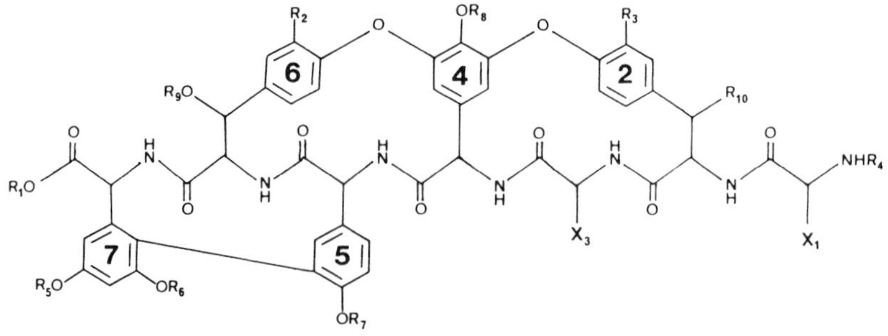

Fig. 1 The general structure (**1**) of the vancomycin group of antibiotics.

general structure shown in Fig. 1 (see, for example, Barna and Williams (1984)).

For a number of years now, we have been engaged not only in the structure elucidation of members of this group, including the structure

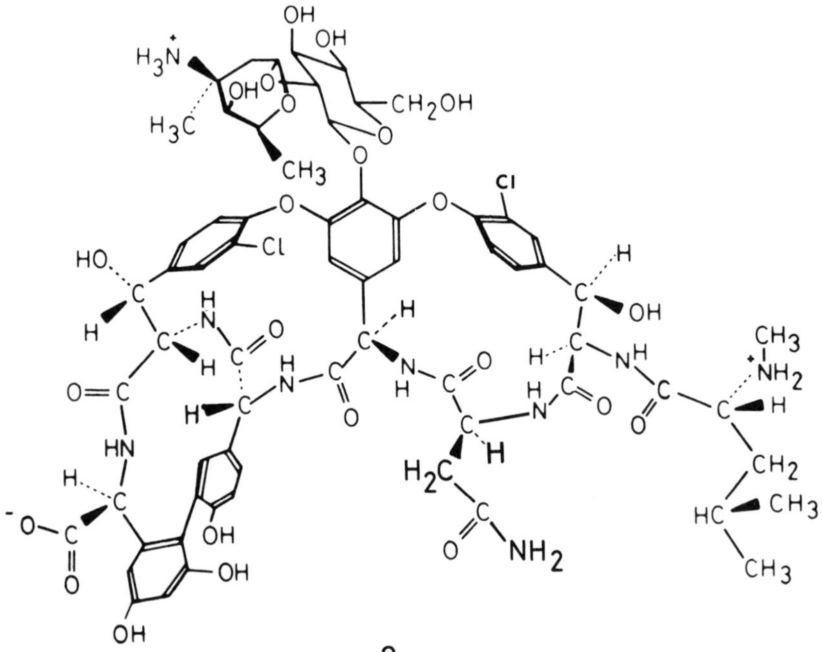

Fig. 2 The structure of vancomycin (**2**).

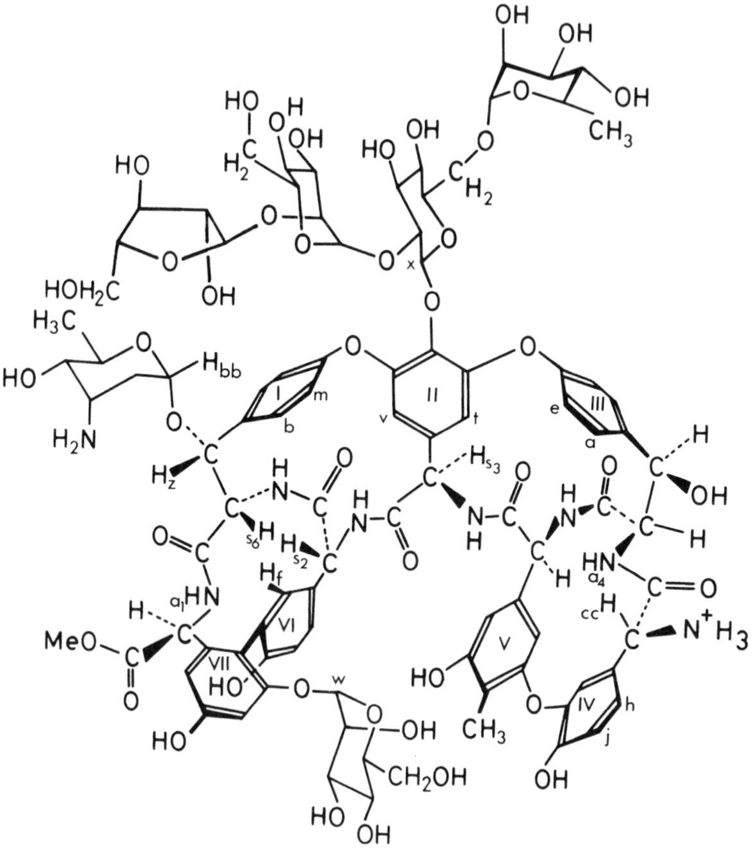

Fig. 3 The structure of ristocetin A (**3**).

elucidation of vancomycin itself, but also in work designed to establish the molecular basis of their mode of action. The latter part of the work has been built on a finding (Perkins, 1969) that vancomycin itself (**2**, Fig. 2) and another member of the group, ristocetin A (**3**, Fig. 3), bind to cell-wall mucopeptide precursors terminating in the peptide –D-Ala–D–Ala. Given this knowledge, we examined the proton magnetic resonance spectra of ristocetin A both in the presence and absence of the cell-wall analogue N-acetyl–D-Ala–D–Ala (hereinafter also referred to as dipeptide) (Kalman and Williams, 1980a,b).

Proton resonances of the antibiotic in its free form, and when bound to the cell-wall analogue were assigned to specific protons in the structure. A similar analysis was carried out for the proton resonances of the dipeptide. With this information in hand, we therefore knew the changes in chemical shift of each proton resonance upon formation of a complex between the antibiotic and the cell-wall analogue. In particular, the changing chemical shift of NH protons of the antibiotic and cell-wall analogue could be used to indicate which of these protons, when they occur as part of a secondary amide unit (–CO–NH–), are involved in hydrogen-bond formation.

This information can be accommodated by proposing that in the complex between the antibiotic and the cell-wall analogue, the cell-wall analogue is oriented relative to the antibiotic as shown in Fig. 4. In the figure, dotted lines indicate hydrogen-bond formation between the carbonyl group of one component and an NH group of the other component. It can be seen that in the proposed complex, the carboxyl group of the C-terminal alanine of the

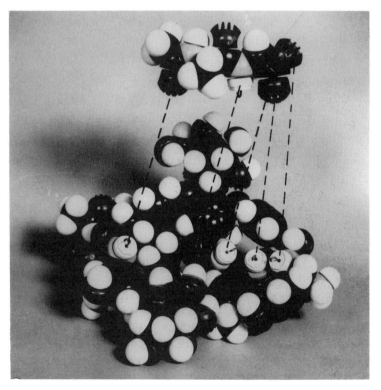

Fig. 4 A model of the interaction between ristocetin A (only the glucose unit of the tetrasaccharide is shown) and the bacterial cell wall analogue *N*-acetyl–D-Ala–D-Ala. The broken lines indicate intermolecular hydrogen bonds formed on complexation.

cell-wall analogue forms no less than three hydrogen bonds to three NH groups which lie in a pocket, bounded by substituted benzene rings, at one end of the antibiotic structure. As these interactions occur, additional hydrogen bonds can be formed between the carbonyl oxygen of the acetyl group of the cell-wall analogue and an NH which is seen at the left-hand part of the antibiotic structure, and between the NH of the C-terminal alanine and a carbonyl group of the antibiotic. The geometry of these hydrogen-bonded interactions allows simultaneously favourable hydrophobic interactions to occur between the two alanine methyl groups of the cell-wall analogue and parts of the benzene rings of the antibiotic.

The above model for the binding interaction has been checked by use of the powerful technique of intermolecular nuclear Overhauser effects (NOE) (Kalman and Williams, 1980b). The NOE data for the ristocetin–dipeptide complex showed that the binding model represented in Fig. 4 is indeed correct in its essential details. Those protons of the antibiotic and cell-wall analogue which are demanded by the binding model to be near in space do give mutual NOEs. Thus, the molecular basis of action of the antibiotics is well founded (Williamson and Williams, 1985).

In addition, by utilizing, and extending, earlier work (Nieto and Perkins, 1971a,b,c), it has been possible to measure the binding constant between the two components by the use of ultraviolet (UV) difference spectroscopy. These measurements were not only carried out for numerous antibiotics of the vancomycin group with N-acetyl–D-Ala–D-Ala, but also for the extended cell-wall analogue, di-N-acetyl–L-Lys–D-Ala–D-Ala (hereafter also called tripeptide). The binding constants in general lie in the range 10^4 to 10^7 l mol^{-1}, with the larger binding constants (by ca. 10^1 to 10^2) normally being found for the more extended cell-wall analogue.

Given the above background, we have been able to explore some of the factors involved in defining the desired antibiotic geometries, and the factors involved in more subtle aspects of binding the cell-wall analogues (Williams and Waltho, 1988). The present chapter is concerned with the analysis of some aspects of the stereoselectivity and thermodynamics of binding, and with considerations of how the derived principles can further our understanding of peptide–peptide interactions and protein folding.

2 Stereoselectivity

The selectivity shown by the antibiotics against peptides containing amino acids of chirality not found in the normal cell-wall mucopeptide precursors is high. Nieto and Perkins (1971) record 'no combination' of di-N-acetyl–L-Lys–D-Ala–L-Ala and of di-N-acetyl–L-Lys–L-Ala–D-Ala to both vancomycin and ristocetin. It is estimated that the method of UV difference spectroscopy employed in these studies would fail to detect an association constant of $<10^3$ 1 mol^{-1}. The data therefore imply that, in the case of vancomycin, the 'wrong' stereochemistry at either alanine residue reduces the binding energy (relative to the 'normal' tripeptide) by at least 18 kJ mol^{-1}, and in the case of ristocetin by at least 15 kJ mol^{-1}. The experiments of Smith *et al.* (1988), using a direct competitive binding assay—and thereby being perhaps more precise—allow a comparison to be made between the binding of C_6H_5CO–D-Ala–D-Ala and C_6H_5CO–D-Ala–L-Ala. In the case of vancomycin, the binding energy of the latter is less than that of the former by 10 kJ mol^{-1}, and in the case of ristocetin by 15–21 kJ mol^{-1}. Although the absolute values of the binding constants derived in these studies are subject to errors estimated to be in the range 5–8 kJ mol^{-1}, the differences in the binding constants are presumably relatively reliable due to the competitive nature of the assay. If this is so, then we can conclude that vancomycin is able to discriminate between a D and an L terminal alanine by a reduction in the binding constant of a factor of ca. 50 and ristocetin by a factor in the range 500–4000.

If the five hydrogen bonds of the normal complex were to continue to be formed, the reduction in binding observed for cell-wall analogues containing L-analine at the C-terminal position could be analysed in the following manner. First, the hydrophobic interaction of a C-terminal D-alanine with the benzene ring of amino acid residue 4 of the antibiotic is lost. Replacement of this residue by glycine indicates that the binding energy lost in this manner lies in the range 3–6 kJ mol^{-1} for vancomycin, and 7–9 kJ mol^{-1} for ristocetin. (In this respect, there is good agreement between the data of Nieto and Perkins (1971) and the data of Smith *et al.* (1988).) Second, C-terminal L-alanine could cause, given the normal hydrogen-bonding pattern, and the geometry of the peptide backbone suggested for the D,D isomer in its bound state, a repulsive interaction between its methyl group and the carbonyl group of the preceding D-alanine. However, molecular modelling studies (unpublished) have so far not given independent support for this possibility; given the experimental facts, this may simply reflect the use of inadequate theory in the modelling studies. In the case of vancomycin, the lower stereoselectivity of binding relative to ristocetin (10 vs. 15–21 kJ mol^{-1}) is possibly due not only to the smaller loss in binding due to removal of the hydrophobic interaction (3–6 vs. 7–9 kJ mol^{-1}) associated with the D-Ala methyl group, but also perhaps due to the greater flexibility of the carboxylate anion binding pocket of the antibiotic in the case of vancomycin. In vancomycin, one wall of the pocket is formed by the 'folding-in' of a flexible N-Me-leucine side chain, whereas in ristocetin, this same wall is constituted from the side chain of a constrained (cross-linked) p-hydroxyphenylglycine. Thus, in the case of vancomycin, the potentially unfavourable steric interaction of the methyl group of the C-terminal L-alanine residue with the carbonyl group of the preceding residue may be more readily relieved by adjusting the position of the carboxylate anion in the more flexible pocket of vancomycin.

3 Peptide–peptide molecular recognition

The problem of protein folding is one of the most important questions of contemporary science. Although enormous progress has been made towards solving this problem during the last two decades, it is still not possible in the general case to take a determined primary sequence of amino acids and from this predict the tertiary structure of the corresponding protein. The challenge to solve this problem is not only intellectually important, but also of great practical relevance in view of the rapidity with which c-DNA sequences may now be obtained, and the corresponding primary amino acid sequences thereby derived.

There is experimental evidence that isolated α-helix and β-sheet structures are, prior to tertiary interactions, populated only to a similar extent as the unfolded structures (see, for example, Wright *et al.* (1988)). Thus, the free energies of such subunits do not differ greatly from those of their unfolded counterparts (i.e. $\Delta G \simeq 0$ kJ mol^{-1}). If it is assumed that the structures of β-sheets do not involve significant van der Waals repulsions, then there appears to be only one important source of unfavourable free-energy change on folding of the backbone into a β-sheet structure. This unfavourable free-energy change is associated with freezing out two rotors for each amino acid to be incorporated in the folded structures. The rotors which must be frozen out are the N–C$_\alpha$ and C$_\alpha$–CO– bonds. For the freezing out of a free rotor, the unfavourable 'entropy' change has been calculated as 4.5–6.0 kJ mol^{-1} (Doig and Williams, unpublished) at room temperature (taken as 300 K). Since we argue that ΔG for formation of a β-sheet is approximately zero per residue, then 9–12 kJ mol^{-1} must be almost exactly counterbalanced by favourable changes. These changes are:

(1) the enthalpy term ($\Delta H(H)$) for the formation of an amide–amide hydrogen bond; and
(2) the entropy term ($T\Delta S(W)$) for the water released in the formation of this hydrogen bond.

Since in the formation of an isolated β-sheet, one hydrogen bond is formed for *two* residues, then:

$$\Delta H(H) - T\Delta S(W) + 18{-}24 \simeq 0 \text{ kJ mol}^{-1} \text{ at } 300 \text{ K} \tag{1}$$

Thus, the intrinsic binding energy (Jencks, 1981) associated with the amide–amide hydrogen-bond formation is calculated to lie in the range 18–24 kJ mol^{-1}. However, for a molecular description of this process, we need to know whether this process is enthalpy or entropy driven (or both). ΔH(H) is available from a comparison of the calorimetric data of Rodriguez-Tebar *et al.* (1986) on the enthalpy of binding of Ac–D-Ala and Ac–Gly–D-Ala to vancomycin and ristocetin A. From our knowledge of the binding sites of the antibiotics for these peptides (Fig. 4), it is known that the enthalpy of binding of the two peptide substrates differs only by the formation of an extra hydrogen bond in the binding of the dipeptide. The ΔH(H) values are -3.4 ± 2.8 in the case of ristocetin, and $+1.4 \pm 2.3$ kJ mol^{-1} in the case of vancomycin, at 25°C. The important point about these values is that they are self-consistently small. We conclude that, in an aqueous environment, the enthalpy change for hydrogen bond formation between amide and amide, adjusted for the unfavourable enthalpy change associated with the release of water molecules from the involved CO and NH units, is near zero.

In contrast, the calorimetric data of Rodriguez-Tebar *et al.* (1986) also show that the entropy change associated with the formation of the same hydrogen bond, and concurrently freezing out the two rotors of glycine necessary to make this hydrogen bond, is (in terms of $T\Delta S$ at 25°C) larger: 11 ± 3 kJ mol^{-1} in the case of vancomycin, and 8 ± 4 kJ mol^{-1} in the case of ristocetin. Since we have calculated that the freezing out of these two rotors is entropically unfavourable by 9–12 kJ mol^{-1} at room temperature (see above), then the total favourable entropy term associated with the formation of the hydrogen bond lies in the range 17–23(± 4) kJ mol^{-1}. We conclude that in these systems (and by extrapolation in isolated β-sheets in general) amide–amide hydrogen-bond formation in aqueous solution is essentially an entropy-driven process, the favourable entropy change being associated with water release from the C=O and NH groups which associate.

The consistency between the intrinsic binding energy (ca. 20 kJ mol^{-1}) for amide–amide hydrogen-bond formation based on experiment coupled to the freezing out of two rotors, with that calculated on the basis of freezing out four rotors alone, supports our estimate for the entropic cost of freezing out the peptide backbone rotors.

4   Approximate binding constants estimated for simple carboxylic acids

We now use the approximate intrinsic binding constant for amide–amide hydrogen-bond formation ($\Delta H \simeq 0$ kJ mol^{-1}, $T\Delta S \simeq 20$ kJ mol^{-1} at 25°C)

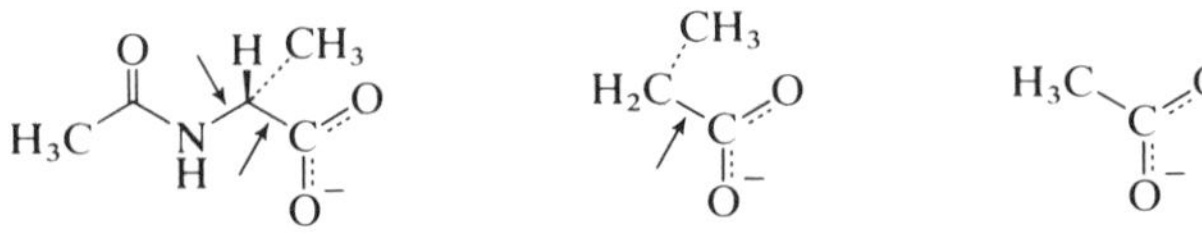

Fig. 5   The structure of N-Ac–D-Ala (4), propionate anion (5) and acetate anion (6).

to estimate the approximate binding constant for acetate and propionate anions to ristocetin A. The thermodynamic data (Rodriguez-Tebar *et al.*, 1986) for the binding of N-Ac–D-Ala 4, (Fig. 5) are $\Delta H = -28.3 \pm 1.4$ kJ mol^{-1} and $\Delta G = -17.4 \pm 0.5$ kJ mol^{-1} at 25°C. The amide NH of 4 is assumed, by analogy to the known mode of binding of N-Ac–D-Ala–D-Ala, to be bound by hydrogen-bond formation to an amide carbonyl of the antibiotic. The intrinsic binding energy of the hydrogen bond is ca. 20 kJ mol^{-1} (see above).

However, upon binding of 4 to the antibiotic, the two rotors indicated by arrows must be frozen out, whereas upon binding of propionate anion (5, Fig. 5) only one such rotor is frozen (see arrow). Since in this system, the freezing out of each rotor is estimated to be unfavourable by $T\Delta S = 5$ kJ mol^{-1} (see earlier), then 5 should bind more weakly than 4 by ca. 15 kJ mol^{-1}. In addition, the methyl of the acetyl group of 4 makes a hydrophobic interaction with the antibiotic which, on the basis of the hydrocarbon–hydrocarbon surface area in contact, is estimated to increase the binding of 4 by ca. 5 kJ mol^{-1}. This binding energy is also lost on passing to 5, and thus ΔG for association of 5 to ristocetin A should be very small and possibly slightly positive ($K = 1$ to 10^{-1}). Moreover, this ΔG value should be constituted from a relatively large negative enthalpy of association (26–30 kJ mol^{-1}), offset by an almost equal or slightly greater unfavourable $T\Delta S$ term at 25°C.

The association constant for acetate anion (6, Fig. 5), can also be estimated similarly. The binding of 6 does not require the freezing out of any of its rotors, so on this basis, and the loss of the hydrogen bond and the hydrophobic interaction of the methyl of the acetyl group relative to the binding of 4,6 should bind less strongly than 4 by ca. 15 kJ mol^{-1}. However, the hydrophobic interaction of the alanine methyl group over the aromatic ring of residue 4 of the antibiotic is also lost on passing from 4 to 6, giving a further reduction in binding of 7–9 kJ mol^{-1} (see earlier). Thus, the total adverse effect is ca. 22–24 kJ mol^{-1}, giving $\Delta G = 5$–7 kJ mol^{-1} ($K = 10^{-1}$ mol^{-1}) for 6. As in the case of the binding of propionate anion, this ΔG value is again estimated to be constituted from a relatively large and negative enthalpy of binding (26–30 kJ mol^{-1}), offset by a slightly greater unfavourable entropy term at 25°C. The very approximate estimates of the binding energies of **5** and **6** are currently being investigated experimentally.

5 A molecular interpretation of the binding process

Following the considerations of Page and Jencks (1971), we can take the unfavourable entropy term for association of propionate anion, or the cell-wall di- or tri-peptides, due to their loss of rotational and translational entropy upon association with ristocetin A as ca. 50–60 kJ mol^{-1} (in terms of $T\Delta S$ at 25°C). Application of the Sackur–Tetrode equation for translational entropy, and of the classical equation for rotational entropy (Atkins, 1986), shows that this term shows a relatively small mass dependence, varying by only 8 kJ mol^{-1} among the three substrates considered (being largest for the substrate of highest molecular mass). Although the equations just cited are, strictly speaking, only applicable to the calculation of the entropy of ideal gases, the values obtained, after adjustment for the decreased entropy of liquids relative to gases (Trouton's rule), give values which are in surprisingly good accord with values obtained from solution experiments.

Given the above estimate, the earlier analysis of the thermodynamics of binding, and noting that the binding of N-acetyl–D-Ala–D-Ala has $\Delta H = -25.4 \pm 1.6$ kJ mol^{-1} and $T\Delta S = 3 \pm 1.8$ kJ mol^{-1} at 25°C, then the following molecular picture of the binding process emerges.

The unfavourable entropy change due to a bimolecular association (50–60 kJ mol^{-1} for $T\Delta S$), and the freezing out of four rotors of the dipeptide (ca. 20 kJ mol^{-1}) is almost exactly balanced by a favourable entropy change. The total unfavourable entropy change at room temperature (70–80 kJ mol^{-1}) is countered by the favourable entropy change associated with: (a) the release of water molecules from the polar groups involved in the binding (approximately 40 kJ mol^{-1} for water released in the formation of two amide bonds, and ca. 30 kJ mol^{-1} for water released from the carboxylate anion and the portion of the antibiotic (three amide NH groups in a cleft) which binds this anion); (b) the hydrophobic interactions involving the two alanine methyl groups and the α-CH of the non-C-terminal alanine ($T\Delta S \simeq 12$ kJ mol^{-1}). In addition, it is known (Williams and Waltho, 1988) that the benzene ring of residue **1** of the antibiotic (see **3**) folds over the carboxylate anion of the bound dipeptide. From our considerations of the thermodynamics of protein folding (Doig and Williams, unpublished), we have calculated that at 25°C, $T\Delta S = 0.125$ kJ mol^{-1} Å^{-2} for such hydrophobic interactions (the driving force in the present case being the removal of the benzene ring from exposure to water in the bound state). The total area of hydrocarbon buried in the binding process is in the region of 150 Å^2 and, therefore, the total favourable entropy-based contribution to binding is estimated to be around 18 kJ mol^{-1}.

The water released in the binding process is, of course, an assembly of water molecules 'attached' (but in a dynamic sense) to each polar group eventually involved in the binding. For pictorial convenience, it may be helpful to regard one water molecule as being detached from each polar group involved in the binding. On the basis of this picture, amide–amide hydrogen-bond formation would be associated with the release of two water molecules. Since the favourable entropy change due to this process is ca. 20 kJ mol^{-1} (see earlier), then the entropy change per water molecule lost is ca. 10 kJ mol^{-1} at room temperature. Thus, seven water molecules would be pictured as being released in the binding process, as in **7** (Fig. 6), to account for $T\Delta S = 70$ kJ mol^{-1} for the water release (see above).

Interestingly, the only favourable enthalpy change involved in the binding in terms of our description lies in the range 25–30 kJ mol^{-1}, and is associated with the intrinsic binding constant for the carboxylate anion into the pocket of three adjacent NH groups. The entropic part of the intrinsic binding constant of the carboxylate anion is also favourable for binding ($T\Delta S$ near 30 kJ mol^{-1} at room temperature, see earlier). Binding constants predicted to be not far from the 10^{-1} to 1 range for acetate and propionate anions are small as a consequence of the above favourable enthalpic and entropic terms for binding being together almost equal and opposite to the loss of rotational and translational entropy on binding.

Finally, we note that it is the sign and order of magnitude of the thermodynamic parameters which we have discussed (rather than their

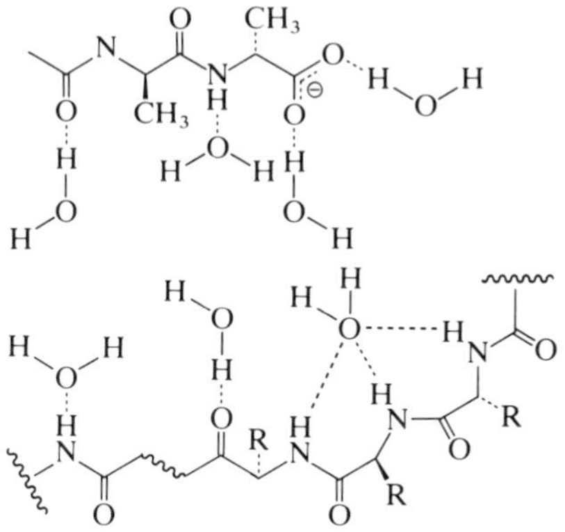

7

Fig. 6   Schematic picture of water molecules released in the binding process.

specific values) which are important. The picture of the binding which has been derived is not yet precise, but the emerging model seems physically reasonable, and helps increase our understanding of peptide–peptide binding in aqueous solution.

Acknowledgements

The SERC and the Upjohn Company (Kalamazoo) are thanked for financial support.

References

Atkins, P. W. (1986). *Physical Chemistry*, 3rd edn, p. 857. Oxford University Press, Oxford.
Barna, J. C. J. and Williams, D. H. (1984). The structure and mode of action of glycopeptide antibiotics of the vancomycin group. *Ann. Rev. Microbiol.* **38**, 339–357.
Jencks, W. P. (1981). On the attribution and additivity of binding energies. *Proc. Natl. Acad. Sci.* **78**, 4046–4050.
Kalman, J. R. and Williams, D. H. (1980a). An NMR study of the structure of the antibiotic ristocetin A. The negative nuclear Overhauser effect in structure elucidation. *J. Am. Chem. Soc.* **102**, 897–905.
Kalman, J. R. and Williams, D. H. (1980b). An NMR study of the interaction between the antibiotic ristocetin A and a cell wall peptide analogue. Negative nuclear Overhauser effects in the investigation of drug binding sites. *J. Am. Chem. Soc.* **102**, 906–912.
Nieto, M. and Perkins, H. R. (1971a). Physicochemical properties of vancomycin and iodovancomycin and their complexes with diacetyl-L-lysyl-D-alanyl-D-alanine. *Biochem. J.* **123**, 773–787.
Nieto, M. and Perkins, H. R. (1971b). Modifications of the Acyl–D-alanyl–D-alanine terminus affecting complex-formation with vancomycin. *Biochem. J.* **123**, 789–803.
Nieto, M. and Perkins, H. R. (1971c). The specificity of combination between ristocetins and peptides related to bacterial cell wall mucopeptide precursors. *Biochem. J.* **124**, 845–852.
Page, M. I. and Jencks, W. P. (1971). Entropic contributions to rate accelerations in enzymic and intramolecular reactions and the chelate effect. *Proc. Natl. Acad Sci. USA* **68**, 1678–1683.
Perkins, H. R. (1969). Specificity of combination between mucopeptide precursors and vancomycin or ristocetin. *Biochem. J.* **111**, 195–205.
Rodriguez-Tebar, A., Vasquez, D., Perez Velazquez, J. L., Laynez, J., and Wadso, I. (1986). Thermochemistry of the interaction between peptides and vancomycin or ristocetin. *J. Antibiot.* **39**, 1578–1583.
Smith, P. W., Chang, G. and Still, W. C. (1988). Molecular complex evaluation. A simultaneous assay of binding using substrate mixtures. *J. Org. Chem.* **53**, 1587–1590.
Williams, D. H. and Waltho, J. P. (1988). Molecular basis of the activity of antibiotics of the vancomycin group. *Biochem. Pharmacol.* **37**, 133–141.

Williamson, M. and Williams, D. (1985). [1]NMR Studies of the structure of ristocetin A and of its complexes with bacterial cell wall analogues in aqueous solution. *J. Chem. Soc., Perkins Trans. I* 949–956.

Wise, R. and Reeves, D. (eds) (1984). Symposium on vancomycin therapy. *J. Antimicrob. Chemother.* **14**, (Suppl. D).

Wright, P. E., Dyson, H. J. and Lerner, R. A. (1988). Conformation of peptide fragments of proteins in aqueous solution: implications for initiation of protein folding. *Biochemistry* **27**, 7167–7125.

7

Recent Developments in the Use of Enzyme-Catalysed Reactions in Organic Synthesis

STANLEY M. ROBERTS

Department of Chemistry, University of Exeter, Stocker Road, Exeter, EX4 4QD, UK

1 Introduction

Over the past 10 years the use of enzymes as catalysts for the preparation of novel organic molecules has received a steadily increasing amount of attention. Before 1980 the employment of enzymes and/or whole cell systems in organic chemistry was localized in a few pioneering laboratories; now many non-specialists are discovering the advantages in utilizing these natural catalysts. There are two easily recognized advantages that may be gained from utilizing enzymes. First the proteins are able to promote reactions under very mild conditions of temperature, pH, and pressure. Secondly, enzymes are chiral catalysts and are often able to produce optically active molecules that can be used as building blocks (synthons) for the preparation of homochiral compounds. These two facets of biotransformations will form recurring themes in this review. Experiments from the Exeter laboratories will be quoted as examples: other texts are available that give a more comprehensive coverage of the earlier literature (Davies *et al.*, 1989).

Two of the most popular areas of biotransformations that have a very great relevance to organic synthesis involve the use of hydrolase enzymes on the one hand and oxidoreductase enzymes on the other. These two areas are

CHIRALITY IN DRUG DESIGN AND SYNTHESIS
ISBN 0-12-136670-7

discussed here in turn. In Section 4 we describe some carbon–carbon bond-forming reactions that are catalysed by enzymes and in the final section future directions of the work in the area of biotransformations are indicated.

2 Recent uses of hydrolase enzymes

Enzymes are available for the hydrolysis of carboxylic acid esters, phosphate esters, amides, and nitriles. The enzyme-catalysed hydrolysis of alkyl carboxylates has been extensively investigated. For example, the acetate (1) is easily prepared and is hydrolysed enantioselectively using *Mucor miehei* lipase or lyophilized yeast cells. The alcohol (2) is obtained (enantiomeric excess (e.e.) = 80–100%) and this synthon is utilized in the preparation of 13-HODE (coriolic acid) (3), a naturally occurring, biologically active compound (Glänzer *et al.*, 1987; Chan *et al.*, 1988). While this chemo-enzymatic synthesis of 13-HODE is interesting and useful for the preparation of selected analogues, the preparation of the natural product itself is more efficiently accomplished using another enzyme-catalysed reaction namely the conversion of linoleic acid into 13-HODE (in 40% yield) using a lipoxygenase enzyme. We have developed this process to allow the production of quantities of material sufficient for further chemical studies (Maguire *et al.*, 1990).

Meso-diacetates such as the compound (4) are very interesting substrates in enzyme-catalysed transformations. Compound (4) is converted into the half-ester (5) using porcine pancreatic lipase. The yield of (5) is almost quantitative and the optical purity is very high (>98% e.e.) (Cox and Roberts, 1990). Compound (5) has been converted into the nucleotide analogue (6) and is being used in various enzyme studies.

Similarly, the dimethyl cyclopentane dicarboxylate (7) is hydrolysed with exquisite selectivity using pig liver esterase to give the mono-ester (8) in a highly pure form (96% yield; 98% e.e.) (Zemlicka *et al.*, 1988; Hutchinson *et al.*, 1990). Note that the 'meso-trick' (where enzyme-catalysed reactions can be applied to conversions such as 4 → 5 and 7 → 8) allows the possibility of forming optically pure products in quantitative yield from the chosen substrates, a process that is very difficult to emulate using conventional chemical catalysts.

$$H\!-\!\!\!\equiv\!\!\!-CH(OCOCH_3)C_5H_{11}$$

(1)

(2)

(3)

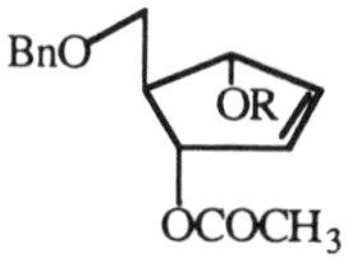

NH$_2$

BnO— OR / OCOCH$_3$

(4) R=COCH$_3$
(5) R=H

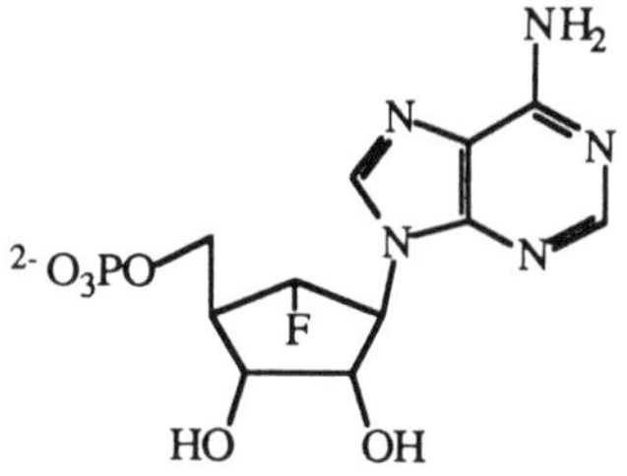

2- O$_3$PO— F

HO   OH

(6)

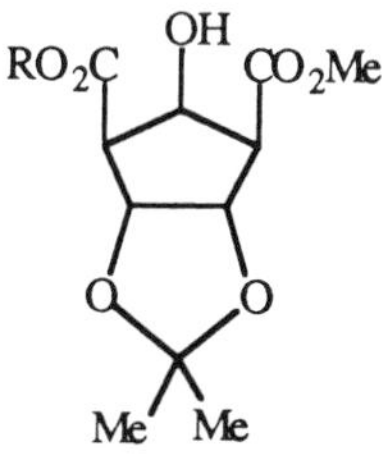

RO$_2$C   OH   CO$_2$Me

Me Me

(7) R=Me
(8) R=H

RO—

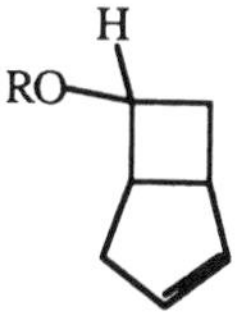

(9) R=H
(10) R=COCH$_3$

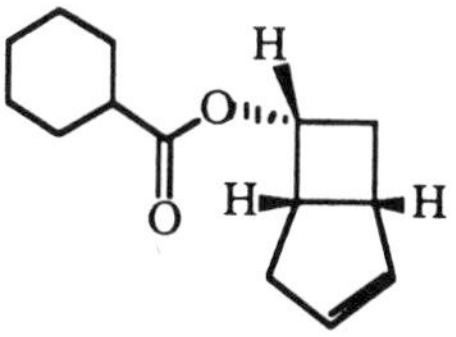

(11)

In recent years the employment of lipases in organic media for the preparation of esters from carboxylic acids and alcohols has been studied by a number of research groups (Roberts, 1989; Riva *et al.*, 1988). For example, the racemic alcohol (9) in hexane is converted into the optically active ester (11) (90% e.e.) and recovered optically enriched bicyclo[3.2.0]-hept-2-en-6*endo*-ol using cyclohexane carboxylic acid and the catalyst Lipozyme (*Mucor miehei* lipase attached to an inert solid support (Cotterill *et al.*, 1988a).) The ester (11) is obtained in even higher optical purity (>99% e.e.) on employing an interesterification reaction involving the acetate (10) and cyclohexane carboxylic acid. The separated esters can be used in syntheses of prostaglandin-F$_{2\alpha}$, a naturally occurring material with a plethora of biological activities (Scheme 1) (Newton and Roberts, 1982; Macfarlane *et al.*, 1990).

The employment of acylases (such as hog kidney acylase) for the cleavage of amide bonds under mild conditions is well known. This type of hydrolysis is commercially important in the preparation of 6-aminopenicillanic acid and in the synthesis of some optically pure amino acids (Wandrey, 1986).

More recently it has been found that a microbial acylase can effect the enantiospecific hydrolysis of the lactam (12) to give the amino acid (13) and recovered starting material. A second micro-organism can effect the

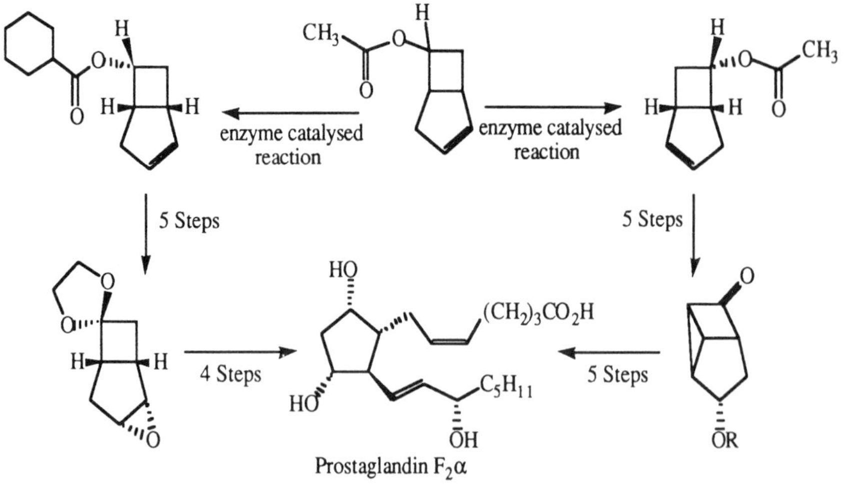

Scheme 1

enantiocomplementary hydrolysis to give the mirror image of compound **13** and recovered lactam (Evans *et al.*, 1990). These optically active amino acids and lactams can be used to prepare the important anti-AIDS agent carbovir (**14**) (Vince and Hua, 1990) in homochiral form.

The synthesis of phosphate esters can be accomplished by kinase enzymes using adenosine triphosphate (ATP) as the phosphate donor. The technique will work with unnatural substrates: for example the racemic nucleoside analogue (**15**) was converted into the racemic nucleotide (**16**) using thymidine kinase and ATP. Enantioselective hydrolysis of the (±)-phosphate (**16**) can be achieved using 5'-nucleotidase from snake venom to give the dextrorotatory carbocyclic nucleoside (+)-**15** which exhibited very powerful anti-herpes activity (Borthwick *et al.*, 1988, 1990).

The hydrolysis of nitrile groups using hydratase enzymes is of great

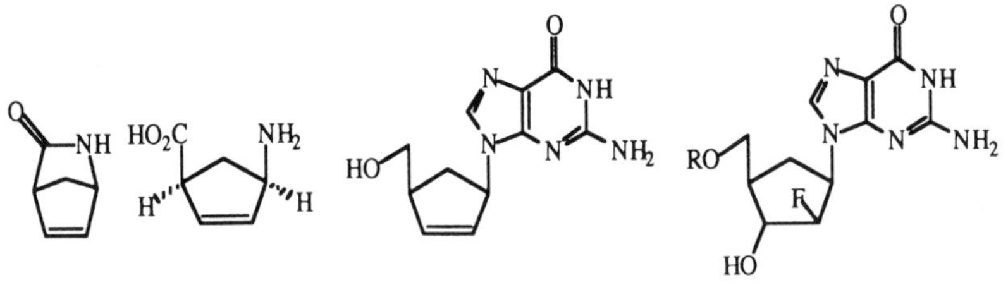

(12)   (13)   (14)   (15) R=H
                                                (16) R=PO$_3$H$_2$

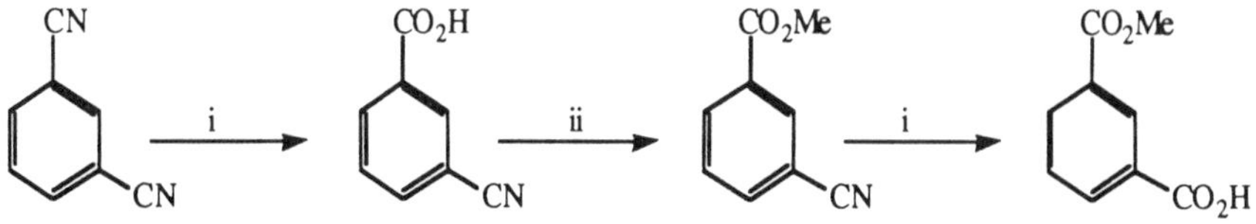

$$\underset{\underset{\text{CN}}{\bigg|}}{\overset{\text{CN}}{\bigg|}} \xrightarrow{\text{i}} \underset{\underset{\text{CN}}{\bigg|}}{\overset{\text{CO}_2\text{H}}{\bigg|}} \xrightarrow{\text{ii}} \underset{\underset{\text{CN}}{\bigg|}}{\overset{\text{CO}_2\text{Me}}{\bigg|}} \xrightarrow{\text{i}} \underset{\underset{\text{CO}_2\text{H}}{\bigg|}}{\overset{\text{CO}_2\text{Me}}{\bigg|}}$$

Scheme 2   Reagents: (i) Nitrile hydratase SP 361, buffer pH 7, 30°C, 12–24 h; (ii) CH_2N_2.

interest to many synthetic organic chemists, principally because the hydrolysis takes place under very mild conditions. The sequence outlined in Scheme 2 illustrates the selectivity of processes of this type (Bengis-Garber and Gutman, 1988; Hwang and Chang, 1989; Endo and Watanabe, 1989; Cohen and Turner, 1990).

The use of hydrolase enzymes by the non-specialist is aided by the availability of models of the active site of enzymes such as pig liver esterase, porcine pancreatic lipase, *Pseudomonas fluorescens* lipase and *Candida cylindraca* lipase (Mohr *et al.*, 1984; Oberhauser *et al.*, 1989; Ohno, 1985; Santianello *et al.*, 1988; Xie *et al.*, 1988).

3   Recent uses of oxidoreductase enzymes

The employment of whole-cell systems (e.g. bakers' yeast) or isolated enzymes for the reduction of carbonyl groups to the corresponding alcohols is well researched. Bakers' yeast has been used to reduce a wide range of simple ketones, β-ketoesters and cyclic diketones (Servi, 1990). The stereoselectivity of the reduction process is predictable and very useful routes to homochiral anti-inflammatory steroids have been explored using this type of biotransformation (Price and Roberts, 1985). Other organisms, such as the fungus *Mortierella ramanniana* can be used in place of bakers' yeast.

More recently partially purified dehydrogenase enzymes have been utilized for the production of optically active secondary alcohols. During the purification of the protein the enzyme cofactor (nicotinamide adenine dinucleotide (phosphate) [NAD(P)H]) is lost and so before the bio-transformation is possible this cofactor must be recoupled to the enzyme. The cofactors NAD(P)H are expensive and cofactor recycling must be set up so that a less-than-stoichiometric amount of the dinucleotide can be employed. Cofactor recycling systems are now well defined thanks to the work of Jones (1986) and others, and are ready for use by non-specialist laboratories.

The ketone (**17**) has been reduced using *M. ramanniana* and by $3\alpha,20\beta$-hydroxysteroid dehydrogenase/NADH. Thus the whole cell reduction gave

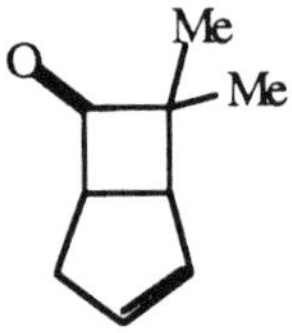

(17) 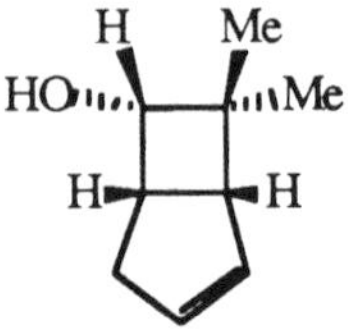   (18) 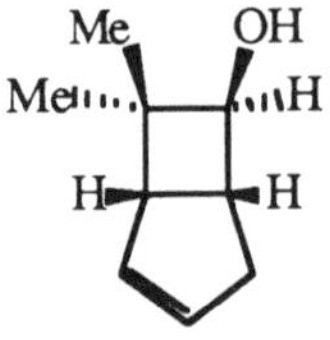   (19)

an equimolar mixture of the 6endo-alcohol (18) and the 6exo-alcohol (19)
(40% yield) (Butt et al., 1985) while the dehydrogenase catalysed an
enantioselective reduction of the ketone (17) by NADH forming the alcohol
(18) in an optically pure state and leaving optically active ketone. The
alcohol (18) has been converted into eldanolide, the pheromone of an
agricultural pest, the sugar cane borer (Scheme 3) (Butt et al., 1987). The
availability of the two enantiomers of the 7,7-dimethylbicyclo[3.2.0]heptane

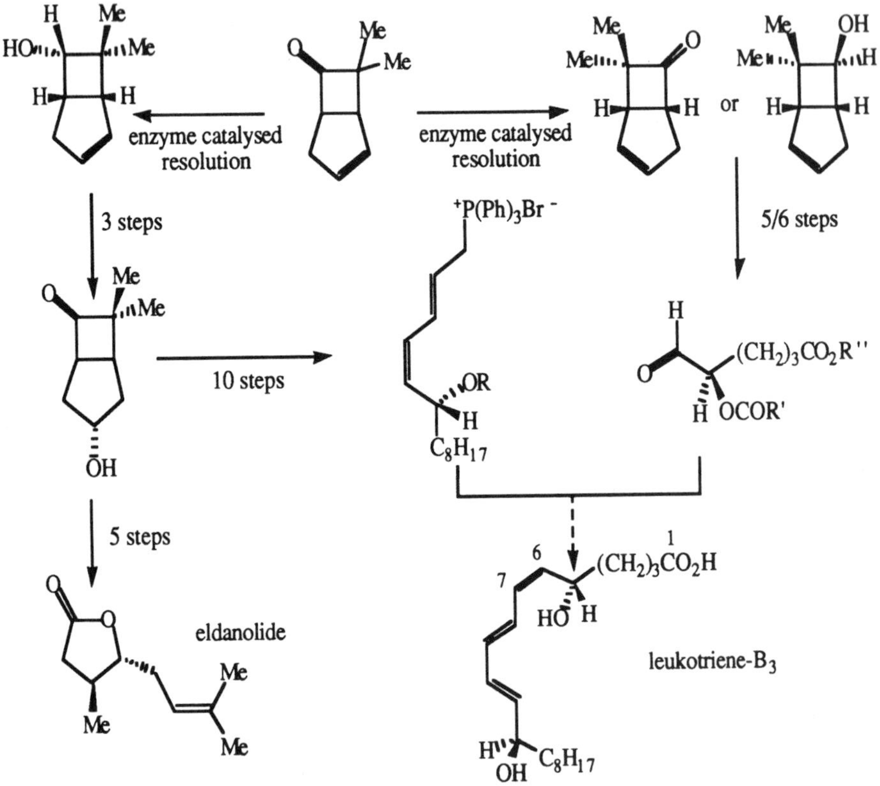

Scheme 3

(20)   (21)

ring system allows the synthesis of biologically interesting leukotriene-B_3.
Note that one enantiomer of the ketone provides the C_1–C_6 section of the
natural product (containing one chiral centre) (Davies *et al.*, 1985) while the
other enantiomer can provide the C_7–C_{20} portion (containing the second
chiral centre (Scheme 3) (Dorman *et al.*, 1989; Cotterill *et al.*, 1990).

Oxidation of aromatic and alicyclic molecules using monooxygenase and
dioxygenase enzymes has attracted a considerable amount of attention
(Sariaslani, 1989). The oxidation of benzene to cyclohexa-3,5-diene-1,2-
cis-diol (20) is a reaction catalysed by *Pseudomonas putida* and substantial
amounts of material can be obtained for further chemical studies.

For example various cycloaddition reactions can be carried out on the
acetonide (21), including Diels–Alder [4 + 2] reactions (to give, for
example the tricyclic compound (22)), [2 + 2] cycloaddition reactions (to
give cyclobutanone derivatives such as 23) and the more unusual [6 + 4]
cycloaddition reactions to give polycyclic compounds such as the ketone (24)
(Cotterill *et al.*, 1988b).

(22)   (23)   (24)

Not only is benzene biotransformed by *Pseudomonads* but so are many
of its derivatives. Often the latter compounds are obtained in an optically
pure form and it is established (at least for some of the compounds) that
these diols have the $1S,2R$ configuration. Trifluoromethylbenzene is
biotransformed into the diol (25); the corresponding acetonide (26) can be
converted into a wide range of derivatives (Scheme 4) through different
chemical reactions (Pittol *et al.*, 1989).

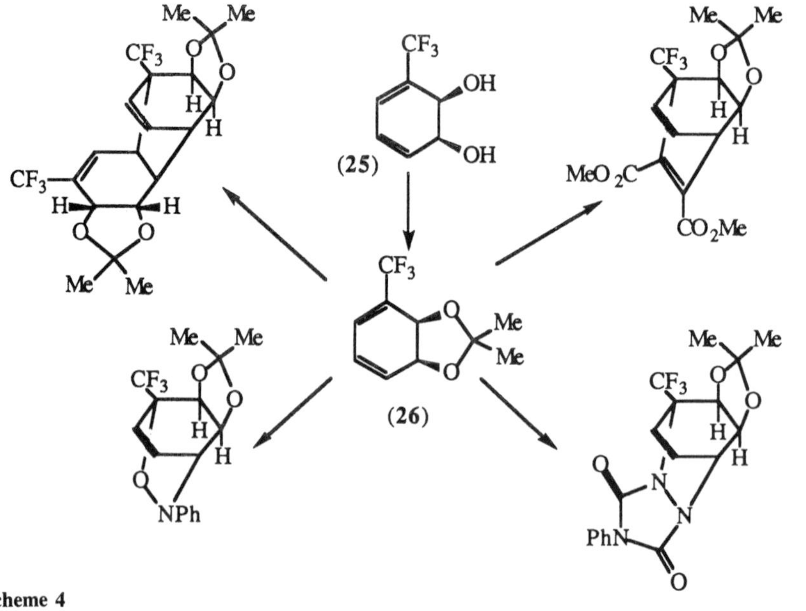

Scheme 4

Interesting conversions involving 3-chlorocyclohexa-3,5-diene-1,2-diol and 3-methylcyclohexa-3,5-diene-1,2-diol have also been described (Hudlicky *et al.*, 1989).

Another oxidation reaction that is gaining an increasing amount of interest is the Baeyer–Villiger catalysed oxidation of a cyclic ketone into a lactone (Walsh and Chen, 1988; Alphand *et al.*, 1989). Recently, we have shown that (±)-7-fluoro-5*endo*-bromo-bicyclo[2.2.1]heptan-2-one is oxidized in an enantioselective manner using the *Acinetobacter* NC1B 9871 to give optically pure lactone (**27**) (30%) and recovered optically active ketone (**28**) (30%). Interestingly oxidation of the ketone (**28**) with the chemical oxidant, *m*-chloroperoxybenzoic acid gave the 3-oxabicyclooctan-

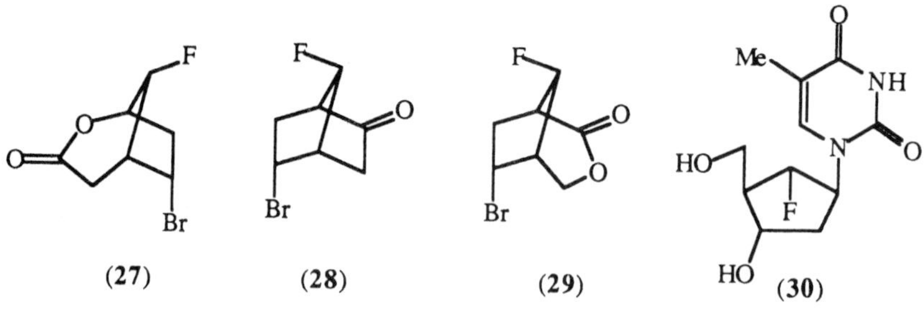

(27)   (28)   (29)   (30)

HO⟍⟋⟍⟋⟍⟋OH   R—⟨⟨⟩⟩
                              N
                              |
                              COPh

(31)   (32) R=H
                            (33) R=OH

2-one (29) as the major product (Levitt *et al.*, 1990). The latter compound was converted into the carbocyclic nucleoside (30), a compound possessing anti-HIV activity (Fletcher *et al.*, 1989).

The ability to derivatize an organic molecule at a position distant from pre-existing functionality is an attractive goal for both organic chemist and microbiologist alike. Some progress has been made towards providing chemical methods for remote hydroxylation (Barton *et al.*, 1990; Dolphin *et al.*, 1989; Fish *et al.*, 1988) but, for the foreseeable future, microbiological methods seem to offer the most likely chances for success. The regioselective hydroxylation of steroids has been investigated in some depth, the formation of 11-hydroxyprogesterone from progesterone being one of the most noteworthy successes (Jones *et al.*, 1976; Iizuka and Naito, 1981). The regioselective (but not regiospecific) oxidation of cyclohexyl-cyclohexane to give the diol (31) using *Cunninghamella blakesleeana* shows that even the most hydrophobic materials can be biotransformed (Davies *et al.*, 1986). Spiro-heterocyclic compounds can be derivatized, often in very high yield, to produce single compounds using *Beauvaria sulfurescens*: for example the azabicycloundecane (32) furnishes the alcohol (33) in 80% isolated yield (Carruthers *et al.*, 1990).

4 Enzyme-catalysed reactions resulting in the formation of carbon–carbon bonds

The stereocontrolled formation of carbon–carbon bonds is at the heart of organic synthesis. The aldol reaction is one popular way of joining together two synthons to give an advanced intermediate in a synthesis, for example, of biologically interesting compounds (Toone *et al.*, 1990).

Impressive progress has been made in controlling base-catalysed aldol reactions (Duplantier *et al.*, 1989) and the recent breakthroughs describe reactions that begin to approach the superb selectivity demonstrated by aldolase enzymes. Rabbit muscle aldolase has been studied in some detail and it has been shown, for example, that the triol monophosphate (34) is formed from phenylethanal and dihydroxyacetone monophosphate using this enzyme (Effenberger and Straub, 1987; Bednarski *et al.*, 1989).

(34)   (35)   (36)

One restriction using this enzyme is that dihydroxyacetone monophosphate can only be replaced as the 'nucleophilic' component of the aldol
reaction by very similar substances. The obvious potential utility of a more
catholic enzyme that is able to catalyse the stereospecific coupling of wide
ranges of carbonyl compounds is the rationale behind on-going research in
this area.

A less aesthetic process, but nevertheless a very useful transformation,
involves the use of lyase enzymes which can catalyse the addition of HCN
to aldehydes to give optically active cyanohydrins. Mandelonitrile lyase
catalyses such an addition of HCN to a variety of aldehydes to afford the
corresponding (R)-cyanohydrins (35) (Effenberger *et al.*, 1987; Brussee
et al., 1988).

Finally Fuganti *et al.* (1984) have explored the use of bakers' yeast for the
controlled addition of acetaldehyde to $\alpha\beta$-unsaturated carbonyl compounds
through an acyloin type of reaction. For example cinnamaldehyde is
converted into (2S,3R)-5-phenylpent-4-ene-2,3-diol (36) in *ca.* 20% yield
and in high diastereoisomeric excess.

5   Future developments in the area of biotransformations

Current trends in the employment of lipases, esterases and amidases for the
preparation of chiral compounds of high optical purity will continue. The
use of these enzymes in non-specialist laboratories will become widespread
and some of the newly found processes will be scaled up to the multikilogram
level. Other hydrolase enzymes, such as the nitrile hydratases will become
increasingly used because of the mild hydrolysis conditions that can be
employed using these enzymes.

The use of micro-organisms, such as bakers' yeast, for bioreduction
processes will also become more widespread. The rate of expansion of this
area of biotransformations will be slower due to the inevitable problems
associated with the use of whole-cell systems (Butt and Roberts, 1987). The
use of dehydrogenase enzymes for the reduction or oxidation of organic
substrates will also become more attractive to the synthetic organic chemist
with further refinement of cofactor recycling systems.

More research work is needed on the use of enzymes for other oxidation
reactions (Baeyer–Villiger type reactions, controlled hydroxylation, *etc.*)

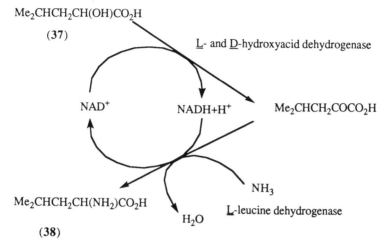

$Me_2CHCH_2CH(OH)CO_2H$

(37)

$\underline{L}$- and $\underline{D}$-hydroxyacid dehydrogenase

NAD^+

$NADH+H^+$

$Me_2CHCH_2COCO_2H$

NH_3

$Me_2CHCH_2CH(NH_2)CO_2H$

H_2O

$\underline{L}$-leucine dehydrogenase

(38)

Scheme 5

before more extensive use is made of these catalysts. In five years time the situation should be different.

Similarly the use of enzymes for the stereocontrolled formation of carbon-carbon bonds will need more attention in research laboratories before the full potential of these catalysts is realized. The exceptions are the enzymes that catalyse the stereoselective formation of cyanohydrins which are now available for more routine use.

The possibility of setting up a cascade of enzyme-catalysed reactions in the same 'pot' is very attractive. The conversion of the racemic hydroxy acid (37) into the amino acid (38) illustrates the sort of coupled process that is feasible (Scheme 5) (Schmidt-Kastner and Egerer, 1984): note that cofactor recycling is nicely accommodated within this sequence. The preparation of unusual sugars, and sugar analogues, using enzyme-catalysed processes will gain prominence. The recent work of Card *et al.* (1986) (Scheme 6) illustrates the elegant way in which fairly complex end-products can be built up without the need for extensive protection-deprotection sequences.

Progress in the field of biotransformations will be matched by equally exciting advances in the area of synthetic organic chemistry. The advances will often be complementary and the use of enzymes for the preparation of materials which are difficult to make by purely chemical methods will remain in vogue for the foreseeable future. Certainly the present problems with the disposal of waste organic solvents, with the consequent focus on reactions that can be conducted in an aqueous environment, concentrate attention on Nature's catalysts which are designed to operate in aqueous

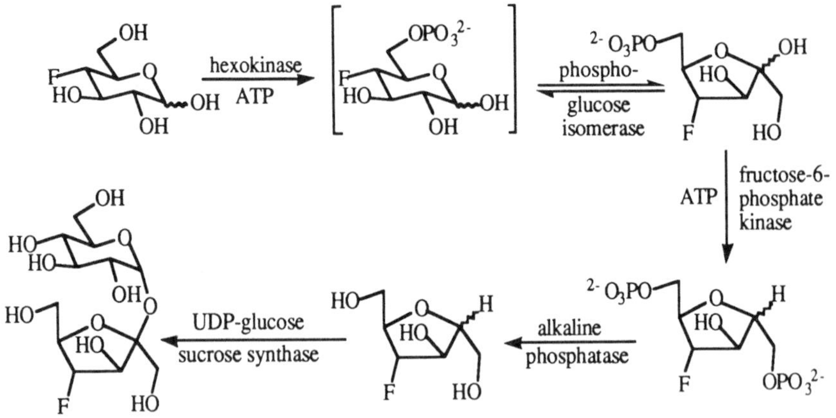

126 Stanley M. Roberts

Scheme 6

solution. Finally it is conceivable that 'man-made' enzymes (*i.e.* catalytic antibodies) will also make a significant impact on research in this area and add to the range of organic reactions that can be catalysed by protein (Kang *et al.*, 1990).

In conclusion the next 10 years should see a lot of exciting developments in the area of biotransformations. Many of the forthcoming investigations will be aimed at producing bulk quantitites of optically active, relatively simple molecules, while an equal volume of work will concentrate on the preparation of more complex, higher value materials in smaller quantities. It promises to be a fascinating decade for those scientists involved in the research and development of processes that have enzyme catalysed reactions as the key step(s).

References

Alphand, V., Archelas, A. and Furstoss, R. (1989). Microbial transformations XVI. One-step synthesis of a pivotal prostaglandin chiral synthon via a highly enantioselective microbiological Baeyer-Villiger type reaction. *Tetrahedron Lett.* **30**, 3663.

Barton, D. H. R., Doller, D., Ozbalik, N., Balavoine, G., Gref, A. and Boivin, J. (1990). On the oxidation of 3-ethylpentane under Gif[IV] and Gif–Orsay conditions. *Tetrahedron Lett.* **31**, 353.

Bednarski, M. D., Simon, E. S., Bischofberger, N., Fessner, W.-D., Kim, M. J., Lees, W., Saito, T., Waldmann, H. and Whitesides, G. M. (1989). Rabbit muscle aldolase as a catalyst in organic synthesis. *J. Am. Chem. Soc.* **111**, 627.

Bengis-Garber, C. and Gutman, A. L. (1988). Bacteria in organic synthesis: selective conversion of 1,3-dicyanobenzene into 3-cyanobenzoic acid. *Tetrahedron Lett.* **29**, 2589.

Borthwick, A. D., Butt, S., Biggadike, K., Exall, A. M., Roberts, S. M., Youds, P. M., Kirk, B. E., Booth, B. R., Cameron, J. M., Cox, S. W., Marr, C. L. P. and Shill, M. D. (1988). Synthesis and enzymatic resolution of carbocyclic 2′-ara-fluoro-guanosine: a potent new antiherpetic agent. *J. Chem. Soc., Chem. Commun.* 656.

Borthwick, A. D., Evans, D. N., Kirk, B. E., Biggadike, K., Exall, A. M., Youds, P. M., Roberts, S. M., Knight, D. J. and Coates, J. A. V. (1990). Fluoro carbocyclic nucleosides: synthesis and antiviral activity of 2′- and 6′-fluoro carbocyclic pyrimidine nucleosides including carbocyclic 1-(2-deoxy-2-fluoro-β-D-arabinofuranosyl)-5-methyluracil and carbocyclic 1-(2-deoxy-2-fluoro-β-D-arabinofuranosyl)-5-iodouracil. *J. Med. Chem.* **33**, 179.

Brussee, J., Roos, E. C. and Van Der Gen, A. (1988). Bio-organic synthesis of optically active cyanohydrins and acyloins. *Tetrahedron Lett.* **29**, 4485.

Butt, S. and Roberts, S. M. (1987). Opportunities for using enzymes in organic synthesis. *Chem. Br.* 127.

Butt, S., Davies, H. G., Dawson, M. J., Lawrence, G. C., Leaver, J., Roberts, S. M., Turner, M. K., Wakefield, B. J., Wall, W. F. and Winders, J. A. (1985). Reduction of bicyclo[3.2.0]hept-2-en-6-one and 7,7,-dimethylbicyclo[3.2.0]hept-en-6-one using dehydrogenase enzymes and the fungus *Mortierella ramanniana*. *Tetrahedron Lett.* **26**, 5077.

Butt, S., Davies, H. G., Dawson, M. J., Lawrence, G. C., Leaver, J., Roberts, S. M., Turner, M. K., Wakefield, B. J., Wall, W. F. and Winders, J. A. (1987). Resolution of 7,7-dimethylbicyclo[3.2.0]hept-2-en-6-one using *Mortierella ramanniana* and 3α,20β-hydroxy-steroid dehydrogenase, photochemistry of 3-hydroxy-7,7-dimethylbicyclo[3.2.0]heptan-6-ones, and the synthesis of (+)-eldanolide. *J. Chem. Soc., Perkin Trans. 1*, 903.

Card, P. J., Hitz, W. D. and Ripp, K. G. (1986). Chemoenzymatic syntheses of fructose-modified sucroses via multienzyme systems. Some topographical aspects of the binding of sucrose to a sucrose carrier protein. *J. Am. Chem. Soc.* **108**, 158.

Carruthers, W., Prail, J. D. and Roberts, S. M. (1990). Site selective oxidation of some azaspiro-undecanes using *Beavaria sulfurescens* ATCC 7159. *J. Chem. Soc. Perkin Trans. 1*, (in press).

Chan, C., Cox, P. B. and Roberts, S. M. (1988). Convergent stereocontrolled synthesis of 13-hydroxy-9Z, 11E-octadecadienoic acid (13-HODE). *J. Chem. Soc., Chem. Commun.* 971.

Cohen, M. A. and Turner, N. J. (1990). Unpublished results.

Cotterill, I. C., Macfarlane, E. L. A. and Roberts, S. M. (1988a). Resolution of bicyclo[3.2.0]hept-2-en-6-ols and bicyclo[4.2.0]oct-2-en-*endo*-7-ol using lipases. *J. Chem. Soc., Perkin Trans. 1*, 3387.

Cotterill, I. C., Roberts, S. M. and Williams, J. O. (1988b). Diels–Alder reactions involving *cis*-1,2-isopropylidenedioxycyclohexa-3,5-diene and enzymatic resolution of one of the adducts. *J. Chem. Soc., Chem. Commun.* 1628.

Cotterill, I. C., Dorman, G., Roberts, S. M., Wakefield, B. J. and Winders, J. A. (1990). Unpublished results.

Cox, P. B. and Roberts, S. M. (1990). Unpublished results.

Davies, H. G., Roberts, S. M., Wakefield, B. J. and Winders, J. A. (1985). Synthesis of (3S,4R)-eldanolide and (5S,12R)-leukotriene-B$_4$ through photolysis of optically active hydroxy-7-7-dimethylbicyclo[3.2.0]heptanones. *J. Chem. Soc., Chem. Commun.* 1166.

Davies, H. G., Dawson, M. J., Lawrence, G. C., Mayall, J., Noble, D., Roberts, S. M., Turner, M. K. and Wall, W. F. (1986). Microbial hydroxylation of cyclo-

128   Stanley M. Roberts

hexylcyclohexane: synthesis of an analogue of leukotriene-B₃. *Tetrahedron Lett.* **27**, 1089.

Davies, H. G., Green, R. H., Kelly, D. R. and Roberts, S. M. (1989). *Biotransformations in Preparative Organic Chemistry: The Use of Isolated Enzymes and Whole–cell Systems in Synthesis.* Academic Press, London.

Dolphin, D., Matsumoto, A. and Shortman, C. (1989). β-Hydrolyalkyl σ-metalloporphyrins: models for epoxide and alkene generation from cytochrome P-450. *J. Am. Chem. Soc.* **111**, 411.

Dorman, G., Roberts, S. M., Wakefield, B. J. and Winders, J. A. (1989). 5-(Z)-oct-2-enyltetrahydrofuran-2-one as a key intermediate in the synthesis of leukotriene B₄. *J. Chem. Soc., Perkin Trans. 1*, 1543 for background references.

Duplantier, A. J., Nantz, M. H., Roberts, J. C., Short, R. P., Somfai, P. and Masamune, S. (1989). Triple asymmetric synthesis for fragment assembly: validity of approximate multiplicativity of the three diastereofacial selectivities. *Tetrahedron Lett.* **30**, 7375.

Effenberger, F. and Straub, A. (1987). A novel convenient preparation of dihydroxyacetone phosphate and its use in enzymatic aldol reactions. *Tetrahedron Lett.* **28**, 1641.

Effenberger, F., Ziegler, T. and Forster, S. (1987). Enzyme-catalysed cyanohydrin synthesis in organic solvents. *Angew. Chem. Int. Ed. Engl.* **26**, 458.

Endo, T. and Watanabe, I. (1989). Nitrile hydratase of *Rhodococcus* sp. N-774: purification and amino acid sequences. *FEBS Lett.* **243**, 61.

Evans, C., Roberts, S. M., Sutherland, A. G. and Thomas, S. (1990). Chemo-enzymatic synthesis of (−)-carbovir utilizing a whole cell catalysed resolution of 2-azabicyclo [2:2.1]hept-5-en-3-one. *J. Chem. Soc. Chem. Commun.* (in press).

Fish, R. H., Fong, R. H., Vincent, J. B. and Cristou, G. (1988). Carbon–hydrogen activation chemistry: hydroxylation of C₂,C₃ and cyclo-C₆ hydrocarbons by manganese cluster catalysts with a mono-oxygen transfer reagent. *J. Chem. Soc., Chem. Commun.* 1504.

Fletcher, C. A., Hilpert, H., Myers, P. L., Roberts, S. M. and Storer, R. (1989). Synthesis of compounds active against HIV: preparation of 6′-fluorocarbocyclic AZT (AZT = 3′deoxy-3′-azidothymidine). *J. Chem. Soc., Chem. Commun.* 1707.

Fuganti, C., Grasselli, P., Spreafico, F. and Zirotti, C. (1984). Synthesis of the enantiomeric forms of α- and β-alkoxy carbonyl compounds from the (2S,3R)-2,3-diol prepared in fermenting bakers' yeast from α-methylcinnamaldehyde. *J. Org. Chem.* **49**, 543 and references therein.

Glänzer, B. I., Faber, K. and Griengl, H. (1987). Enantioselective hydrolyses by bakers' yeast-III. Microbial resolution of alkynyl esters using lyophilised yeast. *Tetrahedron* **43**, 5791.

Hudlicky, T., Luna, H., Price, J. D. and Rulin, F. (1989). An enantiodivergent approach to D- and L-erythrose via microbial oxidation of chlorobenzene. *Tetrahedron Lett.* **30**, 4053.

Hutchinson, E., Pettman, R. B. and Roberts, S. M. (1990). Unpublished results.

Hwang, J. S. and Chang, H. N. (1989). Biotransformation of acrylonitrile to acrylamide using immobilised whole cells of *Brevibacterium* CH1 in a recycle fed-batcher reactor. *Biotechnol. Bioeng.* **34**, 380.

Iizuka, H. and Naito, A. (1981). *Microbial Conversion of Steroids and Alkaloids* University of Tokyo, Press and Springer-Verlag, Berlin.

Jones, J. B. (1986). Enzymes in organic synthesis. *Tetrahedron* **42**, 3351.
Jones, J. B. Sih, C. H. and Perlman, D. (1976). *Applications of Biochemical Systems in Organic Chemistry. Part 1,* p. 58. Wiley, New York.
Kang, A. S., Kingsbury, G. A., Blackburn, G. M. and Burton, D. R. (1990). Catalytic antibodies – designer enzymes. *Chem. Br.* 128.
Levitt, M. S., Newton, R. F., Roberts, S. M. and Willetts, A. J. (1990). Preparation of optically active 6-fluorocarbocyclic nucleosides utilising an enantiospecific enzyme-catalysed Baeyer–Villiger type oxidation. *J. Chem. Soc., Chem. Commun.* 619.
Macfarlane, E. L. A., Roberts, S. M. and Turner, N. J. (1990). Enzyme-catalysed inter-esterification procedure for the preparation of esters of a chiral secondary alcohol in high enantiomeric purity. *J. Chem. Soc., Chem. Commun.* (in press).
Maguire, N., Read, G. and Roberts, S. M. (1990). Unpublished results.
Mohr, P., Waespe-Sarcevic, N., Tamm, C., Gawronska, K. and Gawronska, J. K. (1983). A study of stereoselective hydrolysis of symmetrical diesters with pig liver esterase. *Helv. Chim. Acta* **66**, 2501.
Newton, R. F. and Roberts, S. M. (1982). *Prostaglandins and Thromboxanes: An Introductory Text.* Butterworths, London.
Oberhauser, T., Faber, K. and Griengl, H. (1989). A substrate model for the enzymatic resolution of esters of bicyclic alcohols by *Candida cylindracea* lipase. *Tetrahedron* **45**, 1679.
Ohno, M. (1985). In *Enzymes in Organic Synthesis* (eds R. Porter and S. Clark), p. 171. Pitmans, London.
Pittol, C. A., Pryce, R. J., Roberts, S. M., Ryback, G. and Williams, J. O. (1989). Diels–Alder reactions involving 1,2-isopropylidenedioxy-3-trifluoromethyl-cyclohexa-3,5-diene. *J. Chem. Soc., Perkin Trans. 1*, 1160.
Price, B. J. and Roberts, S. M. (1985). *Medicinal Chemistry: The Rôle of the Organic Chemist in Drug Research,* p. 196 and references therein. Academic Press, Orlando.
Riva, S., Chopineau, J., Kieboom, A. P. G. and Klibanov, A. M. (1988). Protease-catalysed regioselective esterification of sugars and related compounds in anhydrous dimethylformamide. *J. Am. Chem. Soc.* **110**, 584.
Roberts, S. M. (1989). Use of enzymes as catalysts to promote key transformations in organic synthesis. *Phil. Trans. R. Soc. London.* **324**, 577, and references therein.
Santianello, E., Chiari, M., Ferraboschi, P. and Trave, S. (1988). Enhanced and reversed enantioselectivity of enzymatic hydrolysis by simple substrate modifications: the case of 3-hydroxyglutarate diesters. *J. Org. Chem.* **53**, 1567.
Sariaslani, F. S. (1989). Microbial enzymes for oxidation of organic molecules. *Critical Rev. Biotechnol.* **9**, 171.
Schmidt-Kastner, G. and Egerer, P. (1984). In *Biotechnology*, Vol. 6a (ed. K. Kieslich), p. 387. Verlag Chemie, Weinheim.
Servi, S. (1990). Bakers' yeast as a reagent in organic synthesis. *Synthesis* 1.
Toone, E. J., Simon, E. S., Bednarksi, M. D. and Whitesides, G. M. (1989). Enzyme-catalysed synthesis of carbohydrates. *Tetrahedron* **45**, 5365.
Vince, R. and Hua, M. (1990). Synthesis and anti-HIV activity of carbocyclic 2',3'-didehydro-2',3'-dideoxy-2,6-disubstituted purine nucleosides. *J. Med. Chem.* **33**, 17.
Walsh, C. T. and Chen, Y. -C. J. (1988). Enzymic Baeyer–Villiger oxidations by flavin-dependent monooxygenases. *Angew. Chem. Int. Ed. Engl.* **27**, 33.

Wandrey, C. (1986). In *Enzymes as Catalysts in Organic Synthesis* (ed. M. P. Schneider), p. 263. D. Reidel, Dordrecht.

Xie, Z. F., Nakamura, I., Suemune, H. and Sakai, K. (1988). An insight into the enantioselective hydrolysis of cyclic acetates catalysed by *Pseudomonas fluorescens* lipase. *J. Chem. Soc., Chem. Commun.* 966.

Zemlicka, J., Craine, L. E., Heeg, M.-J. and Oliver, J. P. (1988). Enantioselective hydrolysis of dimethyl $2\alpha,3\alpha$-[dimethylmethylene)dioxy]-5-β-hydroxy-1β,4α-cyclopentanedicarboxylate with pig liver esterase. Stereoselective synthesis of methyl $2(R),3(S)$-[(Dimethylmethylene)dioxy]-5(R)-hydroxy-1(S)-carboxy-4(R)-cyclopentanecarboxylate. A cyclopentane synthone with all ring atoms chiral. *J. Org. Chem.* **53**, 937.

8

Recent Progress in Research on the Immunosuppressant FK-506

PHILIP KOCIENSKI and MICHAEL STOCKS
Department of Chemistry, The University, Southampton,
SO9 5NH, UK

DAVID K. DONALD
Fisons Pharmaceuticals PLC, Bakewell Road, Loughborough,
LE11 0RH, UK

1 Isolation, structure determination and stability of FK-506

FK-506 was isolated by researchers at the Fujisawa Pharmaceutical Co. in Japan in 1984 whilst looking for an agent which, like cyclosporin A, inhibited the production of the key intercellular signal interleukin 2 (IL-2) (Okuhara *et al.*, 1986; Kino *et al.*, 1987a; Goto *et al.*, 1987). FK-506 was produced by a hitherto unidentified strain of *Streptomyces* which was subsequently designated *Streptomyces tsukubaensis* after its place of isolation—Tsukuba, Ibaraki Prefecture, Japan. The elucidation of the gross structure of FK-506 with its 23-membered macrolide ring harbouring the unusual masked 1,2,3-tricarbonyl system relied on extensive chemical, degradative and spectroscopic studies (Tanaka *et al.*, 1987). The determination of the relative configuration of the stereogenic centres however was not possible by NMR spectroscopy and came instead from a single-crystal X-ray analysis (Taga *et al.*, 1987). The absolute configuration of FK-506 could then be assigned since acid hydrolysis resulted in the isolation of L-pipecolic acid.

In deuteriochloroform the ^{13}C NMR spectrum of FK-506 shows a doubling of all peaks with a relative intensity of approximately 3:1. This

CHIRALITY IN DRUG DESIGN AND SYNTHESIS
ISBN 0-12-136670-7

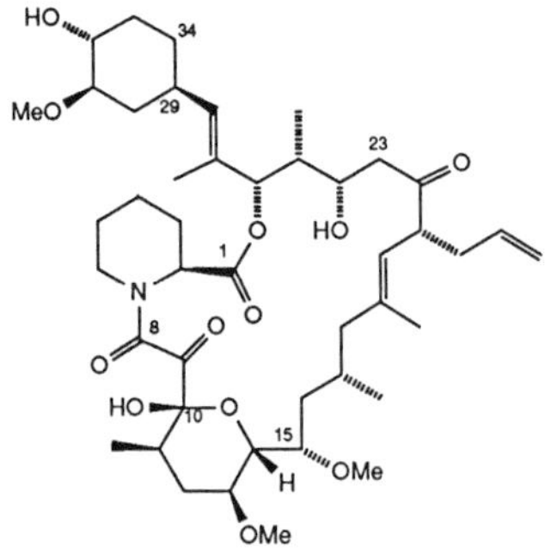

FK-506 (1)

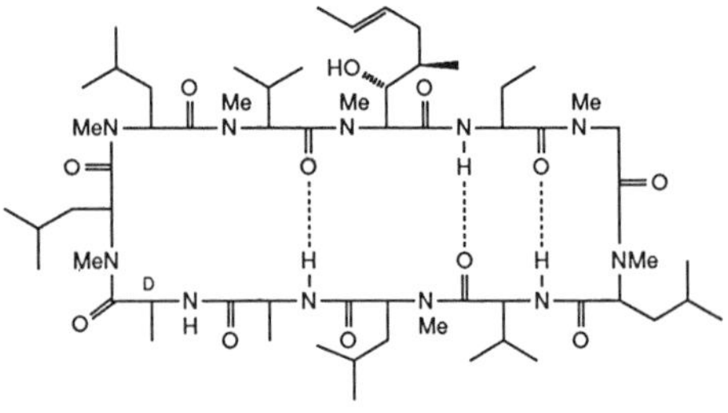

Cyclosporin A (2)

ratio is, however, highly solvent dependent. If FK-506 is dissolved in CD_2Cl_2 at low temperature ($-60°C$) only one rotameric form is seen corresponding to that seen in the X-ray structure. As the temperature is raised another set of signals appears and the calculated energy barrier to this process corresponds to that expected for amide bond rotation (Tanaka *et al.*, 1987; Hunter, 1988).

FK-506 is stable to mild acid (e.g. acetic acid overnight at room temperature); however, dilute nucleophilic base (e.g. aqueous sodium hydroxide) attacks the carbonyl at C9. Subsequent benzilic acid rearrangement then leads to 3 (Askin *et al.*, 1989). With non-nucleophilic base a slower reaction occurs to produce 4 (Donald *et al.*, 1990).

1.1 Related compounds

A number of compounds closely related to FK-506 have been isolated in small amounts from *Streptomyces tsukubaensis* and related strains of

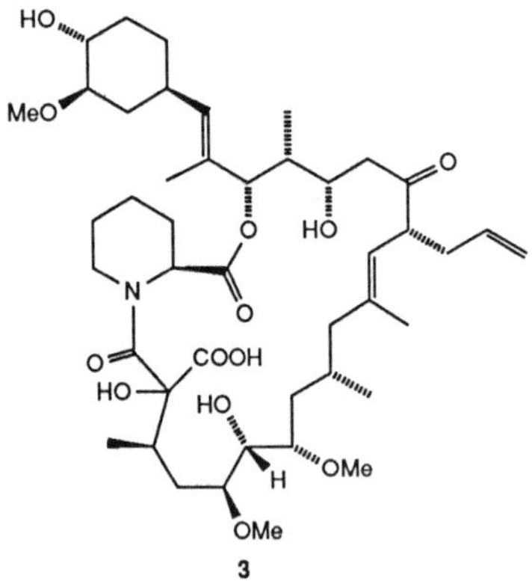

3

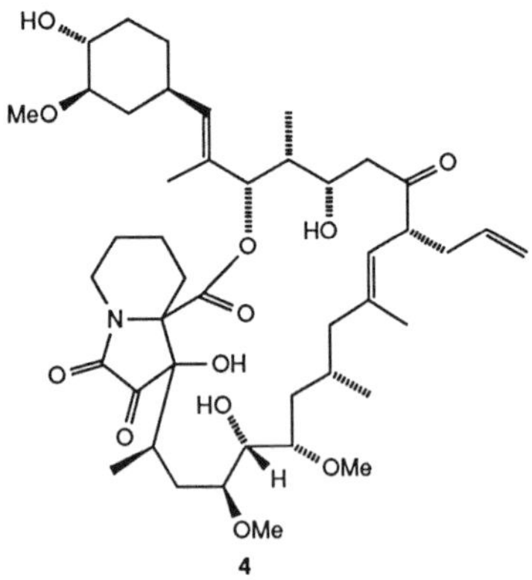

4

Streptomyces. These include the methyl (FR-900523 (**5**)) and ethyl analogues (FR-900520 (**6**)) (Hatanaka *et al.*, 1989) and the proline compound (FR-900525 (**7**)) (Okuhara *et al.*, 1986). These compounds are also immunosuppressive *in vitro* although less so than FK-506 (Hatanaka *et al.*, 1988).

More distantly related compounds are the antifungals rapamycin (**8**) (Vezina *et al.*, 1975; Sehgal *et al.*, 1975a, b) and 29-demethoxy rapamycin (**9**) (Findlay *et al.*, 1982) which are also produced by a strain of *Streptomyces* although the strain is unrelated to *Streptomyces tsukubaensis*. Rapamycin also displays immunosuppressive activity (Martel *et al.*, 1977; Calne *et al.*, 1989). The relationship of this activity to FK-506 is reviewed below.

Rapamycin (**8**) R = OMe
29-Demethoxy rapamycin (**9**) R = H

R = Me FR 900523 (**5**)
R = Et FR 900520 (**6**)

FR 900525 (**7**)

2 Biological activity

Cyclosporin A revolutionized transplantation surgery but its clinical use is complicated by adverse reactions of which nephrotoxicity (Hamilton, 1982) is the most serious. Thus in clinical use cyclosporin A trough levels are usually monitored daily for some time after transplantation and dosage is adjusted accordingly. Efforts to circumvent the problems of clinical toxicity associated with cyclosporin A have focused on the search for alternative agents which would offer an improved therapeutic profile in transplantation surgery as well as other diseases with an autoimmune pathogenic component. These include diabetes mellitus, collagen-vascular diseases, rheumatic and neurological diseases (e.g. rheumatoid arthritis), glomerular disease and inflammatory disease of the eye, skin (e.g. psoriasis) and bowel (e.g. ulcerative colitis). Cyclosporin A has already shown some utility in a number of these conditions (*Lancet*, 1985; Weinblatt *et al.*, 1987). Experiments also indicate that FK-506 is active in animal models of a variety of these conditions (Inamura *et al.*, 1988a,b; Kawashima *et al.*, 1988; Arita *et al.*, 1989; Sandoz AG, 1989; Takabayashi *et al.*, 1989; Takagashi *et al.*, 1989).

In a range of *in vitro* test systems FK-506 was shown to be around 100 times more potent than cyclosporin A. These included its effect on IL-2 and γ-interferon (γ-INF) production, cytotoxic T-cell generation, and in the murine and human mixed lymphocyte reaction (Kino *et al.*, 1987a,b,c). FK-506 was also shown to be 3–10 times more potent than cyclosporin A in a number of *in vivo* correlates such as suppression of plaque-forming cell responses, delayed type hypersensitivity and localized graft-versus-host reaction in mice and in skin allografting in rats (Inamura *et al.*, 1988c). However, differences of opinion quickly became apparent over the toxicity of the compound. Studies in rodents suggest that FK-506 is well tolerated (Lim *et al.*, 1987; Nalesnik *et al.*, 1987; Inagaki *et al.*, 1989; Stephen *et al.*, 1989) although at high doses weight loss and central nervous system effects have been reported (Gudas *et al.*, 1989). Calne and his group reported severe toxicity (particularly vasculitis and anorexia) in dogs (Collier *et al.*, 1987) and low efficacy together with a diabetic type syndrome in baboons (Calne *et al.*, 1987; Thiru *et al.*, 1987). These effects were somewhat disputed by the groups of Ochiai (Ochiai *et al.*, 1987a,b) and Starzl (Todo *et al.*, 1988a,b). In considering these studies it is important to note that different protocols were used—primarily in route of administration—which could have given rise to different bioavailability profiles (Morimoto *et al.*, 1989). Baboon lymphocytes were also subsequently shown to be approximately ten-fold less sensitive than human lymphocytes to the drug (Starzl *et al.*, 1989a). Starzl's animal studies were subsequently extended to human patients suffering from uncontrolled liver allograft rejection and/or other complications related to cyclosporin A (Starzl et al., 1989b). By October 1989, 111 patients had received FK-506 (Thomson, 1990) and a multicentre liver transplant trial is planned to take place in 1990.

2.1 Mechanism of action

Whilst FK-506 is more potent than cyclosporin A, both compounds appear to act in a similar fashion by interfering with an early event in T-cell activation. Once cells are committed to proliferation neither FK-506 nor cyclosporin A has any effect, (Sawada et al., 1987). Although many details of the T-cell activation process are unclear, some parts of the process can be identified albeit only in rather broad outline. Binding of antigen to the T-cell receptor complex leads to activation of phospholipase C and resultant degradation of plasma membrane phosphatidylinositol-4,5-bisphosphate (PIP_2). This generates inositol triphosphate which creates a Ca^{2+} signal in the lymphocyte cytoplasm, and diacylglycerol (DAG) which activates protein kinase C. The subsequent rise in intracellular calcium results in the induction of mRNAs which encode lymphokines which are important in cell activation such as IL-2 and γ-INF. The subsequent interaction of these lymphokines with their receptors then stimulates the cell to proliferate (King, 1988). Evidence for the point of inhibition by FK-506 within this pathway is rapidly growing as outlined below.

(1) *Antigen binding to the T-cell receptor complex.* Stimulation of cells with the combination of calcium ionophore A23187 and PMA is known to bypass this complex. FK-506, however, inhibits cells stimulated with A23187/PMA suggesting that FK-506 acts at a point subsequent to perturbation of the T_i/T_3 complex (Sawada et al., 1987).

(2) *Degradation of PIP_2.* FK-506 has been shown to have no effect on the degradation of PIP_2 induced by concanavalin A (CON A) and levels of PIP_2 that are found in stimulated cells are not reduced in the presence of FK-506 (Fujii et al., 1989).

(3) *Effects through the DAG (diacylglycerol)/protein kinase C pathway.* Phorbol esters such as 12-*O*-tetradecanoylphorbol-13-acetate (TPA) and phorbol 12,13-dibutyrate (PDB) are known to activate protein kinase C that is to mimic the action of DAG. However, the stimulation of lymphocytes that is induced by either PDB or TPA was not inhibited by FK-506 (Kay et al., 1989a). FK-506 has been reported not to inhibit protein kinase C *in vitro* (Gschwendt et al., 1989).

(4) *Effects through the calcium pathway.* In contrast, stimulation of

lymphocytes with calcium ionophores (such as A23187 and ionomycin), which mimic the action of inositol triphosphate, was strongly inhibited by FK-506 (Kay *et al.*, 1989a). FK-506 also inhibits the proliferative response of the D10.G4 T cell clone when induced by IL-1 plus ionomycin (a calcium dependent pathway) but does not inhibit induction by IL-1 plus PMA (a calcium independent pathway) (Dumont, 1990a). The inhibitory effect of FK-506 on CON A-stimulated peripheral blood lymphocytes has been shown to be dependent on the availability of calcium ions in the lymphocyte culture medium (Kay *et al.*, 1989b) FK-506 however has no effect on the concentration of Ca^{2+} within the cell after stimulation (Bierer *et al.*, 1990). Thus its effect seems to be on the calcium signalling pathway and not on calcium mobilization itself.

Like cyclosporin A, FK-506 also has inhibitory effects on B-cell proliferation when the proliferative signal is mediated by the generation of a cytoplasmic Ca^{2+} signal (for example, as in B-cell stimulation with anti-mouse immunoglobulin (Walliser, 1989)).

(5) *Effects on IL-2 receptor expression.* Although inhibition of IL-2 receptor expression has been claimed (Kino *et al.*, 1987b; Sawada *et al.*, 1987), this is likely to have been due to an indirect effect arising from the inhibition of IL-2 production (Tocci *et al.*, 1989).

(6) *Effects on IL-2 and γ-INF production.* The production of both IL-2 and γ-INF have been shown to be strongly inhibited by FK-506. In the mixed lymphocyte reaction (which is taken to be an *in vitro* correlate of organ transplantation), the presence of IL-2 and not γ-INF has been shown to be important for the proliferative response by the use of antibodies which bind specifically to each of the lymphokines. Thus binding to γ-INF had little effect whilst binding to IL-2 was inhibitory (Bucy *et al.*, 1988).

(5) *Effects on gene expression.* Non-specific effects on DNA synthesis can be ruled out—at least within the therapeutic concentration range of the compound (Sawada *et al.*, 1987). In the cell genes are activated in a specific sequence. The three phases of gene activation that are recognized are designated IE (immediate early), E (early) and L (late) depending on their kinetics of appearance and mode of regulation (Reed *et al.*, 1986). It has been shown that FK-506 inhibits the expression of a specific subset of these activation genes. FK-506 appears to affect the expression of E phase activation genes which include mRNAs for IL-2, IL-3, IL-4, γ-INF, TNF-α, GM-CSF and c-myc. No effect was seen on the expression of mRNAs either from genes which are activated before (IE phase) or after (L phase, e.g. IL-2Rα) (Tocci *et al.*, 1989). This is very similar to that reported for cyclosporin A (Kroenke *et al.*, 1984).

The mechanism of action of FK-506 thus appears to be a relatively specific inhibition of the transcriptional activation of the IL-2 gene. How this occurs is not known at present.

2.2 Biological relationship to rapamycin

Biological studies on rapamycin have shown some striking similarities and differences to FK-506. As noted above, rapamycin is also immuno-suppressive (Martel et al., 1977; Calne et al., 1989); yet unlike FK-506 and cyclosporin A, it appears to affect a late stage in T-cell activation. IL-2 production is not inhibited—indeed rapamycin seems to enhance the accumulation of E phase transcripts in activated human T-cells (Tocci et al., 1989). Rapamycin also inhibits both the proliferative response of the D10.G4 T cell clone when induced by IL-1 plus ionomycin (a calcium dependent pathway) and that induced by IL-1 plus PMA (a calcium independent pathway) (Dumont et al., 1990a). The proliferation of CTLL cells mediated by IL-2 which is unaltered by either FK-506 or cyclosporin A is also inhibited by rapamycin (Dumont et al., 1990a). This is surprising since FK-506 and rapamycin appear to bind to the same cytosolic 'receptor' protein (Harding et al., 1989). That the two compounds bind to the same receptor protein but elicit different biological effects is intriguing.

2.3 Cis–trans peptidyl–prolyl isomerase activity and immunosuppression

It has been reported that the FK-506 binding protein (FKBP) has prolyl–peptidyl cis–trans isomerase (PPIase) activity (Harding et al., 1989; Siekierka et al., 1989a)—an activity which has also been reported for the putative cyclosporin 'receptor' cyclophilin (Takahashi et al., 1989; Fischer et al., 1989). The FK-506 binding protein is, however, distinct from cyclophilin (Siekierka et al., 1989b). Neither rapamycin nor FK-506 bind to cyclophilin and cyclosporin A does not bind to FKBP.

The role of cyclophilin in the immunosuppression induced by cyclosporin A is still controversial. Cyclophilin does bind cyclosporin A and its analogues with a structure–function profile consistent with its playing a role in immunosuppression (Quesniaux et al., 1987; Durette et al., 1988; Harding and Handschumacher, 1988). Whether inhibition of the PPIase activity of cyclophilin by cyclosporin A plays a role in immunosuppression is also not clear. Interestingly, although cyclosporin A bound to cyclophilin protects an SH group that is believed to be important in the PPIase activity of cyclophilin, prior blocking of this group with iodoacetamide or N-ethylmaleimide does not compromise cyclosporin A binding (Foxwell et al., 1989).

Schreiber, in an elegant study with synthetic FK-506 labelled with ^{13}C at positions 8 and 9, has also shown that there is no change in hybridization at these positions when FK-506 binds to FKBP (Rosen *et al.*, 1990) as might be expected for the proposed mechanism of PPIase activity (Fischer, 1989). Only one of the two rotamers of FK-506 binds to FKBP in accordance with a specific interaction (Rosen *et al.*, 1990).

The fact that FK-506 and rapamycin both inhibit the PPIase activity of FKBP and yet have different immunological activity suggests that inhibition of PPIase activity is not necessarily linked to immunosuppression. However, it could be that FK-506 and/or rapamycin bind to a range of isomerases and the differential inhibition of these gives rise to their disparate activity. The finding that rapamycin and FK-506 can act as reciprocal antagonists in a number of systems (Dumont *et al.*, 1990b) has strengthened the belief that the true receptor has been found and that another model for the mechanism of immunosuppression is needed. A more convincing model might be a ternary complex model in which a second protein recognizes the FK-506 or rapamycin bound protein. The results of this recognition would then be different for the two cases. The fact that cyclosporin A and FK-506 bind to different receptor proteins yet elicit an identical response is intriguing. It is possible that the common 'true' receptor protein which binds both has not been found. It is equally likely that the cyclophilin/cyclosporin A, FKBP/ FK-506 pairs are but two examples of a family of proteins that, with their natural ligands, regulate gene expression. In this case we will probably not have to wait long before other examples are found.

3   Synthetic approaches to FK-506

Organic synthesis has a crucial role to play in helping define the topographical relationship between FK-506 and its receptor(s). The complexity and novel structure of FK-506 provide a severe test of modern synthetic methodology for achieving enantio- and diastereo-control in a multifunctional substrate. The ensuing discussion attempts to summarize concisely all the synthetic efforts reported as of March 1990. In order to simplify the organization of the large number of reaction schemes, only selected intermediates are assigned a numerical descriptor which defines first the number of the scheme followed by the number of the intermediate in that scheme. After a discussion of the Merck total synthesis of FK-506, the approaches to various fragments will be summarized and these will be grouped according to the position of the fragment in the natural product.

3.1   The Merck total synthesis

Any discussion of the extensive synthetic effort invested in FK-506 must

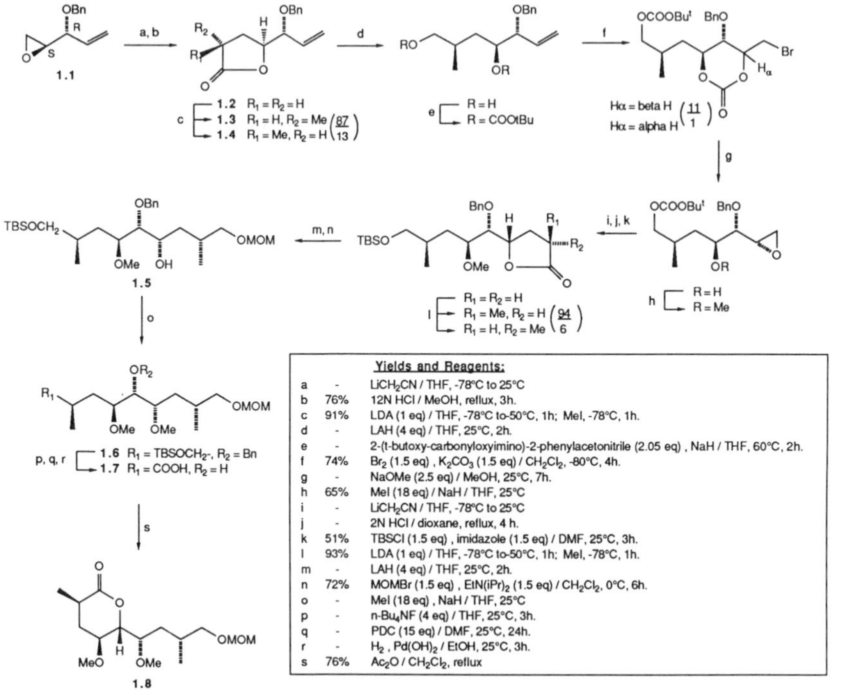

Scheme 1

Structures and reagent labels (Scheme 1):

1.1

c
- 1.2 $R_1 = R_2 = H$
- 1.3 $R_1 = H, R_2 = Me$ (**87**)
- 1.4 $R_1 = Me, R_2 = H$ (**13**)

e
- $R = H$
- $R = COOtBu$

- $H\alpha = beta\ H$ (**11**)
- $H\alpha = alpha\ H$ (**1**)

1.5

m, n

- $R_1 = R_2 = H$
- $R_1 = Me, R_2 = H$ (**94**)
- $R_1 = H, R_2 = Me$ (**6**)

h
- $R = H$
- $R = Me$

p, q, r
- 1.6 $R_1 = TBSOCH_2-, R_2 = Bn$
- 1.7 $R_1 = COOH, R_2 = H$

s

1.8

		Yields and Reagents:
a	-	LiCH₂CN / THF, -78°C to 25°C
b	76%	12N HCl / MeOH, reflux, 3h.
c	91%	LDA (1 eq) / THF, -78°C to-50°C, 1h; MeI, -78°C, 1h.
d	-	LAH (4 eq) / THF, 25°C, 2h.
e	-	2-(t-butoxy-carbonyloxyimino)-2-phenylacetonitrile (2.05 eq) , NaH / THF, 60°C, 2h.
f	74%	Br₂ (1.5 eq) , K₂CO₃ (1.5 eq) / CH₂Cl₂, -80°C, 4h.
g	-	NaOMe (2.5 eq) / MeOH, 25°C, 7h.
h	65%	MeI (18 eq) / NaH / THF, 25°C
i	-	LiCH₂CN / THF, -78°C to 25°C
j	-	2N HCl / dioxane, reflux, 4 h.
k	51%	TBSCl (1.5 eq) , imidazole (1.5 eq) / DMF, 25°C, 3h.
l	93%	LDA (1 eq) / THF, -78°C to-50°C, 1h; MeI, -78°C, 1h.
m	-	LAH (4 eq) / THF, 25°C, 2h.
n	72%	MOMBr (1.5 eq) , EtN(iPr)₂ (1.5 eq) / CH₂Cl₂, 0°C, 6h.
o	-	MeI (18 eq) / NaH / THF, 25°C
p	-	n-Bu₄NF (4 eq) / THF, 25°C
q	-	PDC (15 eq) / DMF, 25°C, 24h.
r	-	H₂ , Pd(OH)₂ / EtOH, 25°C, 3h.
s	76%	Ac₂O / CH₂Cl₂, reflux

begin with the total synthesis reported by organic chemists at the Merck, Sharpe and Dohme laboratories. The first paper in the series culminating in the total synthesis of FK-506 (Askin, 1988) described a synthesis of the C10–C18 segment (**1.8** Scheme 1). The Merck strategy reflected the element of symmetry which is most apparent in the differentially protected diol of intermediate (**1.6**). The sequence began with the homochiral oxiran (**1.1**) which is available in high enantiomeric and diastereoisomeric purity by Sharpless asymmetric epoxidation of 1,4-pentadiene-3-ol using (−)-diisopropyl tartrate. Nucleophilic opening of the oxiran ring by the lithio derivative of acetonitrile and further functional group transformations generated the butyrolactone (**1.2**). Alkylation of **1.2** was diastereoselective giving **1.3** and **1.4** (87 : 13, respectively) in 91% yield. Later in the synthesis, this same sequence of oxiran opening and alkylation (steps i–k) was used to construct the intermediate (**1.5**). Further elaboration gave the C10–C18 lactone (**1.8**).

Removal of two of the five chiral centres in cheap and readily available (−)-quinic acid (Scheme 2) afforded hydroxylactone (**2.1**) which was then converted in 13 steps to the C20–C34 fragment (**2.4**) of FK-506 (Mills *et al.*,

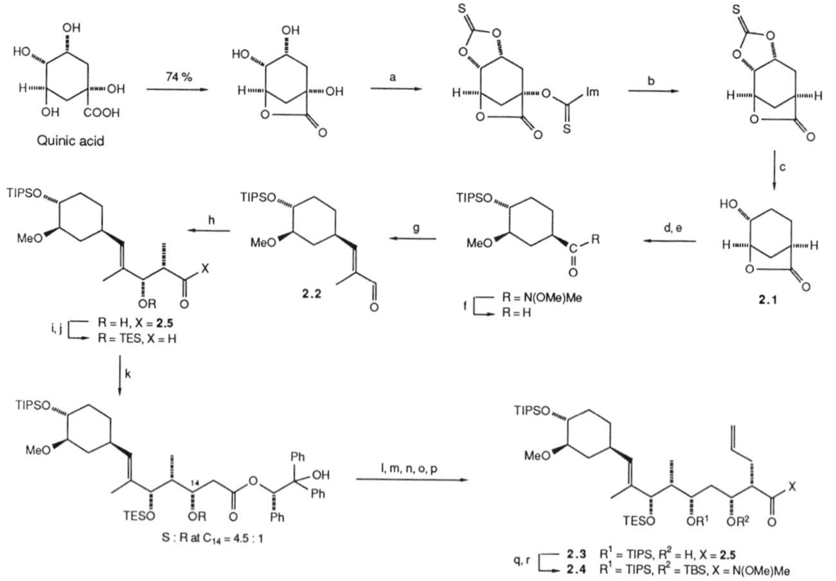

Yields and Reagents

a	-	(imid)$_2$C=S (3 eq) / ClCH$_2$CH$_2$Cl, reflux
b	74%	Bu$_3$SnH (1.5 eq) / xylene, 140°C, 45 min
c	40%	Bu$_3$SnH (2 eq) , AIBN (0.01 eq) / xylene, 140°C, 1 h
d	-	TIPSOTf (1.3 eq) , 2,6-lutidine (2.2 eq) / CH$_2$Cl$_2$, 0°C
e	85%	Me(MeO)NAlCl(Me) (2 eq) / toluene ii) MeOTf , 2,6-di-t-Bu-4-Mepyridine / CH$_2$Cl$_2$, rt
f	85%	DiBAlH (1.5 eq) / THF, -78°C
g	78%	2-Lithio-2-triethylsilylpropanal t-butylamine (2 eq) / THF, -78°C TO -10°C
h	-	(2.6) + n-Bu$_2$BOTf , diisopropylethylamine / CH$_2$Cl$_2$, -78°C to 0°C
i	-	Me(MeO)NAlCl(Me) (2eq) / CH$_2$Cl$_2$, -20°C to 22°C, 12h
j	88%	TESOTf (1.5 eq) , 2,6-lutidine (2.5 eq) / CH$_2$Cl$_2$, 0°C
k	60%	(S)-(-)-2-acetoxy-1,1,2-triphenylethanol (1.5 eq) , LDA (1.5 eq) / THF, -78°C
l	-	NaOMe / methanol, 0°C
m	-	TIPSOTf (1.3 eq) , 2,6-lutidine (2.2 eq) / CH$_2$Cl$_2$, 0°C
n	-	DiBAlH (2.5 eq) / THF, 0°C
o	66%	pyr-SO$_3$, Et$_3$N (4 eq) / DMSO-CH$_2$Cl$_2$, 22°C
p	95%	(2.7) + n-BuOTf , diisopropylethylamine / CH$_2$Cl$_2$, -78°C to 0°C
q	-	Me(MeO)NAlCl(Me) (2 eq) / CH$_2$Cl$_2$, -20°C to 22°C
r	-	TBSOTf (2 eq) / 2,6-lutidine (3 eq) / CH$_2$Cl$_2$, 0°C

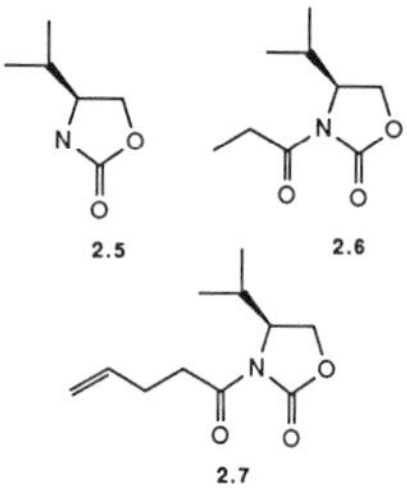

Scheme 2

1988; see also Rama Rao *et al.*, 1990a). The synthetic utility of recent variants of the asymmetric aldol reaction was amply vindicated in the series of three reactions (steps h, k and p) required to extend the chain of aldehyde **2.2** and introduce the remaining five stereogenic centres of the target (**2.4**).

The Merck strategy to form the macrocyclic ring of FK-506 hinged on first constructing the C19–C20 alkene using a Horner–Wittig reaction and thereby securing the bulk of the carbon skeleton of the final product. The phosphine oxide partner (**3.2**) required to implement this strategy was incorporated into the C10–C18 fragment (**3.2**) by modifications (Scheme 3) (T. K. Jones *et al.*, 1989) to the route previously disclosed (Scheme 1).

The aldehyde partner (**4.1**) required for the key Horner–Wittig reaction

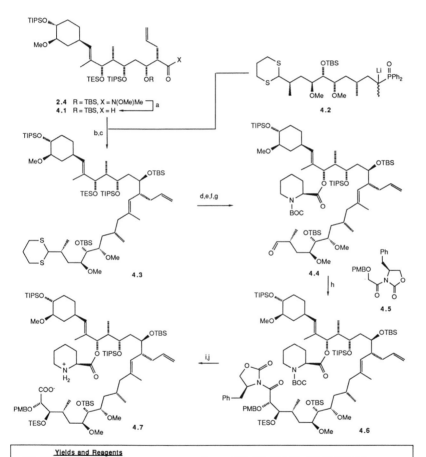

Scheme 3

Scheme 4

Yields and Reagents (Scheme 3)

a	-	Pivaloyl chloride / pyr, 0°C
b	-	NaH , CH₃I / THF, 0°C
c	-	H₂ , Pd(OH)₂ / EtOAc
d	-	TBSOTf / 2,6-lutidine / CH₂Cl₂
e	77%	TFA / H₂O-THF, 20°C
f	-	(COCl)₂ , DMSO / CH₂Cl₂, -78°C; Et₃N
g	-	CH₂(CH₂SH)₂ , BF₃OEt₂ / CH₂Cl₂, 0°C
h	-	TFA / H₂O-THF, 20°C
i	76%	LAH / THF, 0°C
j	-	PhSO₂Cl / pyr, 0°C
k	87%	Ph₂P(O)CH(Li)CH₃ / THF, -78°C.

Yields and Reagents (Scheme 4)

a	96%	DIBAlH / THF, -30°C
b	-	Separation hydroxy phosphine oxides 38% : 39%
c	31%	KHMDS / THF, 0°C
d	-	TFA / H₂O - THF, 20°C
e	-	BOC-pipecolinic acid / DCC , DMAP / CH₂Cl₂, -15°C
f	-	AgNO₃ , NCS , 2,6-Lutidine / CH₃OH - THF, 20°C
g	31%	Glyoxylic acid hydrate / HOAc / CH₂Cl₂, 40°C
h	88%	Et₃N / add 1 / n-Bu₂OTf / toluene, -50°C; add aldehyde at -30°C
i	-	LiOH-H₂O-30% H₂O₂ / THF / H₂O, 0°C
j	80%	TESOTf (4.5 eq) / 2,6-lutidine (6 eq) / CH₂Cl₂, 0°C

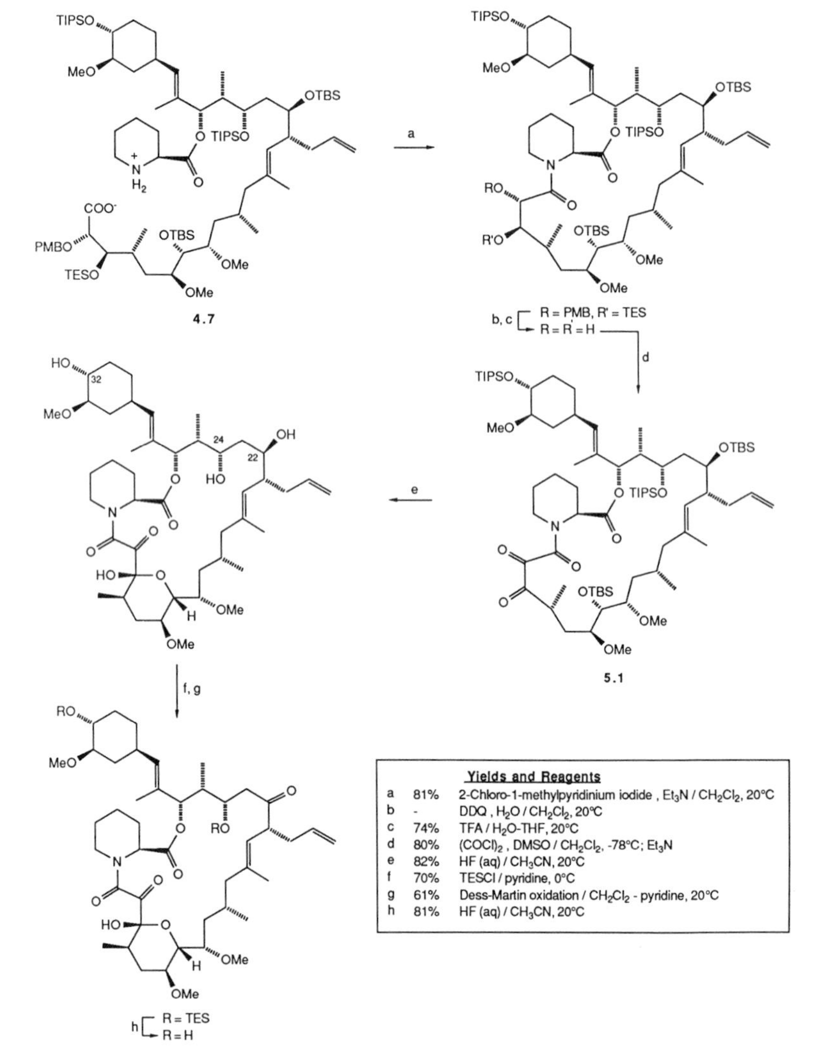

		Yields and Reagents
a	81%	2-Chloro-1-methylpyridinium iodide , Et_3N / CH_2Cl_2, 20°C
b	-	DDQ , H_2O / CH_2Cl_2, 20°C
c	74%	TFA / H_2O-THF, 20°C
d	80%	$(COCl)_2$, DMSO / CH_2Cl_2, -78°C; Et_3N
e	82%	HF (aq) / CH_3CN, 20°C
f	70%	TESCl / pyridine, 0°C
g	61%	Dess-Martin oxidation / CH_2Cl_2 - pyridine, 20°C
h	81%	HF (aq) / CH_3CN, 20°C

Scheme 5

was prepared by reduction of the *N*-methoxyamide (**2.4**) as shown in Scheme 4 (T. K. Jones *et al.*, 1989). The two fragments were then coupled by reaction of the lithiated phosphine oxide (**4.3**) (derived from **3.2**) with aldehyde **4.1** to give a mixture of two hydroxy phosphine oxides (38% and 39%) which were separated chromatographically. On treatment of the less polar diastereoisomer with potassium hexamethyldisilazide, the desired (*E*)-olefin was generated in 82% yield.

The cyclization precursor (**4.7**) was prepared in seven steps from the Horner–Wittig product (**4.3**) as shown in Scheme 4. After selectively removing the triethylsilyl group, BOC-protected pipecolic acid was introduced under standard conditions. Hydrolysis of the terminal dithiane revealed an aldehyde function in **4.4** which underwent a two-carbon homologation (88% yield) using the boron enolate derived from the oxazolidinone (**4.5**) to give the adduct (**4.6**) which incorporated all of the carbon skeleton required to complete the synthesis of FK-506. Hydrolysis of the amide bond and reprotection of the hydroxyl group at C10 then provided the desired macrocyclization precursor (**4.7**).

The macrocyclization reaction (Scheme 5) was achieved in 81% yield using the Mukaiyama reagent 2-chloro-1-methylpyridinium iodide under high dilution conditions. The crucial 1,2,3-tricarbonyl macrocycle (**5.1**) was then produced by a series of selective deprotection and oxidation reactions and the desired tetrahydropyran ring produced by total deprotection of the remaining robust triisopropylsilyl and t-butyldimethylsilyl protection groups. Unfortunately, selective oxidation of the hydroxyl group at C22 required triethylsilylation of the less hindered C32 and C24 hydroxyl groups. Finally, Dess–Martin oxidation of the remaining C22 hydroxyl function and hydrolysis of the triethylsilyl protecting groups gave (−)-FK-506 which was identical to the natural product.

As part of a collaborative effort aimed at the synthesis of FK-506 and analogues thereof, research teams at Southampton University and Fisons Pharmaceuticals have formulated a strategy which requires the synthesis of three major fragments. The first of these, the C1–C15 fragment (**6.7**) was synthesized as outlined in Scheme 6 (Kocieński et al., 1988). The β-keto amide (**6.4**) was prepared from aldehyde (**6.2**) by a three-step sequence

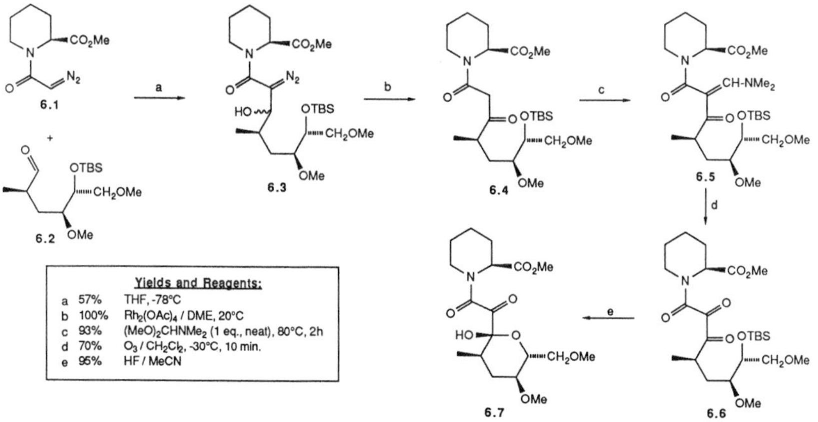

Yields and Reagents:	
a	57%	THF, -78°C
b	100%	Rh₂(OAc)₄ / DME, 20°C
c	93%	(MeO)₂CHNMe₂ (1 eq., neat), 80°C, 2h
d	70%	O₃ / CH₂Cl₂, -30°C, 10 min.
e	95%	HF / MeCN

Scheme 6

beginning with an aldol condensation using the unstable lithiated N-diazo-acetyl-(S)-pipecolinate ester (**6.1**). Successful union of **6.1** and **6.2** was best achieved by adding a solution of lithium diisopropylamide to a mixture of **6.2** and **6.1** in THF at $-78°C$ in which case the anion derived from **6.1** reacted rapidly *in situ* with the aldehyde. Under these conditions a 57% yield of the diastereomeric α-diazo-β-hydroxy amides (**6.3**) was obtained. When **6.3** was treated with a catalytic amount of Rh(II) in dimethoxyethane at room temperature, smooth nitrogen evolution occurred in a remarkably clean reaction to give the desired β-keto amide (**6.4**) in quantitative yield.

The final stage of the synthesis involved the oxidation of **6.4** to the 1,2,3-tricarbonyl intermediate (**6.6**). Thus **6.4** reacted with one equivalent of dimethylformamide dimethylacetal (neat) at 80°C to give a 93% yield of the enamine (**6.5**). Subsequent ozonolysis of **6.5** at $-30°C$ gave the 1,2,3-tricarbonyl intermediate (**6.6**) in 70% yield which was immediately treated with HF in MeCN to give the target (**6.7**; 95%).

A closely related protocol for constructing the 1,2,3-tricarbonyl moiety has also been recently described by Rama Rao and co-workers (Rama Rao *et al.*, 1990b).

The aldehyde (**6.2**) was synthesized (Scheme 7) in six steps (27% overall yield) from the diol (**7.2**) which itself was prepared in three steps (81% overall yield) from commercial tri-O-acetyl-D-glucal (**7.1**). A highly diastereoselective alkylation of the SAMP-hydrazone (**7.3**) gave an inseparable 94 : 6 mixture of diastereoisomers (64% yield) in which the desired product (**7.4**) was the major component. Subsequent ozonolytic cleavage of the hydrazone was achieved without epimerisation of the C11 stereogenic centre to give an inseparable 94 : 6 mixture of diastereoisomeric aldehydes.

A conceptually similar approach to the 1,2,3-tricarbonyl ensemble was applied to the synthesis of the C1–C15 fragment (**8.4**, Scheme 8) (Wasserman *et al.*, 1989). Coupling of the acid chloride (**8.2**) with the

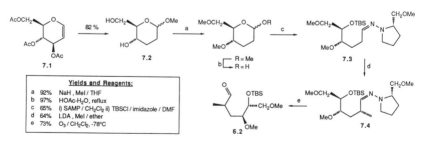

Yields and Reagents:
a 92% NaH , MeI / THF
b 97% HOAc·H₂O, reflux
c 65% i) SAMP / CH₂Cl₂ ii) TBSCl / imidazole / DMF
d 64% LDA , MeI / ether
e 73% O₃ / CH₂Cl₂, -78°C

Scheme 7

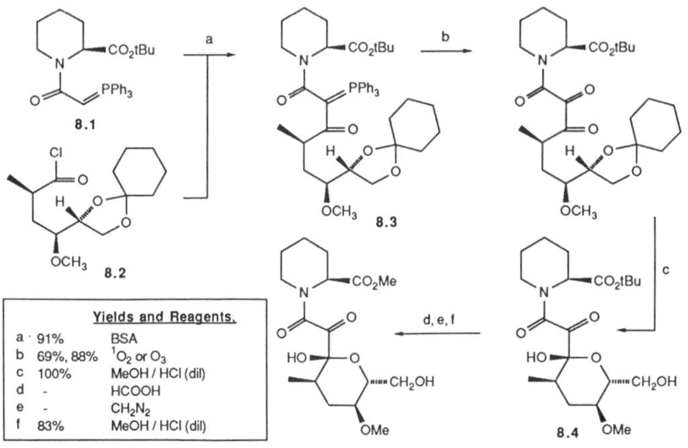

Scheme 8

acylphosphoranylidene (**8.1**) in the presence of bis(trimethylsilyl)-acetamide(BSA) as base gave the keto ylide carboxylate (**8.3**). Unfortunately, a possible limitation of this method to the synthesis of FK-506 derives from the competitive rates of oxidation of trisubstituted double bonds (of which there are two in FK-506) and the keto ylide carboxylate moiety with singlet oxygen.

Williams and Benbow (1988) have described a brief synthesis of the C1–C15 fragment (**8.4**) in which the 1,2,3-tricarbonyl ensemble was prepared by SeO_2 oxidation of a β-ketoamide as outlined in Scheme 9. The single stereogenic centre created in this approach was introduced by diastereoselective addition of the Grignard reagent (**9.2**) to the aldehyde (**9.1**) (derived from D-mannitol) to give a mixture of diastereoisomers (8.4 : 1); the major isomer was transformed to the C1–C15 fragment (**8.4**). The Grignard reagent was prepared from a biotransformation product which is now commercially available.

The Danishefsky group generated the C8–C9 bond of the 1,2,3-tricarbonyl ensemble in model compound **10.6** (Scheme 10) by nucleophilic acylation of the metallated dithiane (**10.3**) with the oxalate ester (**10.4**) (Egbertson and Danishefsky, 1989). Subsequent unmasking of the dithiane moiety in **10.5** generated the desired 1,2,3-tricarbonyl ensemble which was a precursor to the lactol (**10.6**).

Ireland and Wipf (1989) have also generated the C8–C9 bond of the C1–C15 fragment (**11.3**; Scheme 11) by reacting an enolate derived from a protected glycolate ester with the lactone (**11.1**) derived from D-glucose in 14 steps (ca. 24% overall). A useful feature of this approach is in the

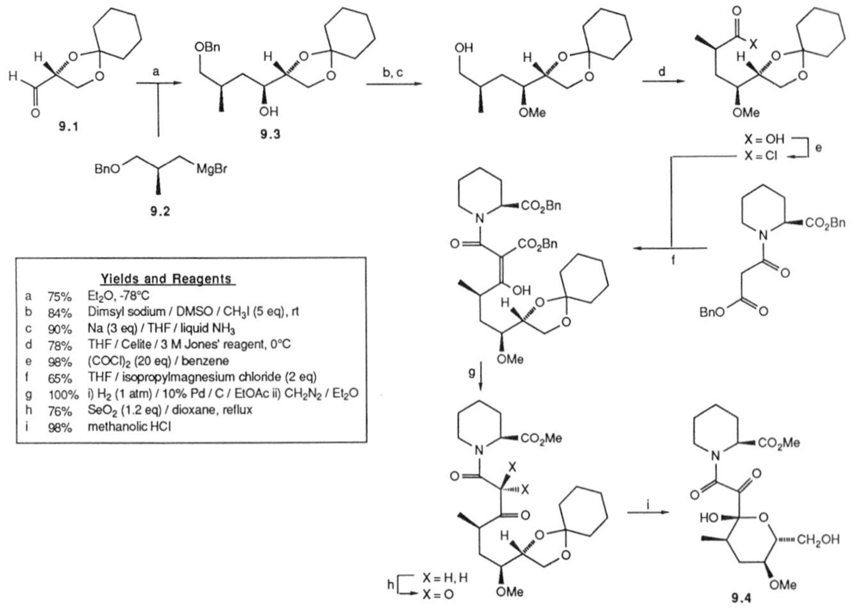

Yields and Reagents

a 75%   Et₂O, -78°C
b 84%   Dimsyl sodium / DMSO / CH₃I (5 eq), rt
c 90%   Na (3 eq) / THF / liquid NH₃
d 78%   THF / Celite / 3 M Jones' reagent, 0°C
e 98%   (COCl)₂ (20 eq) / benzene
f 65%   THF / isopropylmagnesium chloride (2 eq)
g 100% i) H₂ (1 atm) / 10% Pd / C / EtOAc ii) CH₂N₂ / Et₂O
h 76%   SeO₂ (1.2 eq) / dioxane, reflux
i 98%   methanolic HCl

Scheme 9

introduction of the reactive keto-hemiketal functionality in a protected form in order to facilitate subsequent synthetic operations required to fashion the natural product.

Wang (1989) has achieved a synthesis (Scheme 12) of the C10–C24 fragment (**12.2**; seven stereogenic centres) which uses an efficient

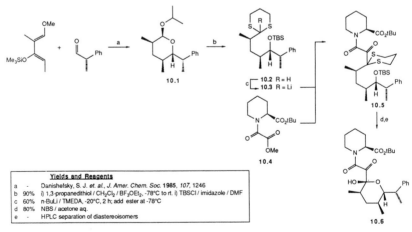

Yields and Reagents

a -   Danishefsky, S. J. *et. al.*, *J. Amer. Chem. Soc.* 1985, *107*, 1246
b 90% i) 1,3-propanedithiol / CH₂Cl₂ / BF₃OEt₂, -78°C to rt. i) TBSCl / imidazole / DMF
c 60% n-BuLi / TMEDA, -20°C 2 h; add ester at -78°C
d 80% NBS / acetone aq.
e -   HPLC separation of diastereoisomers

Scheme 10

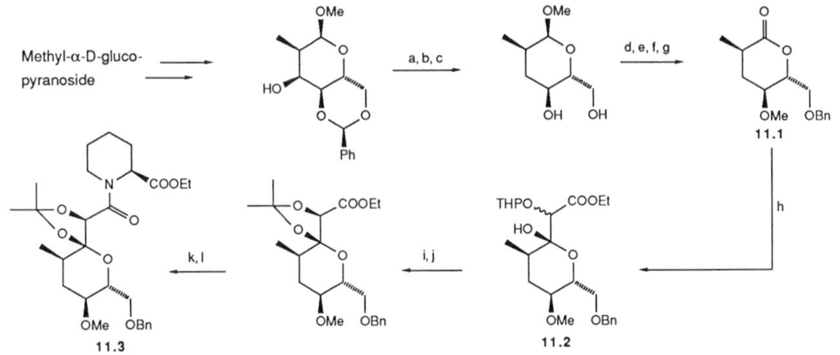

Methyl-α-D-gluco-
pyranoside

Scheme 11

	Yields and Reagents		
a	-	i) n-BuLi / DME / TMEDA, 0°C ii) Cl₂PONMe₂, rt, 4h	
b	-	HNMe₂, rt, 4h	
c	75%	Li / THF - EtOH - EtNH₂, 10°C, 1h	
d	-	NaH , BnBr / THF, 0°C, 36h	
e	-	NaH , CH₃I / THF, rt, 8h	
f	-	HOAc - H₂SO₄ - H₂O, 90°C, 90 min	
g	57%	Ac₂O / DMSO, rt, 24h
h	-	i) LDA / THF / THPOCH₂CO₂C₂H₅, -78°C, 3h ii) EtOH
i	-	PPTs / THF - H₂O, 55°C, 5h
j	69%	CH₃COCH₃ / P₂O₅, rt, 15h
k	-	LiOH / MeOH - H₂O, rt, 6h
l	50%	SOCl₂ / pyridine, rt, 10 min ii) ethyl pipecolinate, rt, 2h

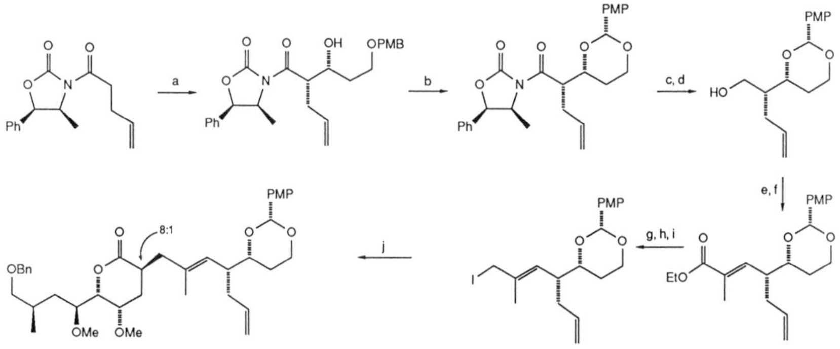

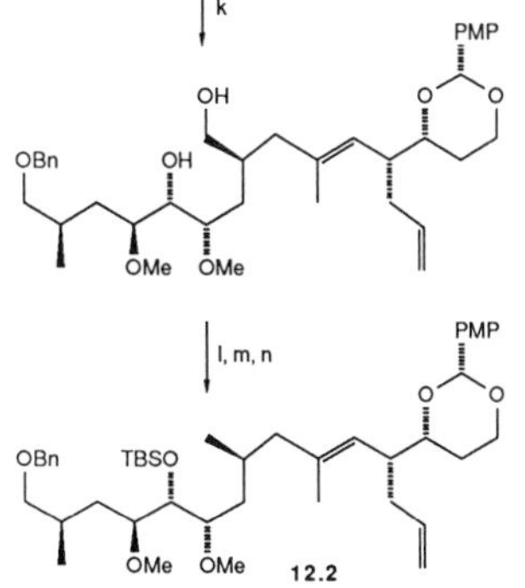

	Yields and Reagents	
a	95%	(c-C₅H₉)₂BOTf / i-Pr₂NEt; add PMBOCH₂CH₂CHO / CH₂Cl₂,-78°C
b	92%	DDQ / CH₂Cl₂
c	-	LiOH , H₂O₂ / THF-H₂O
d	65%	LiAlH₄ / THF, 0°C
e	-	(COCl)₂ , DMSO, Et₃N / CH₂Cl₂, -78°C
f	95%	Ph₃P=C(Me)CO₂Et / THF
g	-	LiAlH₄ / Et₂O, -20°C
h	-	Ph₃P, CBr₄ / CH₂Cl₂
i	84%	NaI / acetone
j	80%	Enolate **12. 3**
k	93%	LiAlH₄ / THF, -20°C
l	-	p-TsCl , Et₃N / CH₂Cl₂
m	-	TBSOTf , 2,6-lutidine / CH₂Cl₂
n	82%	LiEt₃BH / THF

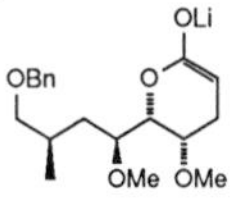

Scheme 12

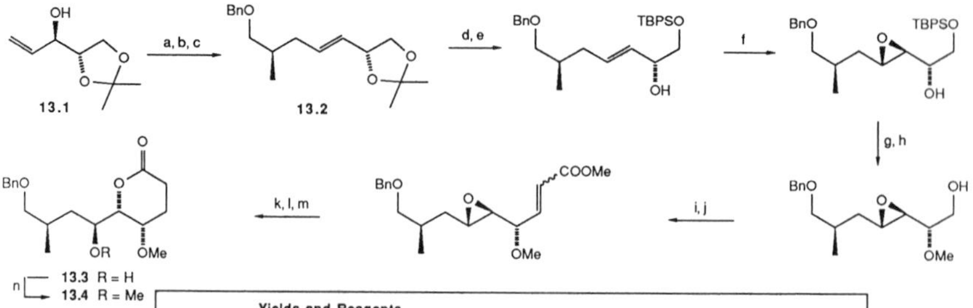

148   Philip Kocieński *et al.*

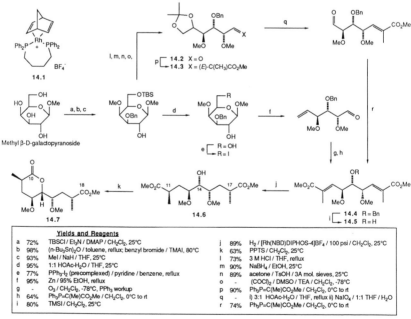

Scheme 13

Diastereoselective alkylation (step j) to unite two principal subunits and generate the stereogenic centre at C17. The adjacent stereogenic centres in the iodide (**12.1**) were generated by an Evans asymmetric aldol reaction (step a). A noteworthy feature of this synthesis is the high degree of stereocontrol achieved in the synthesis of the trisubstituted alkene at

Scheme 14

C19–C20 using a stabilized ylide. Other connective approaches to this functional group have been much less stereoselective (see below). The lactone subunit (**13.4**) which served as the precursor to the enolate (**12.3**) was prepared (Scheme 13) in 14 steps from the allylic alcohol (**13.1**), which itself was prepared in seven steps from L-arabinose in 60% overall yield by a process which did not require chromatographic purification of intermediates. Chain extension of the alcohol (**13.1**) was accomplished by an Ireland–Claisen rearrangement (step b), which also served to introduce the stereogenic centre at C11 in **13.2** with the desired stereochemistry. After deprotection of the vicinal diol in **13.2** and protection of the terminal hydroxyl function, a Sharpless asymmetric epoxidation (step f) was used to construct the remaining two stereogenic centres.

Villalobos and Danishefsky (1989) disclosed a conceptually elegant approach to the C10–C18 fragment (**14.7**; Scheme 14) which exploits the symmetrical disposition of functionality about the central hydroxyl function in the intermediate (**14.4**). The stereogenic centres at C13, C14 and C15 were derived from D-galactose and the stereogenic centres at C11 and C17 were secured by catalytic hydrogenation using a rhodium catalyst (**14.1**) under guidance from the neighbouring homoallylic hydroxyl function in

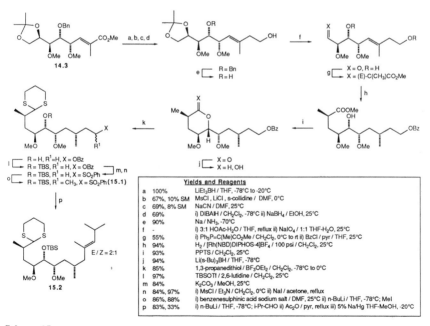

Scheme 15

14.5. The selectivity in the hydrogenation was impressive: of the four possible diastereoisomers, only three were observed and these were formed in the ratio 20 : 2.25 : 1. The major product corresponded to **14.6**. End-group differentiation was then achieved by acid-catalysed lactonization, but the regioselectivity of this process was disappointing (4–6 : 1).

The route depicted in Scheme 14 was modified (Villalobos and Danishefsky, 1989) in order to exploit the end-group differentiation inherent in intermediate **14.3**. An extensive series of functional-group transformations were required in order to transform **14.3** to the penultimate product in Scheme 15 (sulphone **15.1**). In a model study designed to evaluate the Julia olefination for the construction of the C19–C20 trisubstituted double bond, the sulphone (**15.1**) was metallated and condensed with isobutanal but the subsequent reductive elimination produced the alkene (**15.2**) as a mixture of isomers ($E : Z = 2 : 1$).

Schreiber *et al.* (1989) synthesized the C10–C19 fragment (**16.5**) from arabitol (**16.1**) which exploits the efficiency of reaction duplication in a 'two-directional chain synthesis strategy'. This strategy is based on the recognition of a symmetrical disposition of functional groups in the target and intermediates leading to it. Thus arabitol, with its central chirotopic, nonstereogenic centre (marked *, Scheme 16) was elaborated in six steps

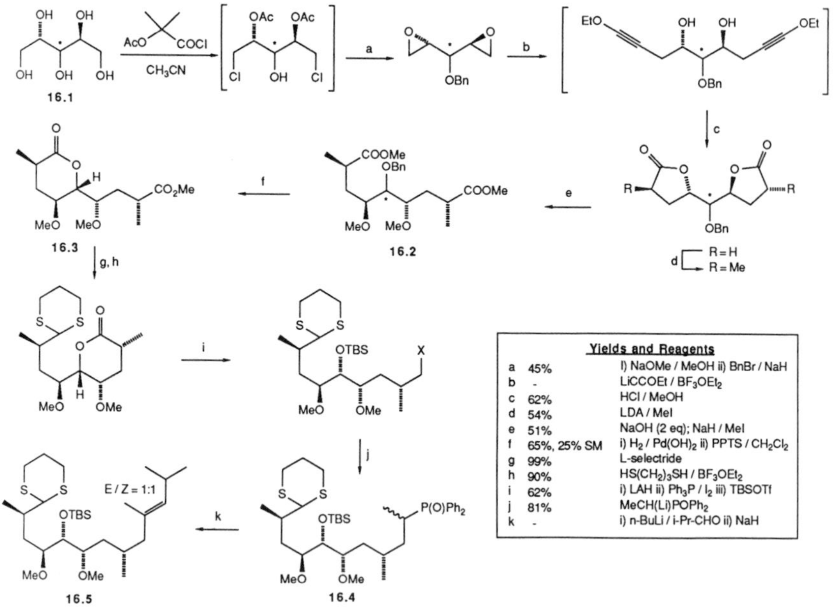

		Yields and Reagents
a	45%	i) NaOMe / MeOH ii) BnBr / NaH
b	–	LiCCOEt / BF₃OEt₂
c	62%	HCl / MeOH
d	54%	LDA / MeI
e	51%	NaOH (2 eq); NaH / MeI
f	65%, 25% SM	i) H₂ / Pd(OH)₂ ii) PPTS / CH₂Cl₂
g	99%	L-selectride
h	90%	HS(CH₂)₃SH / BF₃OEt₂
i	62%	i) LAH ii) Ph₃P / I₂ iii) TBSOTf
j	81%	MeCH(Li)POPh₂
k	–	i) n-BuLi / i-Pr-CHO ii) NaH

Scheme 16

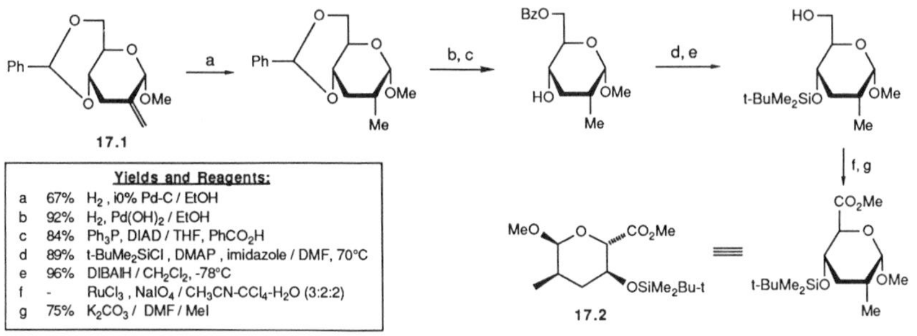

17.1

Yields and Reagents:

a	67%	H_2, i0% Pd-C / EtOH
b	92%	H_2, Pd(OH)$_2$ / EtOH
c	84%	Ph$_3$P, DIAD / THF, PhCO$_2$H
d	89%	t-BuMe$_2$SiCl, DMAP, imidazole / DMF, 70°C
e	96%	DIBAlH / CH$_2$Cl$_2$, -78°C
f	-	RuCl$_3$, NaIO$_4$ / CH$_3$CN-CCl$_4$-H$_2$O (3:2:2)
g	75%	K$_2$CO$_3$ / DMF / MeI

17.2

Scheme 17

(7.7% overall yield) to the benzyl ether (**16.2**) which retained the chirotopic, nonstereogenic centre. Terminus differentiation was then achieved by a diastereotopic group-selective lactonization of the hydroxy diester derived from hydrogenolysis of the benzyl group in **16.2** to give a 6 : 1 mixture of lactones from which the desired diastereoisomer (**16.3**) was obtained in 65% yield.

A further four steps were used to convert **16.3** to the C10–C19 intermediate (**16.4**) in which both termini were activated towards carbanion formation. Chemoselective lithiation at the carbon α to the phosphinoyl group was achieved by treatment of **16.4** with n-BuLi at −78°C. Unfortunately, the Horner reaction between lithiated **16.4** and isobutanal gave the alkene **16.5** as a 1 : 1 mixture of isomers.

Smith and Hale (1989) reported a seven-step synthesis (33% overall yield) of the tetrahydropyran ring (**17.2**) of FK-506 (Scheme 17) from the glycoside (**17.1**) which was prepared from methyl α-D-glucopyranoside in six steps. The ester (**17.2**) served as a key starting material in the synthesis of a C10–C23 fragment (**18.4**) as shown in Scheme 18.

The ester function in **17.2** was condensed with the sulphone **18.1** to complete the carbon skeleton of the target **18.4**. The high stereoselectivity of the Negishi carboalumination reaction (step e) ensured a stereoselective preparation of the C19–C20 trisubstituted alkene. The reductive removal of the sulphone from the β-keto sulphone intermediate **18.2** using a radical process (step k) represents a novel and mild method in place of the more usual reagents (e.g. Al/Hg). The final stereogenic centre at C15 was introduced via a hydroxyl directed reduction of the β-hydroxy sulphone (**18.3**) which resulted in a 20 : 1 mixture of anti and syn 1,3-diols from which the desired major isomer was easily isolated by chromatography.

A salient feature of a synthesis of the C16–C23 fragment (**19.8**; Scheme 19) is the stereoselective construction of the C19–C20 trisubstituted alkene using a novel copper catalysed migratory insertion reaction (Kocieński et al.,

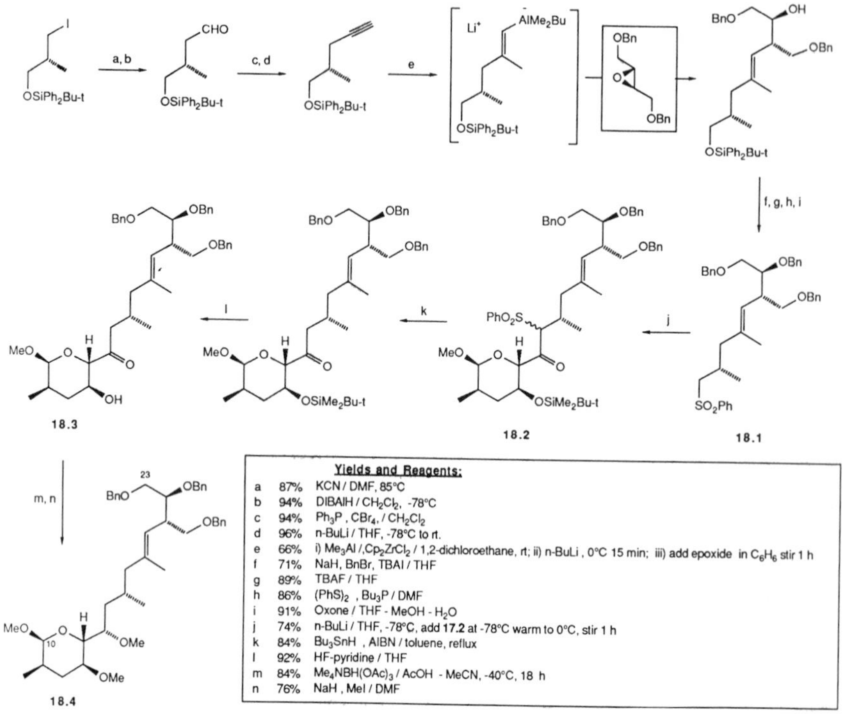

Yields and Reagents:

a	87%	KCN / DMF, 85°C
b	94%	DIBAlH / CH₂Cl₂, -78°C
c	94%	Ph₃P , CBr₄, / CH₂Cl₂
d	96%	n-BuLi / THF, -78°C to rt.
e	66%	i) Me₃Al /,Cp₂ZrCl₂ / 1,2-dichloroethane, rt; ii) n-BuLi , 0°C 15 min; iii) add epoxide in C₆H₆ stir 1 h
f	71%	NaH, BnBr, TBAI / THF
g	89%	TBAF / THF
h	86%	(PhS)₂ , Bu₃P / DMF
i	91%	Oxone / THF - MeOH - H₂O
j	74%	n-BuLi / THF, -78°C, add 17.2 at -78°C warm to 0°C, stir 1 h
k	84%	Bu₃SnH , AIBN / toluene, reflux
l	92%	HF-pyridine / THF
m	84%	Me₄NBH(OAc)₃ / AcOH - MeCN, -40°C, 18 h
n	76%	NaH , MeI / DMF

Scheme 18

1990a). Thus reaction of the metallated dihydrofuran (**19.2**) with the homocuprate (**19.5**) produced a higher order cuprate intermediate (**19.6**) which rearranged with clean inversion of stereochemistry to give the putative higher order oxycuprate (**19.7**). Intermediate **19.7** underwent alkylation with retention of configuration at low temperature to give the trisubstituted alkene (**19.8**) in 57% overall yield from **19.1**.

The synthesis of dihydrofuran (**19.1**) began (Scheme 20) with (+)-tartaric acid which was converted to the oxiran (**20.1**) in 73% overall yield according to known procedures. Nucleophilic scission of the oxiran ring with allylmagnesium bromide gave the alcohol (**20.2**) which was converted to the dihydrofuran (**19.1**) using standard transformations.

(*R*)-Cyclohex-3-enecarboxylic acid (**21.3**; Scheme 21) was a common intermediate in three different approaches to the cyclohexane ring of FK-506. The Southampton–Fisons group prepared **21.3** by two routes (Kocieński *et al.*, 1990b). The first route began with an efficient TiCL₄-catalysed asymmetric Diels–Alder reaction (20 g scale) between butadiene

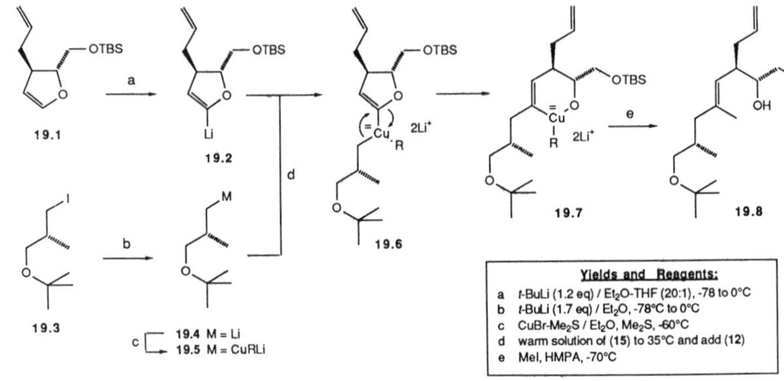
OTBS
19.1
a
Li
19.2
d
2Li+
R
19.6
19.7
e
OH
19.8
M
b
19.3
c
19.4 M = Li
19.5 M = CuRLi
Yields and Reagents:
a t-BuLi (1.2 eq) / Et2O-THF (20:1), -78 to 0°C
b t-BuLi (1.7 eq) / Et2O, -78°C to 0°C
c CuBr-Me2S / Et2O, Me2S, -60°C
d warm solution of (15) to 35°C and add (12)
e MeI, HMPA, -70°C

Scheme 19

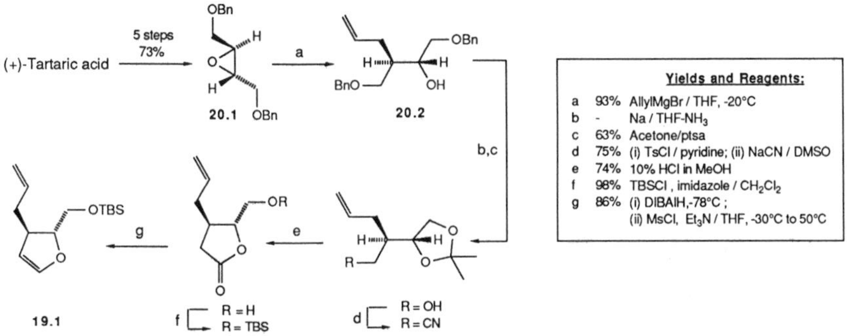
(+)-Tartaric acid
5 steps
73%
OBn
20.1
a
BnO
OH
20.2
b,c
OTBS
g
OR
e
19.1
f
R = H
R = TBS
d
R = OH
R = CN
Yields and Reagents:
a 93% AllylMgBr / THF, -20°C
b - Na / THF-NH3
c 63% Acetone/ptsa
d 75% (i) TsCl / pyridine; (ii) NaCN / DMSO
e 74% 10% HCl in MeOH
f 98% TBSCl, imidazole / CH2Cl2
g 86% (i) DIBAlH,-78°C ;
(ii) MsCl, Et3N / THF, -30°C to 50°C

Scheme 20

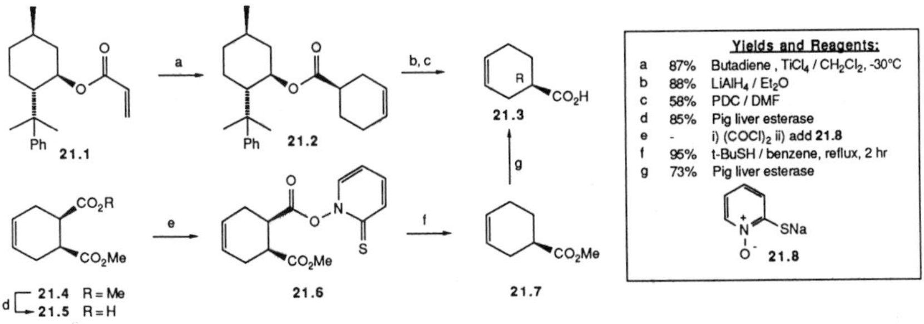
Ph
21.1
a
21.2
b, c
CO2H
21.3
g
CO2R
CO2Me
e
21.6
f
21.7
d
21.4 R = Me
21.5 R = H
Yields and Reagents:
a 87% Butadiene, TiCl4 / CH2Cl2, -30°C
b 88% LiAlH4 / Et2O
c 58% PDC / DMF
d 85% Pig liver esterase
e - i) (COCl)2 ii) add 21.8
f 95% t-BuSH / benzene, reflux, 2 hr
g 73% Pig liver esterase
SNa
21.8

Scheme 21

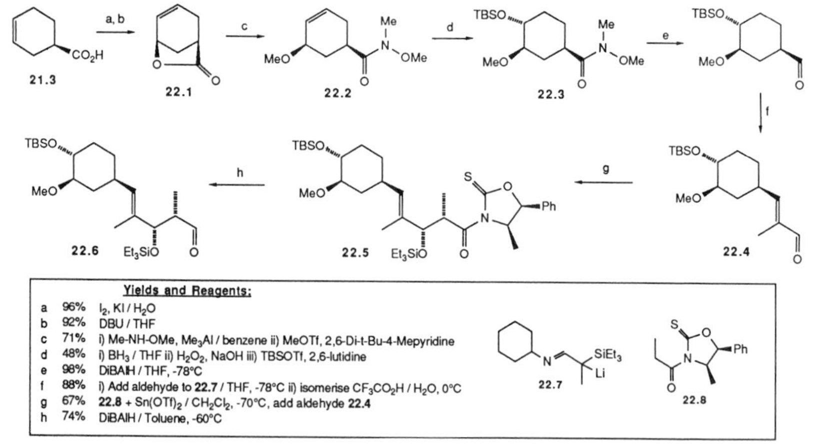

Scheme 22

Yields and Reagents:
a 96% I$_2$, KI / H$_2$O
b 92% DBU / THF
c 71% i) Me-NH-OMe, Me$_3$Al / benzene ii) MeOTf, 2,6-Di-t-Bu-4-Mepyridine
d 48% i) BH$_3$ / THF ii) H$_2$O$_2$, NaOH iii) TBSOTf, 2,6-lutidine
e 98% DiBAlH / THF, -78°C
f 88% i) Add aldehyde to 22.7 / THF, -78°C ii) isomerise CF$_3$CO$_2$H / H$_2$O, 0°C
g 67% 22.8 + Sn(OTf)$_2$ / CH$_2$Cl$_2$, -70°C, add aldehyde 22.4
h 74% DiBAlH / Toluene, -60°C

and the homochiral acrylate ester (21.1). Since attempts to hydrolyse the adduct (21.2) were thwarted by competing racemization, a two-step reduction–oxidation sequence was used to convert the hindered ester (21.2) to the acid (21.3). Owing to the mediocre yield in the final oxidation step in Scheme 21, a second route to 21.3 was examined in which the requisite stereogenic centre was introduced *via* pig liver esterase (ple)-catalysed hydrolysis of the readily available *meso*-diester (21.4). Subsequent decarboxylation of the acid (21.5), followed by a second ple-catalysed ester hydrolysis of the monoester (21.7) gave the desired acid in 59% overall yield from diester 21.4 using reactions which could be easily run on a 40–70 g scale.

Elaboration of the homochiral acid (21.3) to the C24–C34 fragment (22.6) is summarized in Scheme 22 (Kocieński *et al.*, 1990b). A noteworthy feature of the sequence of nine steps (26% overall yield) required to convert 21.3 to the enal (22.4) was the high regio- and stereo-selectivity observed in the hydroboration of the allylic ether (22.2): only minor amounts (< 5%) of stereoisomeric products were obtained. To complete the synthesis of the target aldehyde (22.6), a *syn*-selective aldol condensation between thiazolidinone (22.8) and aldehyde (22.4) in the presence of Sn(OTf)$_2$ gave the adduct (22.5) in 67% yield after silylation. Finally, reduction of the *N*-acylthiazolidinone afforded the aldehyde (22.6) in 74% yield.

Sulphone condensation chemistry played a major role in the construction of the C24–C34 fragment 23.7 (Scheme 23) (Smith *et al.*, 1989). The lactone (23.1), a key intermediate in the Southampton–Fisons synthesis described above, was also prepared by Smith and Hale using an asymmetric Diels–Alder reaction (four steps, 67% overall from butadiene) to create the initial

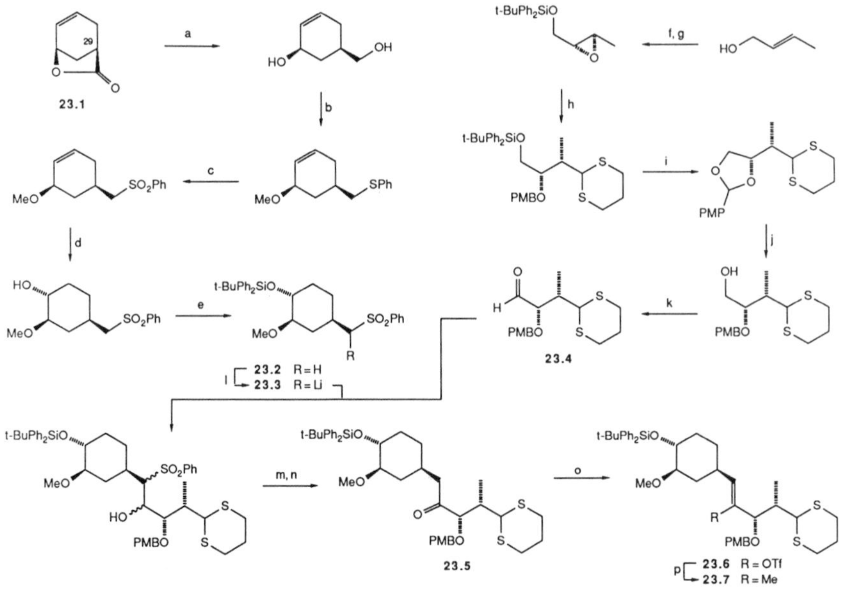

Yields and Reagents

a	93%	LiAlH₄ / Et₂O, 0°C
b	66%	i) Bu₃P , (PhS)₂ / DMF, rt ii) CH₂N₂ / Et₂O / BF₃OEt₂, 0°C
c	87%	Oxone / THF-MeOH-H₂O, 0°C
d	71%	BH₃·THF / NaOH / t-BuO₂H, -78°C to rt
e	70%	t-BuPh₂SiCl / imidazole / DMF, rt
f	-	Sharpless AE / D-(-)-DET / CH₂Cl₂
g	76%	in situ t-BuPh₂SiCl, Et₃N , DMAP / DMF
h	76%	2-lithio-1,3-dithiane , DMU / THF, 0°C
i	95%	i) TBAF / THF, rt ii) p-MeO(C₆H₄)CH(OMe)₂ / DMF / TsOH, 55°C
j	90%	DIBAlH / CH₂Cl₂, -78°C
k	-	SO₃-py , DMSO , Et₃N / CH₂Cl₂, 0°C
l	89%	i) n-BuLi / THF, -78°C ii) add aldehyde (1)
m	84%	i) TFAA , DMSO / CH₂Cl₂, -78°C ii) Et₃N
n	90%	Al(Hg) / THF (aq), reflux
o	70%	LDA , N-Phenyltriflamide / DME - DMPU
p	73%	Me₂CuLi / THF, 0°C

Scheme 23

stereogenic centre at C29. Lactone (**23.1**) was elaborated to the metallated sulphone (**23.3**) which condensed with the aldehyde (**23.4**) to complete the skeleton of the target (**23.7**). The trisubstituted alkene of the target was constructed in two steps from ketone (**23.5**) *via* the Z-enol triflate (**23.6**) (> 99% Z). Coupling of **23.6** with lithium dimethylcuprate afforded two major products (7 : 1) from which the desired E isomer was isolated in 73% yield by column chromatography.

Corey and Huang (1989) have described an elegant synthesis of the C18–C34 model (**24.11**; Scheme 24) which served as a vehicle for demonstrating the efficacy of new enantioselective versions of such major synthetic processes as the Diels–Alder, aldol and carbonyl allylation reactions. Thus, the cyclohexane unit and the C29 stereogenic centre were established by TiCl₄-catalysed Diels–Alder reaction of butadiene with the acrylate ester of (S)-(+)-pantolactone (**24.1**) to give the adduct (**24.2**) in 85% yield and 91% diastereoisomeric excess (de). The second key step in the sequence (step h),

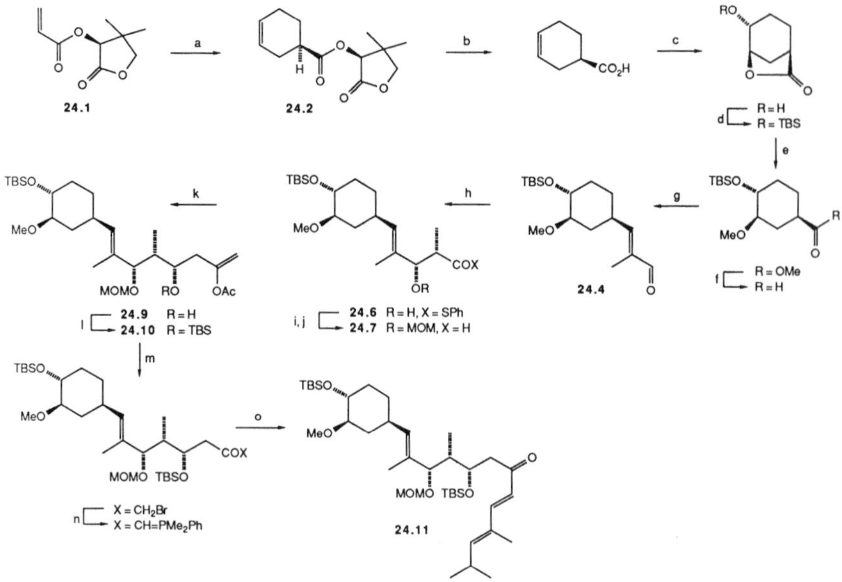

Yields and Reagents

a	85%	Butadiene, $TiCl_4$ (30 eq) / CH_2Cl_2, -32°C, 5 days
b	94%	3.5M $LiOH$-H_2O (3.9 eq) / THF, 23°C
c	95%	i) mcpba (1.1 eq) / CCl_4, 0°C, 4 h ii) Et_3N, 55°C, 3 h
d	92%	TBSCl (1.3 eq), DMAP (1.5 eq) / CH_2Cl_2, reflux 21h
e	88%	i) $NaHCO_3$ (0.5 eq) / MeOH, 25°C ii) MeOTf (3.3 eq) / 2,6-di-t-Bu-4-Mepyr
f	95%	DIBAlH (1.2 eq) / hexane, -78°C
g	-	**24.3** + aldehyde; isomerise with CF_3COOH / H_2O
h	85%	**24.5** + aldehyde / CH_2Cl_2, -78°C, 2h
i	-	MOMBr (6 eq) / diisopropylethylamine / CH_2Cl_2
j	-	DIBAlH / hexane
k	61%	**24.8** + aldehyde / CH_2Cl_2, -78°C
l	100%	TBSOTf (4.2 eq), 2,6-lutidine / CH_2Cl_2, 0°C
m	92%	NBS (1.3 eq) / CH_3CN
n	-	i) dimethylphenylphosphine / CH_3CN ii) 1,4-diazabicyclo[2.2.2]octane
o	87%	(E)-2,4-dimethyl-2-pentenal

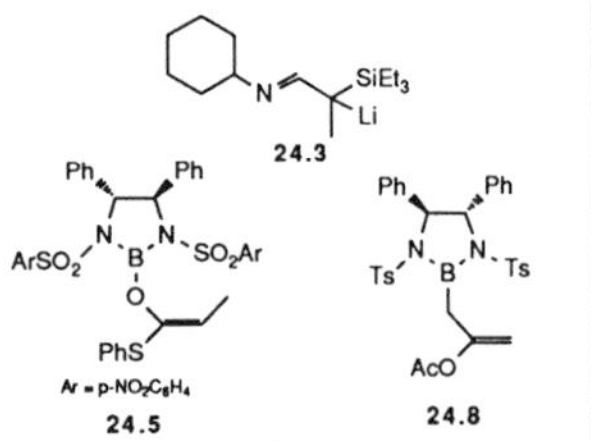

Scheme 24

an asymmetric aldol reaction, depended on a diastereoselective reaction between aldehyde **24.4** and the boronate ester **24.5** prepared by reaction of (*R*,*R*)-1,2-diphenyl-1,2-diaminoethane bis(*p*-nitrobenzenesulphonamide), boron tribromide and (*S*)-phenyl thiopropionate. In the third key step, the thioester (**24.6** 92% de) was converted to aldehyde (**24.7**) which then served as a substrate in an enantioselective 2-acetoxyallylation (89% de) based once again on the 1,2-diphenyl-1,2-diaminoethane controller group.

Schreiber and Smith (1989) prepared the sulphone-activated cyclohexane fragment (**25.7**; Scheme 25; see also Scheme 23) by a route which did not depend on an asymmetric Diels–Alder reaction. Instead, a group- and face-selective epoxidation of 1,4-pentadiene-3-ol (**25.1**) was achieved by the catalytic procedure of Sharpless in which a kinetic resolution coupled with

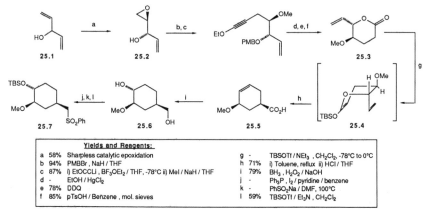

a 58% Sharpless catalytic epoxidation
b 94% PMBBr, NaH / THF
c 87% i) EtOCCLi, BF₃OEt₂ / THF, -78°C ii) MeI / NaH / THF
d - EtOH / HgCl₂
e 78% DDQ
f 85% pTsOH / Benzene , mol. sieves

g - TBSOTf / NEt₃ , CH₂Cl₂, -78°C to 0°C
h 71% i) Toluene, reflux ii) HCl / THF
i 79% BH₃ , H₂O₂ / NaOH
j - Ph₃P , I₂ / pyridine / benzene
k - PhSO₂Na / DMF, 100°C
l 59% TBSOTf / Et₃N , CH₂Cl₂

Scheme 25

the initial asymmetric synthesis resulted in the epoxy alcohol (**25.2**) with a high enantiomeric purity. A subsequent intermediate, lactone (**25.3**), was converted to silyl ketene acetal (**25.4**) which underwent an Ireland–Claisen rearrangement to carbocycle (**25.5**). A regio- and stereo- selective hydroboration of **25.5** and further functional group conversion gave the target C28–C34 sulphone (**25.7**).

Schreiber and Danishefsky have reported a synthesis of the C22–34 fragment (**26.6**; Scheme 26) (A. B. Jones *et al.*, 1989) which features a

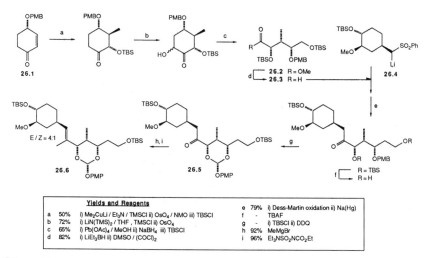

Yields and Reagents
a 50% i) Me₂CuLi / Et₃N / TMSCl ii) OsO₄ / NMO iii) TBSCl
b 72% i) LiN(TMS)₂ / THF , TMSCl ii) OsO₄
c 65% i) Pb(OAc)₄ / MeOH ii) NaBH₄ iii) TBSCl
d 82% i) LiEt₃BH ii) DMSO / (COCl)₂

e 79% i) Dess-Martin oxidation ii) Na(Hg)
f - TBAF
g - i) TBSCl ii) DDQ
h 92% MeMgBr
i 96% Et₃NSO₂NCO₂Et

Scheme 26

multistep conversion of (−)-quinic acid to the aldehyde (**26.3**) *via* enone (**26.1**) and its union with the lithiated sulphone (**26.4**; Scheme 26) to form the C27–C28 bond of ketone (**26.5**). Introduction of the trisubstituted alkene was accomplished in two steps by diastereoselective dehydration of a tertiary alcohol to give the target (**26.6**) as a 4 : 1 mixture of diastereoisomers.

A detraction of the route outlined in Scheme 26 is the excessive number of steps required to convert (−)-quinic acid to the aldehyde fragment **26.3**. Consequently, an alternative route to a series of more complex aldehyde fragments (e.g. **27.5**) was investigated as shown in Scheme 27. An asymmetric catalytic hydrogenation of the β-keto ester (**27.1**) was accomplished with 1% $Ru_2Cl_4[(S)\text{-binap}]_2$ in 90% yield and the resultant stereogenic centre used to relay stereogenicity to other sites of the target. Thus the newly created stereogenic centre was used first to influence the stereochemistry of the alkylation reaction that yielded **27.2** and then to control the stereochemistry of chelation-controlled addition of triphenyl-crotylstannane to the aldehyde (**27.3**). A second 'Cram-type' nucleophilic addition of vinylmagnesium bromide (steps i and j) proceeded with only modest diastereoselectivity to give a 3 : 1 mixture of stereoisomers from which the major isomer (**27.5**) was isolated by chromatography.

The Schreiber group (Ragan *et al.*, 1989) accomplished the synthesis of an advanced intermediate (**28.7**; Scheme 28) which incorporates all but two of

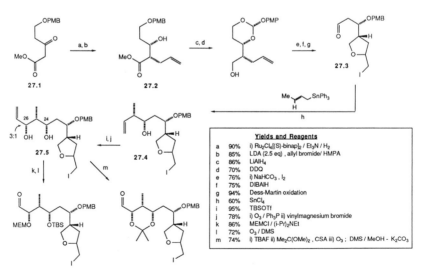

Scheme 27

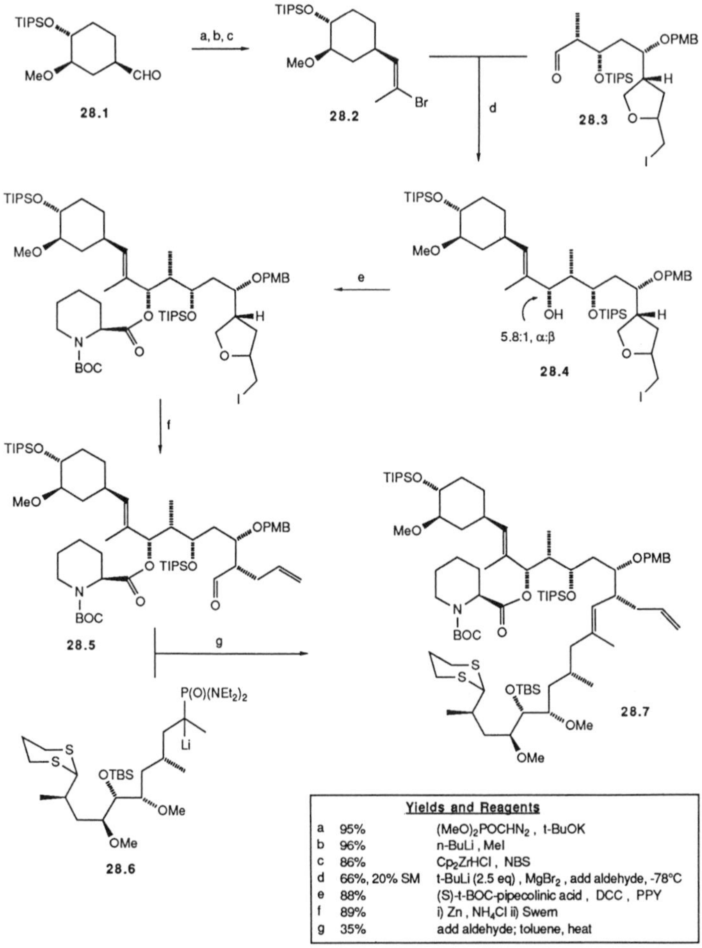

Compounds in Scheme 28: **28.1**, **28.2** (Br), **28.3**, **28.4** (5.8:1, α:β), **28.5**, **28.6**, **28.7**.

Reagents in scheme: a, b, c; d; e; f; g. Other labels: TIPSO, MeO, CHO, OPMB, OTIPS, OH, N–BOC, O, P(O)(NEt₂)₂, Li, OTBS, OMe, OTBS.

Yields and Reagents		
a	95%	(MeO)₂POCHN₂ , t-BuOK
b	96%	n-BuLi , MeI
c	86%	Cp₂ZrHCl , NBS
d	66%, 20% SM	t-BuLi (2.5 eq) , MgBr₂ , add aldehyde, -78°C
e	88%	(S)-t-BOC-pipecolinic acid , DCC , PPY
f	89%	i) Zn , NH₄Cl ii) Swern
g	35%	add aldehyde; toluene, heat

Scheme 28

the carbon atoms of FK-506. The starting materials in this sequence, aldehydes **28.1** and **28.3**, were prepared from intermediates described previously (see Schemes 25 and 27, respectively). Aldehyde **28.1** was converted in three steps (78% overall yield) to the alkenyl bromide (**28.2**) from which an organomagnesium reagent was prepared by a halogen–metal exchange using t-BuLi followed by transmetallation. The resultant vinylmagnesium halide added stereoselectively to aldehyde (**28.3**) to give the allylic alcohol (**28.4**) as a 5.8 : 1 mixture of diastereoisomers. Further elaboration produced the aldehyde (**28.5**) which reacted with the lithiated phosphonamide (**28.6**) to produce a separable mixture (2 : 1) of β-hydroxy-phosphonamides. The major diastereoisomer underwent stereospecific elimination on heating in toluene to produce the C19–C20 trisubstituted alkene of the target (**28.7**) which has recently been converted to FK-506 (Nakatsuka, 1990).

References

Arita, C., Hotokebuchi, T., Miyahara, H., Arai, K., Sugioka, Y., Takagishi, K. and Kaibara, N. (1989). Effect of FK-506 (FR 900506) on collagen arthritis in rats: a preliminary report. *Transpl. Proc.* **21**, 1056–1058.

Askin, D., Volante, R. P., Reamer, R. A., Ryan, K. M. and Shinkai, I. (1988). A diastereoselective synthesis of the C.10–C.18 segment of FK-506. *Tetrahedron Lett.* **29**, 277–280.

Askin, D., Reamer, R. A., Jones, T. K., Volante, R. P. and Shinkai, I. (1989). Chemistry of FK-506: benzilic acid rearrangement of the tricarbonyl system. *Tetrahedron Lett.* **30**, 671–674.

Bieret, B. E., Schreiber, S. L. and Burakoff, S. J. (1990). Mechanisms of immunosuppression by FK-506. *Transplantation* **49**, 1168–1170.

Bucy, R. P., Hanto, D. W., Berens, E. and Schreiber, R. D. (1988). Lack of an obligate role for γ-INF in the primary *in vitro* mixed lymphocyte response. *J. Immunol.* **140**, 1148–1152.

Calne, R. Y., Collier, D. St. J. and Thiru, S. (1987). Observations about FK-506 in primates. *Transpl. Proc.* **19** (Suppl. 6), 63.

Calne, R. Y., Collier, D. St. J., Lim, S., Pollard, S. G., Samaan, A., White, D. J. G. and Thiru, S. (1989). Rapamycin for immunosuppression in organ allografting. *Lancet* **ii**, 227.

Collier, D. St. J., Thiru, S. and Calne, R. Y. (1987). Kidney transplantation in the dog receiving FK-506. *Transpl. Proc.* **19**, (Suppl. 6), 62.

Corey, E. J. and Huang, H.-C. (1989). Enantioselective synthesis of the C(18)–C(35) segment of immunosuppressant FK-506 using efficient new methodology. *Tetrahedron Lett.* **30**, 5235–5238.

Donald, D. K., Birkinshaw, T. N., Cooper, M. E. and Furber, M. (1990). Department of Medicinal Chemistry, Fisons Pharmaceuticals. Unpublished studies.

Dumont, F. J., Staruch, M. J., Koprak, S. L., Melino, M. R. and Sigal, N. H. (1990a). Distinct mechanisms of suppression of murine T-cell activation by the related macrolides FK-506 and Rapamycin. *J. Immunol.* **144**, 251–258.

Dumont, F. J., Melino, M. R., Staruch, M. J., Koprak, S. L., Fischer, P. A. and Sigal, N. H. (1990b). The immunosuppressive macrolides FK-506 and rapamycin act as reciprocal antagonists in murine T-cells. *J. Immunol.* **144**, 1418–1424.

Durette, P. L., Boger, P., Dumont, F. J., Firestone, R., Frankshun, R. A., Koprak, S. L., Lin, C. S., Melino, M. R., Pessolano, A. A. and Pisano, J. (1988). A study of the correlation between cyclophilin binding and *in vitro* immunosuppressive activity of Cyclosporin A and analogues. *Transpl. Proc.* **20** (Suppl. 2), 51–57.

Egbertson, M. and Danishefsky, S. J. (1989). Synthetic route to the 'tricarbonyl' region of FK-506. *J. Org. Chem.* **54**, 11–12.

Findlay, J., Liu, J.-S., Burnell, D. and Nakashima, T. (1982). The structure of demethoxy rapamycin. *Can. J. Chem.* **60**, 2046–2047.

Fischer, G. (1989). Slow conformational changes and their enzymology. *Nova Acta Leopoldina* **269**, 35–53.

Fischer, G., Wittmann-Liebold, B., Lang, K., Kiefhaber, T. and Schmid, F. X. (1989). Cyclophilin and peptidyl–prolyl *cis–trans* isomerase are probably identical proteins. *Nature* **337**, 476–478.

Foxwell, B. M. J., Wong, W.-C., Borel, J.-F. and Ryffel, B. (1989). A comparison of cyclosporine binding by cyclophilin and calmodulin. *Transpl. Proc.* **21**, 873–875.

Fujii, Y., Fujii, S. and Kaneko, T. (1989). Effect of a novel immunosuppressive agent, FK-506, on mitogen-induced inositol phospholipid degradation in rat thymocytes. *Transplantation* **47**, 1081–1082.

Goto, T., Kino, T., Hatanaka, H., Nishiyama, M., Okuhara, M., Kohsaka, M., Aoki, H. and Imanaka, H. (1987). Discovery of FK-506, a novel immunosuppressant isolated from *Streptomyces tsukubaensis*. *Transplantation Proceedings* **19** (Suppl. 6), 4–8.

Gschwendt, M., Kittstein, W. and Marks, F. (1989). The immunosuppressant FK-506, like cyclosporins and Didemnin B, inhibits calmodulin-dependent phosphorylation of the elongation factor 2 *in vitro* and biological effects of the phorbol ester TPA on mouse skin *in vivo*. *Immunobiology* **179**, 1–7.

Gudas, V. M., Carmichael, P. G. and Morris, R. E. (1989). Comparison of the immunosuppressive and toxic effects of FK-506 and cyclosporine in xenograft recipients. *Transpl. Proc.* **21**, 1072–1073.

Hamilton, D. V., Evans, D. B. and Thiru, S. (1982). In *Cyclosporin A* (ed. D. J. G. White), p. 393. Elsevier Biomedical, Amsterdam.

Harding, M. W. and Handschumacher, R. E. (1988). Cyclophilin, a primary molecular target for cyclosporine. Structural and functional implications. *Transplantation* **46** (Suppl. 2), 29S–35S.

Harding, M. W., Galat, A., Uehling, D. E. and Schreiber, S. L. (1989). A receptor for the immunosuppressant FK-506 is a *cis–trans* peptidyl–prolyl isomerase. *Nature* **341**, 758–760.

Hatanaka, H., Kino, T., Miyata, S., Inamura, N., Kuroda, A., Goto, T., Tanaka, H. and Okuhara, M. (1988). FR-900520 and FR-900523, novel immuno-suppressants isolated from a streptomyces. II. Fermentation, isolation and physico-chemical and biological characteristics. *J. Antibiot. (Tokyo)* **41**, 1592–1601.

Hatanaka, H., Kino, T., Asano, M., Goto, T., Tanaka, H. and Okuhara, M. (1989). FK-506 related compounds produced by *Streptomyces tsukubaensis* No. 9993. *J. Antibiot. (Tokyo)* **42**, 620–622.

Hunter, D. (1988). Unpublished studies. Physical Chemistry Department, Fisons Pharmaceuticals.

Inagaki, K., Fukuda, Y., Sumimoto, K., Matsuno, K., Ito, H., Takahashi, M. and Dohi, K. (1989). Effects of FK-506 and 15-Deoxyspergualin in rat orthotopic liver transplantation. *Transpl. Proc.* **21**, 1069–1071.

Inamura, N., Hashimoto, M., Nakahara, K., Nakajima, Y., Nishio, M., Aoki, H., Yamaguchi, I. and Kohsaka, M. (1988a). Immunosuppressive effect of FK 506 on experimental allergic encephalomyelitis in rats. *Int. J. Immunopharmacol.* **10**, 991–995.

Inamura, N., Hashimoto, M., Nakahara, K., Aoki, H., Yamaguchi, I. and Kohsaka, M. (1988b). FK-506 in collagen induced arthritis in rats. *Clin. Immunol. Immunopathol.* **46**, 82–90.

Inamura, N., Nakahara, K., Kino, T., Goto, T., Aoki, H., Yamaguchi, I., Kohsaka, M. and Ochiai, T. (1988c). Prolongation of skin allograft survival in rats by FK-506 and its comparison to Cyclosporin A. *Transplantation* **45**, 206–209.

Ireland, R. E. and Wipf, P. (1989). Studies directed toward the total synthesis of FK-506. Preparation of a C(1) to C(15) segment. *Tetrahedron Lett.* **30**, 919–922.

Jones, A. B., Yamaguchi, M., Patten, A., Danishefsky, S. J., Ragan, J. A., Smith, D. B. and Schreiber, S. L. (1989). Studies relating to the synthesis of the immunosuppressive agent FK-506: coupling of fragments *via* a stereoselective trisubstituted olefin forming reaction sequence. *J. Org. Chem.* **54**, 17–19.

Jones, T. K., Reamer, R. A., Desmond, R., and Mills, S. G. (1990). Chemistry of tricarbonyl hemiketals and applications of Evans' technology to the total synthesis of the immunosuppressant (−)-FK-506. *J. Am. Chem. Soc.* **112**, 2998–3017.

Kawashima, H., Fujino, Y. and Mochizuki, M. (1988). Effects of a new immunosuppressive agent, FK-506, on experimental autoimmune uveoretinitis in rats. *Invest. Opthalmol. Vis. Sci.* **29**, 1265–1271.

Kay, J. E., Doe, S. E. A. and Benzie, C. R. (1989a). The mechanism of action of the immunosuppressive drug FK-506. *Cell. Immunol.* **124**, 175–181.

Kay, J. E., Benzie, C. R., Goodier, M. R., Wick, C. J. and Doe, S. E. A. (1989b). Inhibition of T-lymphocyte activation by the immunosuppressive drug FK-506. *Immunology* **67**, 473–477.

King, S. L. (1988). An assessment of phosphoinositide hydrolysis in antigenic signal transduction in lymphocytes. *Immunology* **65**, 1–7.

Kino, T., Hatanaka, H., Hashimoto, M., Nishiyama, M., Goto, T., Okuhara, M. Kohsaka, M., Aoki, H. and Imanaka, H. (1987a). FK-506, a novel immunosuppressant isolated from a streptomyces. Fermentation, isolation, and physicochemical and biological characteristics. *J. Antibiot. (Tokyo)* **40**, 1249–55.

Kino, T., Hatanaka, H., Miyata, S., Inamura, N., Nishiyama, M., Yajima, T., Goto, T., Okuhara, M., Kohasaka, M., Aoki, H. and Imanaka, H. (1987b). FK-506, a novel immunosuppressant isolated from a streptomyces. II. Immunosuppressive effect of FK-506 *in vitro*. *J. Antibiot. (Tokyo)* **40**, 1256–1265.

Kino, T., Inamura, N., Sakai, F., Nakahara, K., Goto, T., Okuhara, M., Kohsaka, M., Aoki, H. and Ochiai, T. (1987c). Effect of FK-506 on human mixed lymphocyte reaction *in vitro*. *Transpl. Proc.* **19**, (Suppl. 6), 36–39.

Kocieński, P., Stocks, M., Donald, D., Cooper, M. and Manners, M. (1988). A synthesis of the C(1)–C(15) segment of Tsukubaenolide (FK-506). *Tetrahedron Lett.* **29**, 4481–4484.

Kocieński, P., Stocks, M. and Donald, D. (1990a). A synthesis of the C(16)–C(23) segment of FK-506. *Tetrahedron Lett.* **31**, 1637–1640.

Kocieński, P., Stocks, M., Donald, D. and Perry, M. (1990b). A synthesis of the C(24)–C(34) segment of FK-506. *Synlett.*, 38–39.

Kroenke, M., Leonard, W. J., Depper, J. M., Arya, S. K., Wong-Staal, F., Gallo, R. C., Waldmann, T. A. and Greene, W. C. (1984). Cyclosporin A inhibits T cell growth factor gene expression at the level of mRNA transcription. *Proc. Natl. Acad. Sci. USA* **81**, 5214–5218.

Lancet (Editorial). (1985). Cyclosporin in autoimmune disease. *Lancet* **i**, 909–911.

Lim, S. M. L., Thiru, S. and White, D. J. G. (1987). Heterotopic heart transplantation in the rat receiving FK-506. *Transpl. Proc.* **19** (Suppl. 6), 68–70.

Martel, R., Klicius, J. and Galet, S. (1977). Inhibition of the immune response by Rapamycin, a new antifungal antibiotic. *Can. J. Physiol. Pharmacol.* **55**, 48–51.

Mills, S., Desmond, R., Reamer, R. A., Volante, R. P. and Shinkai, I. (1988). Diastereoselective, non-racemic synthesis of the C.20–C.34 segment of the novel immunosuppressant FK-506. *Tetrahedron Lett.* **29**, 281–284.

Morimoto, T., Yamada, F., Kobayashi, T., Iwasaki, K., Sunada, M., Sakamoto, J., Miyaishi, S. and Takagi, H. (1989). Blood levels of FK-506 after intramuscular and intravenous administration in dogs. *Transpl. Proc.* **21**, 1059–1063.

Nakatsuka, M., Ragan, J. A., Sammakia, T., Smith, D. B., Uehling, D. E. and Schreiber, S. L. (1990). Total synthesis of FK-506 and FKBP probe reagents, (C_8, C_9–$^{13}C_2$)-FK-506. *J. Am. Chem. Soc.* **112**, 5583–5601.

Nalesnik, M. A., Todo, S., Murase, N., Gryzan, S., Lee, P. -H., Makowka, L. and Starzl, T. E. (1987). Toxicology of FK-506 in the Lewis rat. *Transpl. Proc.* **19** (Suppl. 6), 89–92.

Ochai, T., Nagata, M., Nakajima, K., Sakamoto, K., Asano, T. and Isono, K. (1987a). Prolongation of canine renal allograft survival by treatment with FK-506. *Transpl. Proc.* **19** (Suppl. 6), 53–56.

Ochai, T., Nagata, M., Nakajima, K., Suzuki, T., Sakamoto, K., Enomoto, K., Gunji, Y., Uematsu, T., Goto, T. and Hori, S. (1987b). Studies of the effects of FK-506 on renal allografting in the beagle dog. *Transplantation* **44**, 729–733.

Okuhara, M., Tanaka, H., Goto, T., Kino, T. and Hatanaka, H. (1986). Tricyclo compounds and a pharmaceutical composition containing them. *EP 184162. Fujisawa Pharmaceutical Co. Ltd., Japan.*

Quesniaux, V. F., Schreier, M. H., Wenger, R. M., Hiestand, P. C., Harding, M. W. and Vanregenmortel, M. H. V. (1987). Cyclophilin binds to the region of cyclosporine involved in its immunosuppressive activity. *Eur. J. Immunol.* **17**, 1359–1365.

Ragan, J. A., Nakatuka, M., Smith, D. B., Uehling, D. E. and Schreiber, S. L. (1989). Studies of the immunosuppressive agent FK-506: synthesis of an advanced intermediate. *J. Org. Chem.* **54**, 4267–4268.

Rama Rao, A. V., Chakraborty, T. K. and Laxma Reddy, K. (1990a). Studies directed toward the synthesis of immunosuppressive agent FK-506: construction of the tricarbonyl moiety. *Tetrahedron Lett.* **31**, 1439–1442.

Rama Rao, A. V., Chakraborty, T. V. and Purandare, A. V. (1990b). Studies directed toward the synthesis of immunosuppressive agent FK-506: synthesis of the C20 to C27 moiety. *Tetrahedron Lett.* **31**, 1443–1446.

Reed, J. C., Alpers, J. D., Nowell, P. C. and Hoover, R. G. (1986). Sequential expression of protooncogenes during lectin-stimulated mitogenesis of normal human lymphocytes. *Proc. Natl. Acad. Sci. USA* **83**, 3982–3986,

Rosen, M. K., Standaeth, R. F., Galat, A., Nakatsuka, M. and Schreiber, S. L. (1990). Inhibition of FKBP Rotamase activity by immunosuppressant FK-506: twisted amide surrogate. *Science* **248**, 863–866.

Sandoz, AG (1989). Use of 11,28-dioxa-4-azatricyclo[22.3.1.0^{4,9}]octacosene derivatives as topical agents for treating inflammatory agents. *EP-315978-A.* Sandoz AG, FRG.

Sawada, S., Suzuki, G., Kawase, Y. and Takaku, F. (1987). Novel immuno-suppressive agent, FK-506. *In vitro* effects on the cloned T-cell activation. *J. Immunol.* **139**, 1797–1803.

Schreiber, S. L. and Smith, D. B. (1989). Studies relating to the synthesis of the immunosuppressive agent FK-506: synthesis of the cyclohexyl moiety via a group-selective epoxidation. *J. Org. Chem.* **54**, 9–10.

Schreiber, S. L., Sammakia, T. and Uehling, D. E. (1989). Studies relating to the synthesis of the immunosuppressive agent FK-506: application of the two-directional chain synthesis strategy to the pyranose moiety. *J. Org. Chem.* **54**, 15–16.

Sehgal, S. N., Baker, H. and Vezina, C. (1975a). Rapamycin (AY-22,989), a new antifungal antibiotic. II. Fermentation, isolation, and characterisation. *J. Antibiot. (Tokyo)* **28**, 727–732.

Sehgal, S. N., Blazekovic, T. M. and Vézina, C. (1975b). Rapamycin, a new antibiotic. U.S. 3,929,992 (30 December 1975), U. S. application 293,699 (29 September 1972).

Siekierka, J. J., Yung, S. H. Y., Poe, M., Lin, C. S. and Sigal, N. H. (1989a). A cytosolic binding protein for the immunosuppressant FK-506 has peptidyl–prolyl isomerase activity but is distinct from cyclophilin. *Nature* **341**, 755–757.

Siekierka, J. J., Staruch, M. J., Yung, S. H. Y. and Sigal, N. H. (1989b). FK-506, a potent novel immunosuppressive agent, binds to a cytosolic protein which is distinct from the cyclosporin A—binding protein cyclophilin. *J. Immunol.* **143**, 1580–1583.

Smith, A. B. and Hale, K. J. (1989). An enantioselective synthesis of the C(10) to C(23) backbone of the potent immunosuppressant FK-506. *Tetrahedron Lett.* **30**, 1037–1040.

Smith, A. B., Hale, K. J., Laakso, L. M., Chen, K. and Riera, A. (1989). FK-506 synthetic studies. 3. An efficient asymmetric synthesis of the C(24)–C(34) fragment of FK-506, FR-900520, and FR-900523. *Tetrahedron Lett.* **30**, 6963–6966.

Starzl, T. E., Todo, S., Tzakis, A. G., Gordon, R. D., Makowka, L. Steiber, A. Podesta, L., Yanaga, K., Concepcion, W. and Iwatsuki, S. (1989a). Liver transplantation: an unfinished product. *Transpl. Proc.* **21**, 2197–2200.

Starzl, T. E., Todo, S., Fung, J., Demetris, A. J., Venkataraman, R. and Jain, A. (1989b). FK-506 for liver, kidney, and pancreas transplantation. *Lancet* **ii**, 1000–1004.

Stephen, M., Woo, J., Hassan, N. U., Whiting, P. H. and Thomson, A. W. (1989). Immunosuppressive activity, lymphocyte subset analysis, and acute toxicity of FK-506 in the rat. *Transplantation* **47**, 60–65.

Taga, T., Tanaka, H., Goto, T. and Tada, S. (1987). Structure of a new macrocylic antibiotic. *Acta. Crystallogr., Sect. C.* **43**, 751–753.

Takabayashi, K., Koike, T., Kurasawa, K., Matsumura, R., Sato, T., Tomioka, H., Ito, I., Yoshiki, T. and Yoshida, S. (1989). Effect of FK-506, a novel immunosuppressive drug on murine systemic lupus erythematosus. *Clin. Immunol. Immunopathol.* **51**, 110–117.

Takagashi, K., Yamamoto, M., Nishimura, A., Yamasaki, G., Kanazawa, N., Hotokebuchi, T. and Kaibara, N. (1989). Effects of FK-506 on collagen arthritis in mice. *Transpl. Proc.* **21**, 1053–1055.

Takahasi, N., Hayano, T. and Suzuki, M. (1989). Peptidyl–prolyl *cis–trans* isomerase is the cyclosporin A binding protein cyclophilin. *Nature* **337**, 473–475.

Tanaka, H., Kuroda, A., Marusawa, H., Hatanaka, H., Kino, T., Goto, T., Hashimoto, M. and Taga, T. (1987). Structure of FK-506: a novel immunosuppressant isolated from streptomyces. *J. Am. Chem. Soc.* **109**, 5031–5033.

Thiru, S., Collier, D. St. J. and Calne, R. (1987). Pathological studies in canine and baboon renal allograft recipients immunosuppressed with FK-506. *Transpl. Proc.* **19** (Suppl. 6), 98–99.

Thomson, A. W. (1990). FK-506 enters the clinic. *Immunol. Today* **11**, 35–36.

Tocci, M. J., Matkovich, D. A., Collier, K. A., Kwok, P., Dumont, F., Lin, S., Degudicibus, S., Siekierka, J. J., Chin, J. and Hutchinson, N. I. (1989). The immunosuppressant FK-506 selectively inhibits expression of early T cell activation genes. *J. Immunol.* **143**, 718–726.

Todo, S., Podesta, L., Chap, P., Kahn, D., Pan, C.-E., Ueda, Y., Okuda, K., Imventarza, O., Casavilla, A., Demetris, A. J., Makowka, L. and Starzl, T. E. (1987). Orthotopic liver transplantation in dogs receiving FK-506. *Transpl. Proc.* **19** (Suppl. 6), 64–67.

Todo, S., Ueda, Y., Demetris, J. A., Imventarza, O., Nalesnik, M., Venkataraman, R., Makowka, L. and Starzl, T. E. (1988). Immunosuppression of canine, monkey and baboon allografts by FK-506: with special reference to synergism with other drugs and to tolerance induction. *Surgery* **104**, 239–249.

Vezina, C., Kudelski, A. and Sehgal, S. N. (1975). Rapamycin (AY-22,989), a new antifungal antibiotic. I. Taxonomy of the producing streptomycete and isolation of the active principle. *J. Antibiot. (Tokyo)* **28**, 721–726.

Villalobos, A. and Danishefsky, S. J. (1989). Stereoselective syntheses of FK-506 subunits by the rhodium(I)-catalyzed hydrogenation of dienes. The synthesis and coupling of a C10–C19 fragment. *J. Org. Chem.* **54**, 12–15.

Walliser, P., Benzie, C. R. and Kay, J. E. (1989). Inhibition of murine B-lymphocyte proliferation by the novel immunosuppressive drug FK-506. *Immunology* **68**, 434–435.

Wang, Z. (1989). Stereoselective synthesis of the C(10)–C(24) fragment of FK-506. *Tetrahedron Lett.* **30**, 6611–6614.

Wasserman, H. H., Rotello, V. M., Williams, D. R. and Benbow, J. W. (1989). Synthesis of the 'tricarbonyl' region of FK-506 through an amidophosphorane. *J. Org. Chem.* **54**, 2785–2786.

Weinblatt, M. E., Coblyn, J. S., Fraser, P. A., Anderson, R. J., Spragg, J., Trentham, D. E. and Austen, K. F. (1987). Cyclosporin A treatment of refractory rheumatoid arthritis. *Arthr. Rheum.* **30**, 11–17.

Williams, D. R. and Benbow, J. W. (1988). Synthesis of the α,β-diketo amide segment of the novel immunosuppressant FK-506. *J. Org. Chem.* **53**, 4643–4644.

9

A Practical, Enantioselective Synthesis of [R-(R*,S*)]-β-[(2-Carboxyethyl)thio]-α-hydroxy-2-(8-phenyloctyl)-benzenepropanoic Acid (SK&F 104353), a Potent LTD$_4$ Antagonist

IVAN LANTOS and VANCE NOVACK

Chemical Development, Smith Kline Beecham Pharmaceuticals, Research and Development, P.O. Box 1539, King of Prussia, PA 19406, USA

---

1 Introduction

The leukotrienes have been the focus of intensive chemical investigation, as their physiological role has been implied in bronchoconstriction of human lung tissue, mediation of muscular permeability, and diseases of immediate hypersensitivity. Smith Kline Beecham Pharmaceuticals (formerly Smith Kline & French Laboratories) has had an interest in developing therapeutic agents capable of alleviating conditions responsible for human asthma. Hence, the discovery of agents capable of antagonizing selective activities of leukotrienes, specifically LTD$_4$, became a natural goal.

In this chapter a historical overview will be given of the discovery and chemical development of a highly effective LTD$_4$ antagonist, SK&F 104353

CHIRALITY IN DRUG DESIGN AND SYNTHESIS
ISBN 0-12-136670-7

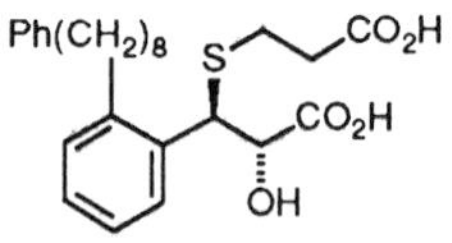

1
SK&F 104353

Fig. 1   The chemical structure of SK&F 104353, showing the 2S,3R absolute stereochemistry.

(1, Fig. 1), from the perspective of a synthetic chemist. The design of this compound and its analogues, as well as pharmacological data, has been described elsewhere (Gleason et al., 1987). An important feature of SK&F 104353 is the 2S,3R stereochemistry, which provides optimal pharmacological activity. Due to this design constraint, a synthesis of **1** which was amenable to large-scale production became a significant challenge.

2 Background

The synthesis of SK&F 104353 originally discovered by medicinal chemists is shown in Fig. 2 (Gleason et al., 1987). 2-(Phenyloctyl)benzaldehyde (**2**), prepared by one of two methods (see below), was transformed to epoxide **3** via a Darzens condensation with methyl chloroacetate. After purification of **3** by chromatography, the epoxide was opened with methyl-3-mercapto-propionate to afford the desired diester **4** together with its regioisomer **5** (ca. 1:1). Separation of these compounds required an arduous chromatography, and thus purification of **4** was not effected at this stage. Instead, the mixture was treated with sodium methoxide to promote a retroaldol fragmentation of **5**. This procedure afforded the starting aldehyde **2** and the sulphur containing fragment **6**, both of which could be readily removed from **4** by chromatographic means. Further elaboration of the diester to the final target was accomplished by alkaline hydrolysis, and resolution of the racemic diacid with an optically active benzylamine. In order to determine the absolute configuration of the final product, the medicinal chemists reduced the enantiomer of SK&F 104353 to the corresponding triol. This material was identical to a (2R,3S)-triol prepared via Sharpless asymmetric epoxidation (Katsuki and Sharpless, 1980) of 2-(phenyloctyl)cinnamyl alcohol with t-butylhydroperoxide in the presence of d-(−)-diethyl tartrate, followed by reaction with methyl mercaptopropionate and subsequent reduction. The 2S,3R configuration of SK&F 104353 has since been confirmed by X-ray crystallography.

   While the above chemistry was useful for the preparation of several grams of **1**, the multi-hundred gram quantities needed for preclinical studies

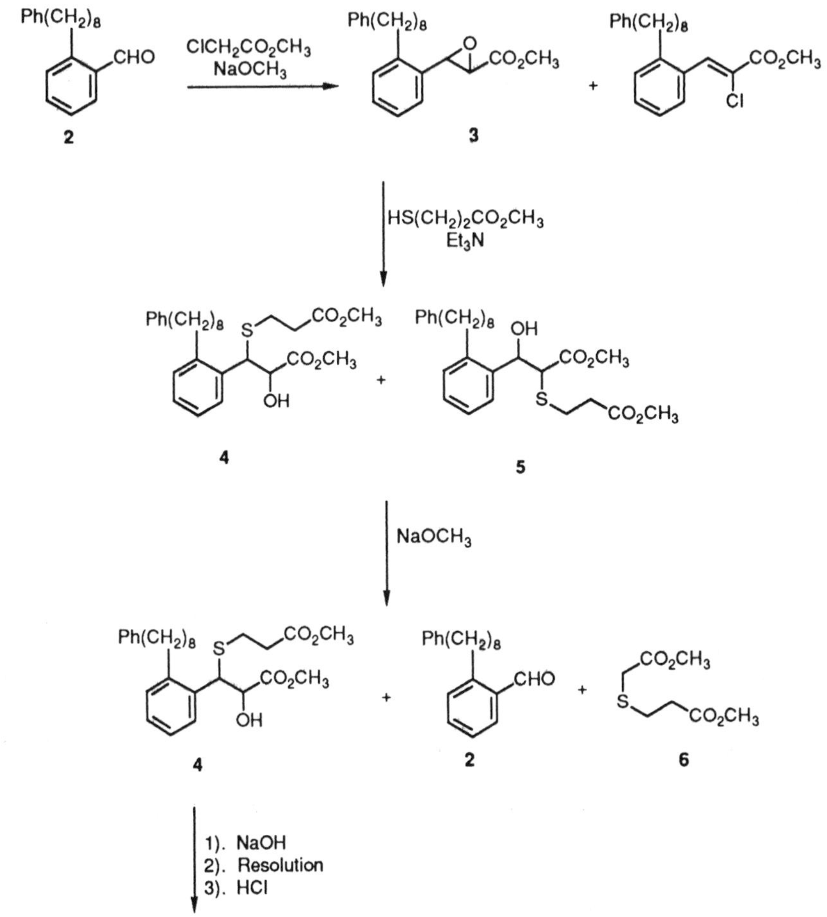

Fig. 2   The original route to SK&F 104353, which was discovered by the Medicinal Chemistry Department and used to prepare preclinical supplies of final product (Gleason *et al.*, 1987).

required an intensive effort from both the Medicinal Chemistry and Synthetic Chemistry Groups at Smith Kline Beecham. The chemistry in Fig. 2 required two chromatographies, and the overall yield was low (the yield was 50% on each of two steps). The optically active amine used in the resolution was also extremely expensive, and unavailable in quantities that would support late-stage clinical trials on **1**.

In addition, problems were encountered with the preparation of 2-(phenyloctyl)benzaldehyde (**2**). Two routes to this key intermediate

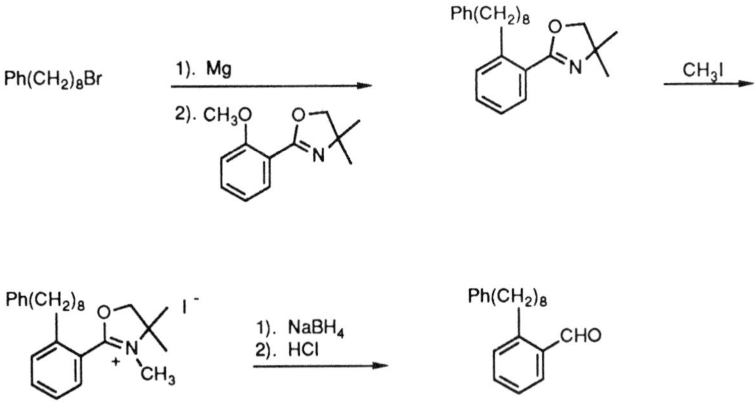
Ph(CH2)8Br
1). Mg
2). CH3O
Ph(CH2)8
CH3I
I-
CH3
1). NaBH4
2). HCl
CHO

2

Fig. 3 An early route to 2-(phenyloctyl)benzaldehyde, using the Meyers oxazoline methodology (Perchonock *et al.*, 1985).

have been published (Perchonock *et al.*, 1985), as outlined in Figs 3 and 4. While the Meyers oxazoline methodology (Meyers and Mihelich, 1975) in Fig. 3 appeared amenable to large scale, the route was plagued by the high cost and low availability of phenyloctyl bromide. The Takahashi methodology (Takahashi *et al.*, 1980) in Fig. 4 was also expensive, and required the use of unacceptable reaction conditions (in particular, the need for HMPA).

Thus, in order to synthesize the multi-kilogram quantities of SK&F 104353 that would be required for clinical development, major modi-

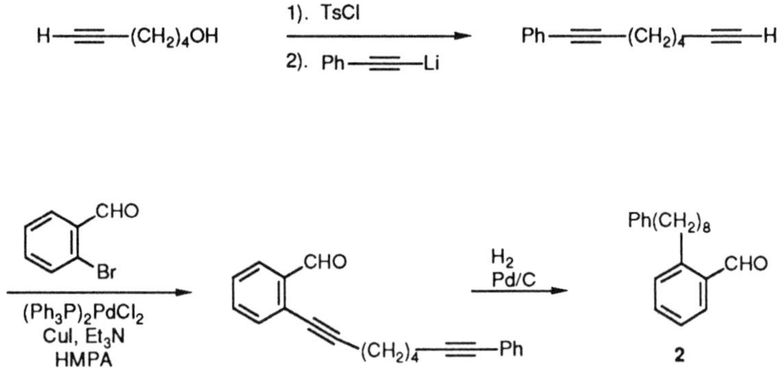
H—≡—(CH2)4OH
1). TsCl
2). Ph—≡—Li
Ph—≡—(CH2)4—≡—H
CHO
Br
(Ph3P)2PdCl2
CuI, Et3N
HMPA
(CH2)4—≡—Ph
H2
Pd/C
Ph(CH2)8

2

Fig. 4 An early route to 2-(phenyloctyl)benzaldehyde, using the Takahashi methodology (Perchonock *et al.*, 1985).

fications were needed in some key aspects of the chemistry:

(1) a less-expensive, large-scale synthesis of 2-(phenyloctyl)-benzaldehyde was required;
(2) the regioselectivity of the epoxide opening had to be improved, or a different intermediate had to be chosen; and
(3) the need for a resolution had to be eliminated, i.e. an enantioselective synthesis of a chiral epoxide intermediate had to be devised.

3 Improvements in the synthesis of 2-(phenyloctyl)benzaldehyde

Since the only major drawback to the oxazoline methodology in Fig. 3 was the availability of phenyloctyl bromide, our efforts were initially focused on this problem. The result was the synthesis depicted in Fig. 5, which was the first route to **2** that was adaptable to multi-kilogram scale processing. Unfortunately, the demand for 2-(phenyloctyl)benzaldehyde rapidly outpaced our ability to produce sufficient material by this rather lengthy sequence.

Further development of this chemistry depended upon two major findings. First, we found that the alkylation of *ortho* stabilized tolyl anions

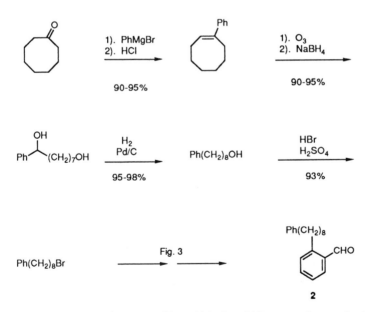

Fig. 5 An early route to 2-(phenyloctyl)benzaldehyde, which was used to synthesize this key intermediate in multi-hundred gram quantities.

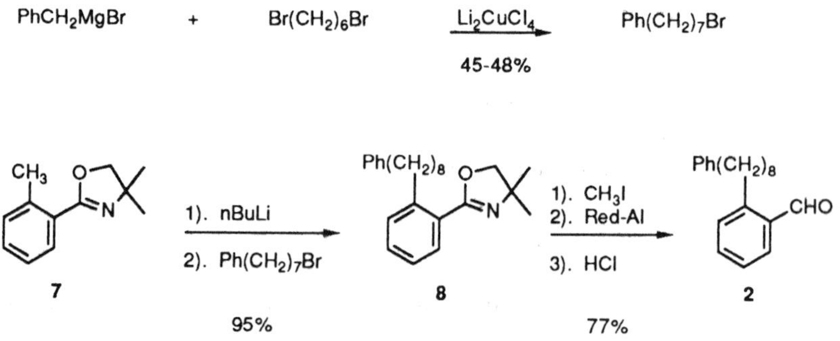
PhCH2MgBr
+
Br(CH2)6Br
Li2CuCl4
45-48%
Ph(CH2)7Br
CH3
O
N
7
1). nBuLi
2). Ph(CH2)7Br
95%
Ph(CH2)8
O
N
8
1). CH3I
2). Red-Al
3). HCl
77%
Ph(CH2)8
CHO
2

Fig. 6 A synthetic route to 2-(phenyloctyl)benzaldehyde, which was capable of producing this compound in multi-kilogram quantities.

(Creger, 1970) afforded cleaner products than did the Grignard aryl substitution process. This led to our second discovery, that phenylheptyl halides were much more readily available from inexpensive starting materials than were phenyloctyl halides.

Figure 6 depicts the incorporation of these advances that finally produced a conveniently short synthesis of **2**. Phenylheptyl bromide was readily prepared by coupling benzylmagnesium chloride with 1,6-dibromohexane in the presence of a catalytic amount of dilithium tetrachlorocuprate (Friedman and Shani, 1974). The yield for this process was approximately 50%, which reflected the statistical nature of the reaction. According to the procedure of Gschwend and Hamdan (1975), the oxazoline of *o*-toluic acid (**7**) was lithiated with n-butyllithium, then treated with phenylheptyl bromide to afford oxazoline **8** in better than 90% yield. Transformation of the oxazoline functionality into an aldehyde was accomplished via formation of a quaternary salt, reduction, and hydrolysis (Nordin, 1966). Thus, we had available a short synthesis of **2**, which was capable of producing very large quantities of material from relatively inexpensive precursors.

4 Regioselective epoxide opening

We felt that a regioselective epoxide opening was critical to the commercial success of any epoxide-based approach to SK&F 104353. In an attempt to accomplish this with the glycidic ester intermediate **3**, a great number of reaction conditions and Lewis acid catalysts were examined. Unfortunately, regioisomeric and/or diastereomeric mixtures were always obtained.

Sharpless has reported that glycidic acids and amides are regioselectively cleaved in the β position with nucleophiles in the presence of titanium tetraisopropoxide (Chong and Sharpless, 1985). We found that this protocol

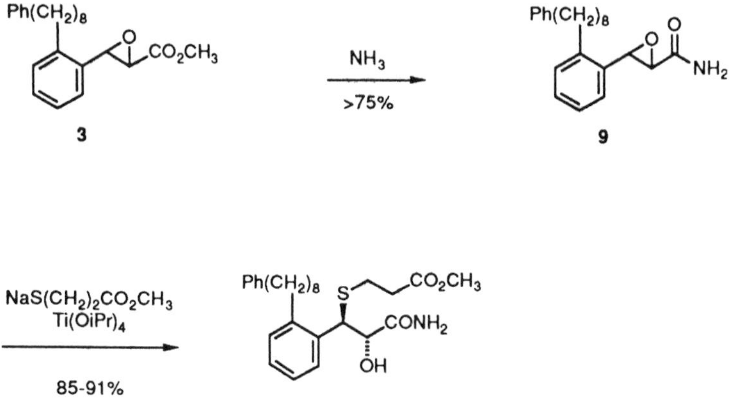

Fig. 7   After conversion of 3 to amide 9, the racemic epoxide could be cleaved under conditions developed by Chong and Sharpless (1985).

could be applied to our current situation. Because glycidic acids in general are prone to decarboxylation, we decided to focus our efforts on an appropriate glycidic amide intermediate. Furthermore, we felt that a primary epoxy-amide would be easier to hydrolyse and more economical to prepare than the secondary amides typically used by Sharpless. Consequently, we chose to apply the Sharpless procedure to glycidic amide 9 (Fig. 7). This crystalline amide was prepared in >75% yield by reacting 3 with ammonia. Treatment of 9 with the sodium salt of methyl-3-mercaptopropionate in the presence of titanium tetraisopropoxide afforded the desired racemate 10 in 85–91% yields. Only the desired regioisomer was detected by ^{1}H NMR spectroscopy (400 MHz).

With this result in hand, we were then in a position to address the last major synthetic problem: the development of an enantioselective synthesis. Given the absolute stereochemistry of SK&F 104353, this task was reduced to finding an efficient enantioselective preparation of a glycidic amide with a 2R,3S configuration.

5   Enantioselective synthesis of an epoxide intermediate

Whenever an optically active epoxide is required, practitioners of organic synthesis frequently resort to the asymmetric epoxidation procedure discovered by Sharpless and coworkers (Katsuki and Sharpless, 1980). We examined this methodology within the context of SK&F 104353, but found that it was not as satisfactory for our purposes as originally anticipated

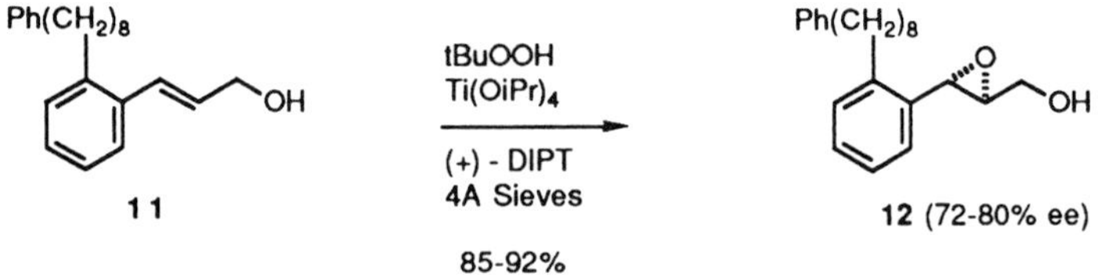

Fig. 8 The Sharpless asymmetric oxidation of 2-(phenyloctyl)cinnamyl alcohol.

(Fig. 8). While oxidation of the requisite cinnamyl alcohol **11** proceeded with good yields (85–92%), the optical yields were somewhat disappointing (72–80% enantiomeric excess (ee)). Unfortunately, the epoxy-alcohol **12** was an oil, which precluded any chance of enhancing the optical activity by recrystallization. Furthermore, we discovered that clean conversion of **12** to the necessary glycidic amide was extremely difficult under a variety of

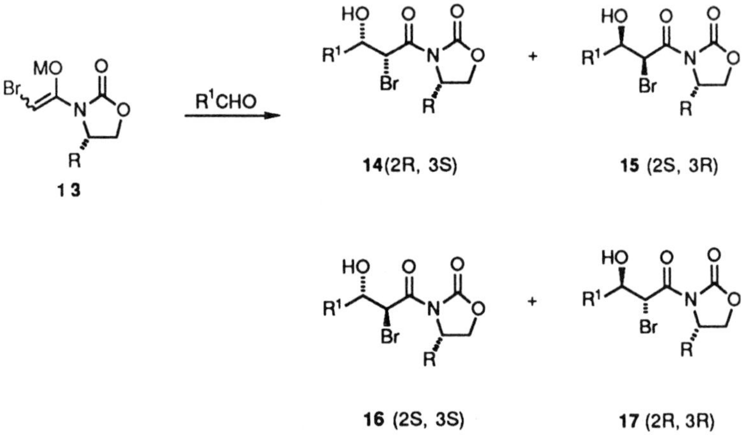

R	R¹CHO	M	Syn:Anti (14+15):(16+17)	Enantioselection 14:15	16:17	Yield (%)
iPr	CH₃(CH₂)₄CHO	Zn(II)	3:1	5:1	1:4	61
iPr	"	Sn(II)	3:1	1:6	3:2	73
iPr	"	B	>20:1	<1:20	N.D.	62
iPr	(CH₃)₂CHCHO	Zn(II)	7:1	9:1	3:1	72
iPr	"	Sn(II)	15:1	1:6	1:1	65
iPr	"	B	>20:1	<1:20	N.D.	51
iPr	2	Zn(II)	1:2	2:1	1:1.6	76
iPr	"	Sn(II)	1:2.7	3:1	16 only	67
*Ph	"	Sn(II)	1:19	14 only	16 only	79
iPr	"	B	>20:1	1:19	17 only	60

N.D. = not determined

Fig. 9 The Darzens condensation of chiral enolate **13** with various aldehydes, including 2-(phenyloctyl)benzaldehyde (**2**).

oxidative conditions. The nickel peroxide methodology of Nakagawa *et al.* (1966) was the most efficient method we could find for transforming **12** to a glycidic amide, and even then only low yields ($\leq 50\%$) were obtained. In our search for alternative routes to enantiomerically pure epoxides, two approaches were explored. The first dealt with a chiral modification of the Darzens glycidic ester formation. In particular, the expansion of the Darzens reaction to include substrates containing the Evans chiral oxazolidinone auxiliary (Evans *et al.*, 1981a,b) seemed an intriguing idea. Accordingly, bromoimidate enolates such as **13** were prepared and condensed with various aldehydes as shown in Fig. 9.

While condensations of **13** (R = *i*Pr) with aliphatic aldehydes uniformly provided the expected *erythro* or *syn* products (**14** and **15**; Abdel-Magid *et al.*, 1984, 1986), similar condensations with 2-(phenyloctyl)benzaldehyde (**2**) afforded predominantly *threo* or *anti* products (**16** and **17**) with Zn(II) and Sn(II) enolates (Pridgen *et al.*, 1989). This *anti* selectivity was particularly high (nearly 20 : 1) with the Sn(II) enolate if the chiral auxiliary was derived from phenylglycine (R = Ph, see * in the table in Fig. 9). In this instance, the *anti* 2*S*,3*S* stereoisomer was highly favoured over the *anti* 2*R*,3*R* isomer, and could be isolated in 79% yield after silica-gel chromatography. This result was of obvious importance to our current problem, as exposure of **16** to basic conditions should result in ring closure to an epoxide with the desired 2*R*,3*S* stereochemistry. As shown in Fig. 10, imide **16** (R = Ph, R^1 = 2-(phenyloctyl)phenyl) was converted directly to the desired chiral epoxy-amide **18** in 86% yield (>98% ee) upon exposure to ammonium hydroxide. Amide **18** was highly crystalline and readily isolated from large-scale preparations.

Our second approach to optically active epoxides focused on methodology developed by Julia and coworkers (Julia *et al.*, 1980; Colonna *et al.*, 1983). Julia *et al.* demonstrated that substituted benzylidene acetophenones undergo enantioselective epoxidations in triphasic systems consisting of NaOH/aqueous H_2O_2, an organic solvent, and a polyamino acid. We felt that the epoxy-ketone arising from such a procedure could be converted to a useful optically active ester via Baeyer–Villiger oxidation,

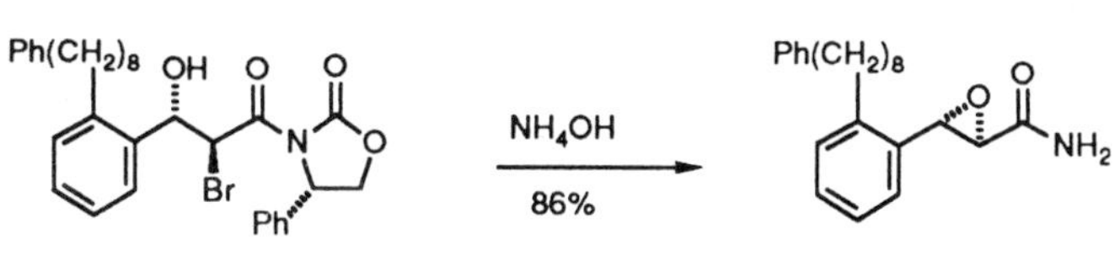

16   **18** (>98% ee)

Fig. 10   Ring-closure of **16** to afford glycidic amide **18**, with high selectivity for the 2*R*,3*S* configuration.

although regioselectivity for this oxidation on α,β-epoxy-ketones had not been documented in the literature.

In choosing a specific substrate for the Julia epoxidation, we considered the very practical problem of designing intermediates which were easy to isolate and purify (i.e. crystalline). After considerable experimentation, we decided that ketone **19** (Fig. 11) was the most judicious choice, as the 2-naphthyl substituent imparted high crystallinity to the intermediates in the sequence. The unsaturated ketone (**19**) was readily prepared in 89% yield by condensing 2-(phenyloctyl)benzaldehyde with inexpensive 2-aceto-naphthone in the presence of sodium ethoxide.

Application of the methodology of Julia *et al.* to the epoxidation of **19** was evaluated with a number of commercially available polyamino acids, and we concluded that poly-L-leucine consistently gave the highest yields and optical purities. While commercial poly-L-leucine is expensive, it can be readily prepared by the polymerization of L-leucine-*N*-carboxyanhydride (leucine-NCA). A number of methods for polymerizing leucine-NCA are

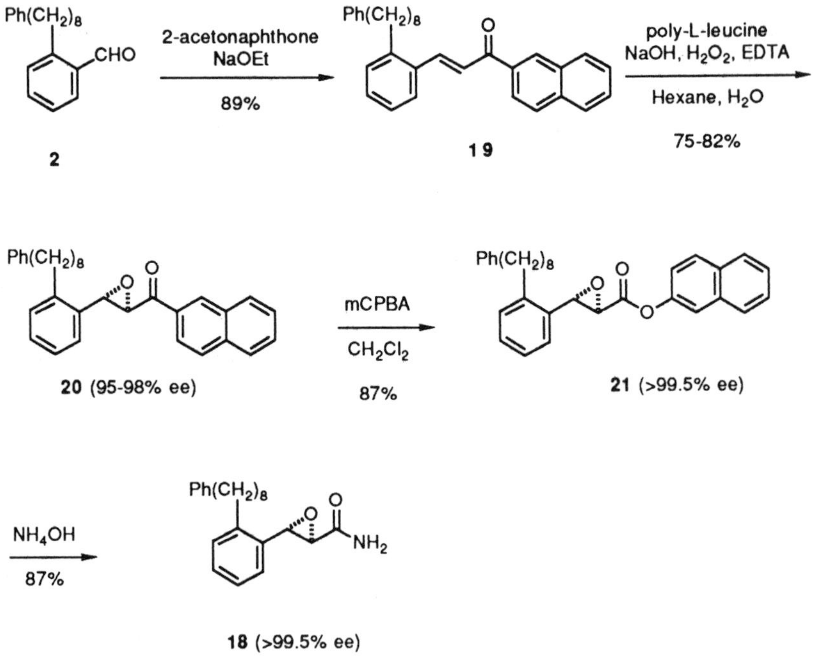

Fig. 11   A second route to optically pure glycidic amide **18**. After asymmetric epoxidation of **19** according to Julia's methodology, a regioselective Baeyer–Villiger reaction was performed.

described in the literature (Katchalski and Sela, 1958). However, we found that a solid-state procedure was the most convenient (Shionoya *et al.*, 1974). Freshly prepared leucine-NCA was placed in large trays to a depth of 6–8 cm, and then left at ambient temperature in a humidity chamber at 70–75% relative humidity. The progress of the polymerization was conveniently monitored by infra-red (IR) spectroscopy for the disappearance of carbonyl stretches for leucine-NCA (1780 and 1830 cm^{-1}) and the appearance of an amide carbonyl stretch (1655 cm^{-1}, indicative of an α-helix conformation).

Under optimal reaction conditions, unsaturated ketone 19 and an equal weight of poly-L-leucine were combined in a mixture of hexane/water with approximately 12 molar equivalents of sodium hydroxide. The heterogeneous mixture was stirred for 24 h at ambient temperature (to allow the polymer to swell), and then treated with 20 equivalents of aqueous hydrogen peroxide. To control the decomposition of the peroxide under the basic reaction conditions, a few mole% of EDTA was also added. Generally, the reaction proceeded to completion within 20–24 h; if starting ketone still remained after this period, additional base and hydrogen peroxide were added.

Following this procedure (Fig. 11), naphthyl ketone (19) was routinely converted to epoxy-ketone 20 in good yield (75–82%) and with high asymmetric induction (94–96% ee). Optical purity was ascertained by chiral high-performance liquid chromatographic (HPLC) analysis and comparison with racemic epoxide, which was obtained by alkaline hydrogen peroxide oxidation in the absence of poly-L-leucine. The crystalline nature of the product allowed us to isolate 20 in 95–98% ee by a single recrystallization.

Treatment of epoxy-ketone 20 with *m*-chloroperbenzoic acid in dichloromethane at reflux temperature resulted in a smooth Baeyer–Villiger oxidation to afford 2-naphthyl glycidic ester 21 in 87% yield (Fig. 11). This conversion was completely regioselective, as we were unable to detect any by-products arising from migration of the epoxide. After a single crystallization, the ester was obtained in >99.5% ee (Flisak *et al.*, 1990). Treatment of 21 with ammonium hydroxide afforded optically pure glycidic amide 18 in 87% yield (>99.5% ee).

6 Final elaboration to SK&F 104353

In parallel with results on racemic amide 9, amide 18 was readily cleaved with the sodium salt of methyl-3-mercaptopropionate in the presence of titanium tetraisopropoxide (Fig. 12). The product, amide-ester 22, was obtained as a single regioisomer as shown by ^{1}H NMR spectroscopy (400 MHz). However, isolation difficulties were encountered in this series of optically pure intermediates. While racemic amide-ester 10 was a highly

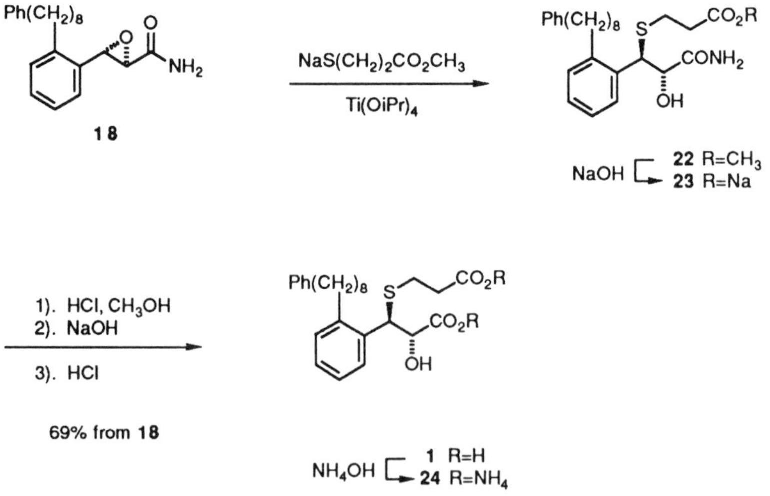

Ph(CH$_2$)$_8$

18

$$\text{Nas(CH}_2)_2\text{CO}_2\text{CH}_3 \xrightarrow{\text{Ti(OiPr)}_4}$$

Ph(CH$_2$)$_8$

Ph(CH$_2$)$_8$ S~CO$_2$R / CONH$_2$, OH

NaOH ⌐ **22** R=CH$_3$
      └► **23** R=Na

1). HCl, CH$_3$OH
2). NaOH
3). HCl
$$\xrightarrow{\hspace{2cm}}$$

69% from **18**

Ph(CH$_2$)$_8$ S~CO$_2$R / CO$_2$R, OH

NH$_4$OH ⌐ **1** R=H
        └► **24** R=NH$_4$

Fig. 12   The final elaboration of epoxy-amide **18** to SK&F 104353.

crystalline product, the 2S,3R enantiomer (**22**) was a low-melting solid and could not be crystallized directly from the reaction mixture. As a result, excess thiol (required for optimal yields of **22**) was not easily removed, and conversion of unpurified **22** to SK&F 104353 afforded final product of low purity. In order to overcome this difficulty, **22** was converted into monosodium salt **23** with sodium hydroxide, then extracted into organic solvents and isolated as a non-crystalline solid. This removed the excess thiol, which presumably remained in the aqueous layer as sodium 3-mercaptopropionate.

The conversion of **23** to the final product, SK&F 104353, was finally achieved by a multistage hydrolysis: **23** was converted to a dimethyl ester (HCl, CH$_3$OH), which was then hydrolysed to SK&F 104353 (1. NaOH; 2. HCl). In order to achieve a high level of purity, SK&F 104353 was converted to diammonium salt **24** (NH$_4$OH, H$_2$O, acetone), which was readily isolated as a crystalline monohydrate in 69% yield from chiral glycidic amide **18**. The molecular composition of **24**, as well as the *anti* configuration, was confirmed by ^{1}H and ^{13}C NMR, Fourier transform IR, HPLC retention time, and elemental analysis. Examination of the material by chiral HPLC, with comparison with authentic samples of SK&F 104353 and the corresponding racemate, indicated that the desired 2S,3R enantiomer had been synthesized with >99.5% ee.

Thus, an enantioselective synthesis of SK&F 104353 had been achieved. Of the two methods developed for introduction of the optically active epoxide, that via the Julia methodology (Fig. 11) has been the most amenable to scale-up. In its longest linear sequence, this process proceeds via 13 isolated intermediates in an overall yield of approximately 20–25%. Efforts continue in our laboratories to enhance the overall yield and reduce the number of steps.

Acknowledgements

I. L. and V. N. are indebted to the diligent efforts of a number of individuals within the Synthetic Chemistry Department: J. Flisak, L. Gillyard, K. Gombatz, M. Holmes, A. Jarmas, C. Labaw, W. Mendelson, L. Pridgen, J. Remich, S. Shilcrat, M. Sienko, L. Snyder, A. Tickner, A. Tremper and D. Tuddenham. We are also indebted to members of the Analytical Chemistry and Physical & Structural Chemistry Departments for analytical support. Finally, we would like to acknowledge K. Kopple and Professors T. Cohen, P. Gassman and L. Overman for helpful discussions.

References

Abdel-Magid, A., Lantos, I. and Pridgen, L. N. (1984). Aldol condensations of chiral α-haloimidates. A chiral Darzens condensation procedure. *Tetrahedron Lett.* **25**, 3273–3276.

Abdel-Magid, A., Pridgen, L. N., Eggleston, D. S. and Lantos, I. (1986). Metal assisted aldol condensation of chiral α-halogenated imide enolates: a stereo-controlled chiral epoxide synthesis. *J. Am. Chem. Soc.* **108**, 4595–4602.

Chong, J. M. and Sharpless, K. B. (1985). Nucleophilic openings of 2,3-epoxy acids and amides mediated by $Ti(OiPr)_4$. Reliable C-3 selectivity. *J. Org. Chem.* **50**, 1560–1563.

Colonna, S., Molinari, H., Banfi, S., Julia, S., Masana, J. and Alvarez, A. (1983). Highly enantioselective epoxidation by means of polyaminoacids in a triphase system: influence of structural variations within the catalysts. *Tetrahedron* **39**, 1635–1641.

Creger, P. L. (1970). Metalated carboxylic acids. II. Monoalkylation of metalated toluic acids and dimethyl benzoic acids. *J. Am. Chem. Soc.* **92**, 1396–1397.

Evans, D. A., Bartroli, J. and Shih, T. L. (1981a). Enantioselective aldol condensations. 2. Erythro-selective chiral aldol condensations via boron enolates. *J. Am. Chem. Soc.* **103**, 2127–2129.

Evans, D. A., Takacs, J. M., McGee, L. R., Ennis, M. D., Mathre, D. J. and Bartroli, J. (1981b). Chiral enolate design. *J. Pure Appl. Chem.* **53**, 1109–1127.

Flisak, J. R., Gombatz, K., Lantos, I., Mendelson, W. and Remich, J. (1990). An efficient asymmetric synthesis of substituted phenyl glycidic esters. *Tetrahedron Lett.* (in preparation).

Friedman, L. and Shani, A. (1974). Halopolycarbon homologation. *J. Am. Chem. Soc.* **96**, 7101–7103.

Gleason, J. G., Hall, R. F., Perchonock, C. D., Erhard, K. F., Frazee, J. S., Ku, T. W., Kondrad, K., McCarthy, M. E., Mong, S., Crooke, S. T., Chi-Rosso, G., Wasserman, M. A., Torphy, T. J., Muccitelli, R. M., Hay, D. W., Tucker, S. S. and Vickery-Clark, L. (1987). High-affinity leukotriene receptor antagonists. Synthesis and pharmacological characterization of 2-hydroxy-3-[(2-carboxyethyl)thio]-3-[2-(8-phenyloctyl)phenyl]propanoic acid. *J. Med. Chem.* **30**, 959–961.

Gschwend, H. W. and Hamdan, A. (1975). Ortho-lithiation of aryloxazolines. *J. Org. Chem.* **40**, 2008–2009.

Julia, S., Masana, J. and Vega, J. C. (1980). 'Synthetic enzymes'. Highly stereoselective epoxidation of chalcone in a triphasic toluene-water-poly[(S)-alanine] system. *Angew. Chem. Int. Ed. Engl.* **19**, 929–931.

Katchalski, E. and Sela, M. (1958). Synthesis and chemical properties of poly-α-amino acids. In *Advances in Protein Chemistry* (eds C. B. Afinsen, M. L. Anson, K. Bailey and J. T. Edsall), Vol. 13, pp. 243–492. Academic Press, New York.

Katsuki, T. and Sharpless, K. B. (1980). The first practical method for asymmetric epoxidation. *J. Am. Chem. Soc.* **102**, 5974–5976.

Meyers, A. I. and Mihelich, E. D. (1975). Oxazolines. XXII. Nucleophilic aromatic substitution on aryl oxazolines. An efficient approach to unsymmetrically substituted biphenyls and o-alkyl benzoic acids. *J. Am. Chem. Soc.* **97**, 7383–7385.

Nakagawa, K., Onoue, H. and Minami, K. (1966). Oxidation with nickel peroxide. A new synthesis of amides from aldehydes or alcohols. *J. Chem. Soc., Chem. Commun.* 17–18.

Nordin, I. C. (1966). Reduction of oxazolinium salts to oxazolidines: a new route from carboxylic acids to aldehydes. *J. Heterocycl. Chem.* **3**, 531–532.

Perchonock, C. D., McCarthy, M. E., Erhard, K. F., Gleason, J. G., Wasserman, M. A., Muccitelli, R. M., DeVan, J. F., Tucker, S. S., Vickery, L. M., Kirchner, T., Weichman, B. M., Mong, S., Crooke, S. T. and Newton, J. F. (1985). Synthesis and pharmacological characterization of 5-(2-dodecylphenyl)-4,6-dithianonanedioic acid and 5-[2-(8-phenyloctyl)phenyl]-4,6-dithianonanedioic acid: prototypes of a novel class of leukotriene antagonists. *J. Med. Chem.* **28**, 1145–1147.

Pridgen, L. N., Abdel-Magid, A. and Lantos, I. (1989). A predominantly antistereoselective chiral metal directed aldol condensation with aromatic aldehydes. *Tetrahedron Lett.* **30**, 5539–5542.

Shionoya, G., Furukawa, T. and Akamatsu, A. (1974). Method for manufacturing polyamino acid by the solid-phase method. *Japanese Kokai Patent* No. SHO 49[1974]-38995.

Takahashi, S., Kuroyama, Y., Sonogashira, K. and Hagihara, N. (1980). A convenient synthesis of ethynylarenes and diethynylarenes. *Synthesis* 627–630.

10

Chirality Recognition in Synthesis

STEPHEN G. DAVIES

The Dyson Perrins Laboratory South Parks Road,
Oxford OX1 3QY, UK

1 Introduction

The search for novel general methods for the preparation of homochiral (enantiomerically pure) organic molecules is at the forefront of modern synthetic endeavour. The combination of two chiral, racemic, fragments generally gives two product diastereoisomers each of which is racemic. If one of the fragments is homochiral, two product diastereoisomers will still be produced, although each will now be homochiral. Hence the generally accepted strategy for the efficient synthesis of large molecules involves the combination of several fragments each of which is homochiral. In this way only the desired diastereoisomer is produced, at the cost of preparing each fragment in homochiral form. However, in the reaction of a homochiral reagent with a racemic substrate a single diastereoisomer may result from a chirality recognition process, that is if the homochiral reagent reacts very much faster with one enantiomer of the substrate than with the other. This is feasible, in principle, due to the diastereoisomeric nature of the two transition states involved. Some chirality recognition processes involving the iron chiral auxiliary [$(C_5H_5)Fe(CO)(PPh_3)$] are described below.

2 Structure of the chiral iron acetyl complex [$(C_5H_5)Fe(CO)(PPh_3)COCH_3$]

Figure 1 shows the X-ray crystal structure (Bernal *et al.*, 1988) of the acetyl complex [$(C_5H_5)Fe(CO)(PPh_3)COCH_3$] (**1**). The geometry about the iron atom is close to octahedral with three of the sites being occupied by the

CHIRALITY IN DRUG DESIGN AND SYNTHESIS
ISBN 0-12-136670-7

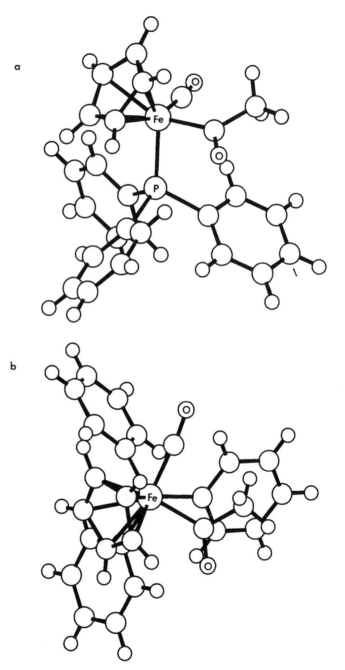

Fig. 1 X-ray crystal structure of R,S-[(C$_5$H$_5$)Fe(CO)(PPh$_3$)COCH$_3$] (**1**) (Bandy, Davies and Prout, unpublished data. (a) Newman projection from Fe to CO. (b) Newman projection from Fe to P.

cyclopentadienyl ligand, while carbon monoxide, triphenylphosphine and the acetyl ligand each occupy one of the remaining, mutually orthogonal, positions. The triphenylphosphine is by far the largest ligand and interactions with the phenyl groups of the triphenylphosphine rotor control the conformation of the acetyl ligand (Davies *et al.*, 1986). The acetyl ligand lies roughly parallel to the face of one phenyl group with the acetyl oxygen orientated towards the edge of a second proximate phenyl group (Fig. 1) (Davies *et al.*, 1986). The acetyl ligand thus prefers the conformation that places its methyl group in the space between the cyclopentadienyl and the carbon monoxide ligands. In this conformation, which minimizes interaction with the triphenylphosphine and the cyclopentadienyl ligands, one face of the acetyl ligand is effectively blocked to the approach of reagents and reactants (Blackburn *et al.*, 1989).

The acetyl complex (**1**) is chiral and configurationally stable. The two enantiomers *R*-(−)-**1** and *S*(+)-**1** are illustrated in Fig. 2 as projections from iron to phosphorus in order to emphasize the orientation of the acetyl ligand (acetyl oxygen *anti* to carbon monoxide) and the blocking effect of the triphenylphosphine. Both enantiomers are commercially available in homochiral form (Oxford Chirality, P.O. Box 412, Oxford, OX1 3QW, UK).

3 Stereoselective enolate alkylation reactions

Treatment of the iron acetyl complex (*R*)-**1** with butyllithium in tetrahydrofuran at −78°C generates the corresponding enolate (Baird and Davies, 1983; Brown *et al.*, 1986). Quenching this enolate at −78°C with methyl or ethyl iodide generates the corresponding propanoyl (*R*)-**2** and butanoyl (*R*)-**3** complexes, respectively, in quantitative yields (Scheme 1). No starting material or dialkylated compounds are obtained indicating that enolate exchange reactions do not occur readily. Ethylation of the lithium enolate derived from the propanoyl complex (**2**) occurs completely

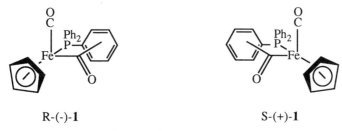

R-(-)-**1**   S-(+)-**1**

Fig. 2   The two enantiomers of $[(C_5H_5)Fe(CO)(PPh_3)COCH_3]$.

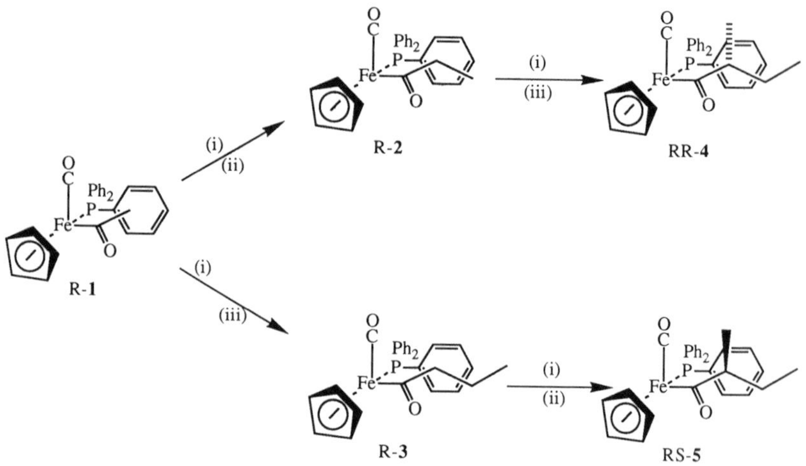

Scheme 1   Reagents: (i) BuLi, (ii) MeI, (iii) EtI.

stereoselectively to generate the R,R diastereoisomer of the 2-methyl-butanoyl complex (**4**). Methylation of the lithium enolate derived from the butanoyl complex (**3**) also occurs completely stereoselectively to give the other diastereoisomer, (R,S)-**5**.

Decomplexation of the products **4** and **5** is readily achieved by oxidation with bromine, N-bromosuccinimide, or by ceric or ferric salts. In the presence of water, alcohols or amines, decomplexation releases the

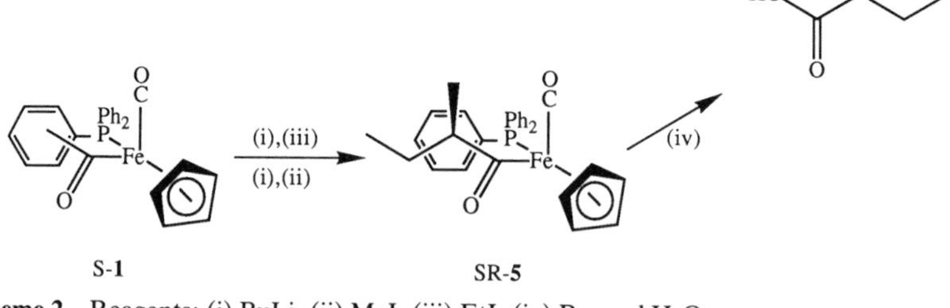

Scheme 2   Reagents: (i) BuLi, (ii) MeI, (iii) EtI, (iv) Br$_2$ and H$_2$O.

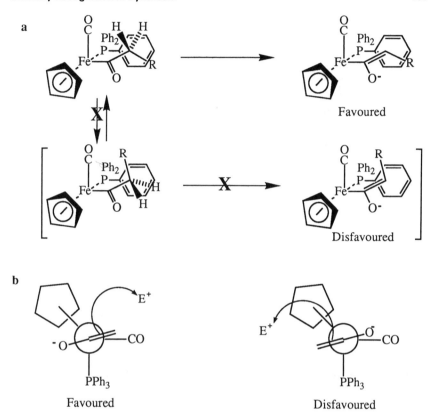

Fig. 3 (a) Favoured formation of (*E*)-enolates. (b) Favoured alkylation of enolates in the *anti* (O^- to CO) conformation

corresponding acids, alcohols or amides, respectively, without compromising the newly formed α-chiral centre. Thus for example, to make (*R*)-2-methyl butanoic acid two routes are available, either sequential methylation and ethylation of (*R*)-**1** or sequential ethylation and methylation of (*S*)-**1** (Scheme 2).

The origin of the stereoselectivity observed in the above alkylation reactions may be attributed to two factors. Firstly, deprotonation of the acyl ligands $COCH_2R$ is completely stereoselective for formation of the (*E*)-enolates (iron *trans* to R). Secondly, alkylation of the (*E*)-enolates occurs only from the unhindered face (away from the triphenylphosphine) in the conformation with the enolate oxygen *anti* to the carbon monoxide ligand (Baird *et al.*, 1983; Baird and Davies, 1986; Davies *et al.*, 1986; Brown *et al.*, 1986). Deprotonation by base approaching from the

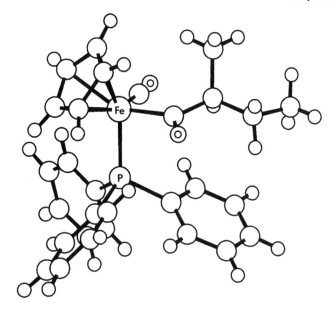

Fig. 4 X-ray crystal structure of (RS,SR)-[(C$_5$H$_5$)Fe(CO)(PPh$_3$)COCH(Me)Et] (**5**).

unhindered face requires the CH$_2$R group to assume a conformation that places the C–H bond to be broken parallel to the p orbital on the acyl carbonyl carbon. Such a conformation may be easily attained for formation of the (E)-enolates but is energetically disfavoured for formation of the corresponding (Z)-enolates due to severe steric interactions between the R group and the carbon monoxide ligand (Fig. 3(a)). In the *anti* (enolate oxygen to carbon monoxide) conformation approach of the electrophile is blocked by the triphenylphosphine for one face while approach is unrestricted to the other face. In the *syn* conformation, however, both faces are blocked, one by the triphenylphosphine the other by the cyclopentadienyl ligand (Fig. 3(b)). Figure 4 shows the X-ray crystal structure of (RS,SR)-**5** where the chiral centre was formed by methylation of the enolate with O$^-$ *cis* to the ethyl group in the *anti* conformation (O$^-$ to CO) from the face away from the triphenylphosphine ligand (Baird *et al.*, 1983).

4 Asymmetric synthesis of captopril and *epi*captopril
(Bashiardes and Davies, 1987)

The angiotensin-converting-enzyme inhibitor captopril, $S,S(-)$-1-(3-mercapto-2-methyl-1-oxypropyl)-L-proline (S,S)-**6** is the amide derived from (*S*)-3-mercapto-2-methylpropionic acid and L-proline (Ondetti *et al.*, 1977; Cushman *et al.*, 1977; Shimazaki *et al.*, 1982; Nam *et al.*, 1984; Hassall *et al.*, 1984; Andrews *et al.*, 1985). In general, synthetic routes to captopril generate it as a mixture with its epimer (−)-*epi*Captopril ((*S,R*)-**7**) (Ondetti

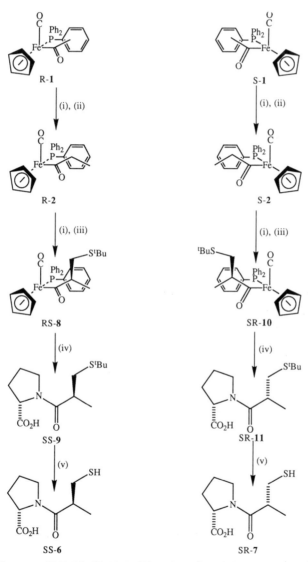

Scheme 3   Reagents: (i) BuLi, (ii) MeI, (iii) BrCH₂ SᵗBu, (iv) Br₂, L-proline ᵗbutyl ester, (v) Hg(OAc)₂,CF₃CO₂H and H₂S.

et al., 1977; Cushman *et al.*, 1977; Shimazaki *et al.*, 1982; Nam *et al.*, 1984). However, use of the chiral iron auxiliary [(C₅H₅)Fe(CO)(PPh₃)] to achieve the asymmetric synthesis of the (*S*)-t-butyl protected 3-mercapto-2-methyl-propanoyl fragment followed by direct coupling to L-proline-t-butyl ester generates, after deprotection, either (*S,S*-captopril or (*S,R*)-*epi*captopril (Scheme 3) (Bashiardes and Davies, 1987).

Methylation of the homochiral parent acetyl complex (*R*)-**1** generates the propanoyl complex (*R*)-**2**. Alkylation of the enolate derived from (*R*)-**2** with bromomethyl-t-butylsulphide generates (*R,S*)-**8** as a single diastereoisomer. Decomplexation of (*R,S*)-**8** with bromine followed by the addition of L-proline t-butyl ester generates the doubly protected derivative of captopril (*S,S*)-**9**. The diastereoisomeric purity of (*S,S*)-**9** confirmed the stereoselectivity of the enolate alkylation reaction and demonstrates that the α-chiral centre is not compromised during the decomplexation procedure. Deprotection was achieved by treatment with mercuric acetate and trifluoroacetic acid followed by hydrogen sulphide gas to yield *S,S*-(−)-captopril (**6**). The overall yield of (−)-captopril was 59% and this material was identical in all respects to an authentic sample. (*S,R*)-*epi*Captopril was similarly obtained by the same synthetic sequence starting from homochiral (*S*)-**1** (Scheme 3).

5   Asymmetric synthesis of differentially protected α-alkylsuccinates

Treatment of the lithium enolate derived from the racemic iron acetyl complex (*R,S*)-**1** at −78°C with racemic t-butyl-2-bromopropionate gave a 40 : 1 mixture of the β-methylsuccinoyl complexes (*RS,SR*)-**12** and (*RR,SS*)-**13** (Scheme 4) (Collingwood *et al.*, 1990). The diastereoselectivity observed in this reaction is the result of a chiral recognition process, one enantiomer of the enolate preferring to react 40 times faster with one of the enantiomers of the α-bromoester than with the other. Competitive debromination of the α-bromoester results in the yield being only moderate (29%).

The origin of the chiral recognition is believed to arise from lithium chelation (Fig. 5). For the (*R*)-enolate reacting with the (*S*)-bromoester

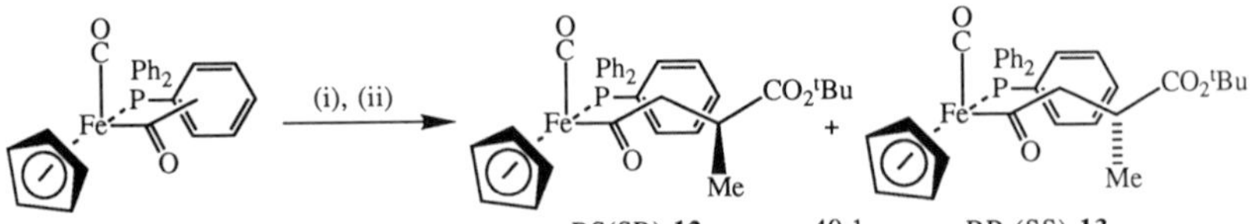

$$\text{R(S)-1} \qquad \text{RS(SR)-12} \quad 40:1 \quad \text{RR,(SS)-13}$$

Scheme 4   Reagents: (i) BuLi, (ii) MeCH(Br)CO₂ᵗBu.

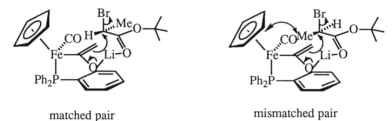

matched pair   mismatched pair

Fig. 5 Chelation controlled α-bromoester displacements. (a) Matched pair of (R)-iron and (S)-bromoester. (b) Mismatched pair of (R)-iron and (R)-bromoester.

initial chelation of lithium between the enolate oxygen and the ester carbonyl should allow delivery of the α-carbon of the ester to the enolate carbon in the correct orientation for an S_N2 displacement. However, for the (R)-enolate and (R)-bromoester this chelation-controlled delivery involves significant steric interactions of the α-methyl group with the cyclopentadienyl ligand.

This analysis predicts the matched pair to be the (R)-enolate with the (S)-bromoester and hence after inversion of configuration in the S_N2 reaction the major diastereoisomer to be RS,SR. This was confirmed by a single-crystal X-ray structure analysis on the major diastereoisomer, (RS,SR)-**12** (Fig.6) (Davies and Wills, unpublished results).

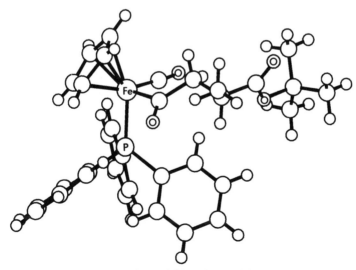

Fig. 6 X-ray crystal structure of (RS,SR)-$[(C_5H_5)Fe(CO)(PPh_3)COCH_2CH(Me)CO_2{}^tBu]$ (**12**).

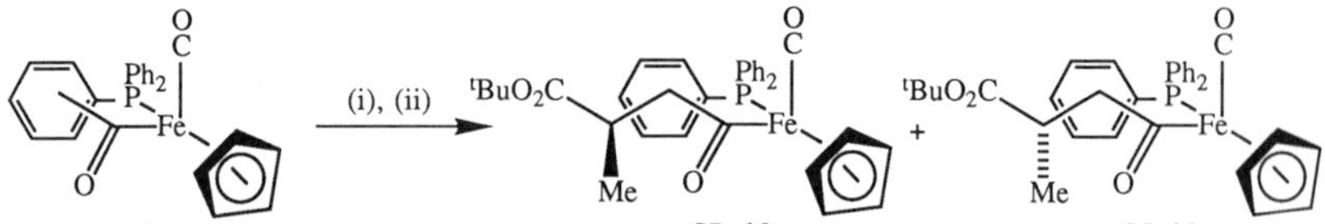

E⁺	ratio	d.e.

E^+	ratio	d.e.
RS-MeCH(Br)CO$_2$^{t}Bu	97.5 : 2.5	95%
R-MeCH(Br)CO$_2$^{t}Bu	100 : 0	100%
S-MeCH(Br)CO$_2$^{t}Bu	50 :50	0%

Scheme 5   Reagents: (i) BuLi, (ii) E^+.

Treatment of the lithium enolate from homochiral (S)-**1** with excess racemic or homochiral (R)- or (S)-t-butyl 2-bromopropionate gave (S,R)-**12** in 95%, 100% and 0% diastereomeric excesses, respectively (Scheme 5). These results establish the S_N2 character of the reaction. In the last reaction liberated bromide partially racemizes the mismatched (S)-t-butyl-2-bromo-propionate.

Alkylation of the lithium enolate derived from (R)-**1** with t-butylbromo-acetate gave the parent succinoyl derivative (R)-**14** (Scheme 6) (Bashiardes *et al.*, 1989). Treatment of the succinoyl complex (R)-**14** with butyllithium and methyl iodide gave a 4 : 1 mixture of (R,S)-**12** and (R,R)-**13** from which pure (R,S)-**12** could be easily isolated (Bashiardes *et al.*, 1989). Similar treatment of (S)-**1** generated (S,R)-**12** (Scheme 6).

Elaborated succinoyl derivatives such as **12** represent differentially protected succinic acid derivatives and may be decomplexed to homochiral succinate half esters, half amides and ester amides (Bashiardes *et al.*, 1989).

Scheme 6   Reagents: (i) BuLi, (ii) BrCH$_2$CO$_2$^{t}Bu, (iii) MeI.

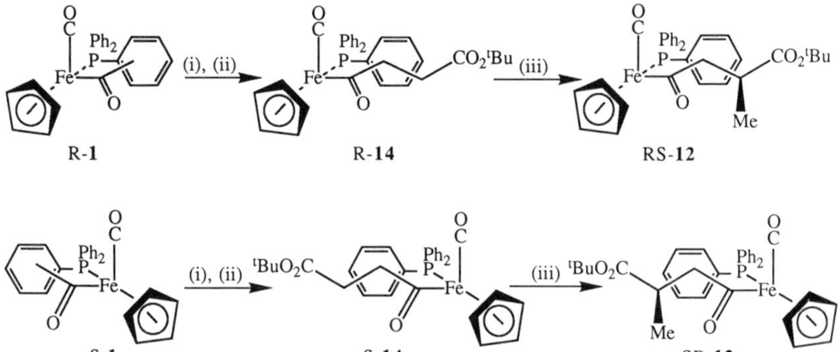

6 Asymmetric synthesis of actinonin and *epi*actinonin

Actinonin (**15**) has been shown to have some antibiotic activity against Gram-positive and Gram-negative bacteria. More importantly, actinonin exhibits high anticollagenase activity (Faucher *et al.*, 1987). Our approach to the synthesis of actinonin (Scheme 7) (Bashiardes and Davies, 1988; Davies, 1989) involves the coupling of an amino acid derived fragment with an α-pentyl-succinate derivative derived by asymmetric synthesis using the iron chiral auxiliary [(C$_5$H$_5$)Fe(CO)(PPh$_3$)].

The synthesis of the required protected amino acid derived fragment **16** is shown in Scheme 8. The starting materials are *N*-Boc protected L-valine (**17**) and L-prolinol (**18**).

The homochiral succinoyl derivates (*S,R*)-**19** and (*R,S*)-**19** were prepared from (*S*)-**1** and (*R*)-**1**, respectively, by both methods described above. For example, alkylation of (*S*)-**14** with butyllithium and pentyl iodide gave (*S,R*)-**19** (>91% diastereomeric excess (de)) and one crystallization furnished pure (*S,R*)-**19**. Decomplexation of (*S,R*)-**19** with bromine in the presence of *N,O*-dibenzylhydroxylamine gave (*R*)-**20**, the t-butylester protecting group being removed by the hydrogen bromide released in the decomplexation reaction. Coupling of the two fragments **16** and (*R*)-**20** then gave (*S,S,R*)-**21**. The stereochemical integrity of (*S,S,R*)-**21** confirms the homochirality of the succinoyl fragment (*R*)-**20**. Reductive removal of the three benzyl protecting groups gave (*S,S,R*)-(−)-actinonin ((*S,S,R*)-**15**) identical in all respects to an authentic sample (Scheme 9) (Bashiardes and

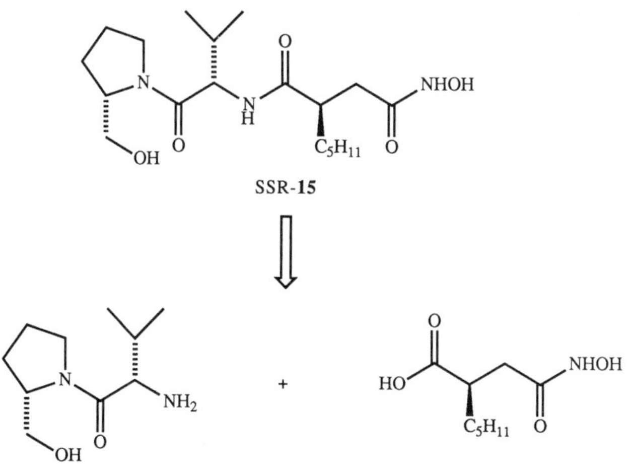

SSR-**15**

Scheme 7   Retrosynthetic analysis for (−)-actinonin (**15**).

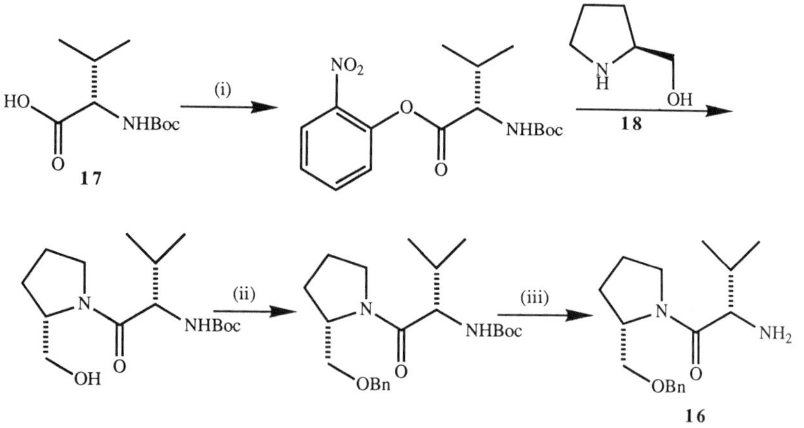

Scheme 8   Reagents: (i) DCC, *o*-nitrophenol, (ii) NaH and BnBr, (iii) TFA.

Davies, 1988). The overall yield of actinonin throughout the whole sequence is 41%. *epi*Actinonin ((S,S,S)-**22**) was similarly prepared from $R(-)$-**1** in 42% overall yield.

7 Asymmetric synthesis of butyrolactones

No reaction occurs at $-78°C$ between the lithium enolate from the racemic acetyl complex (R,S)-**1** and racemic propene oxide. In the presence of the Lewis acid, boron trifluoride, however, smooth opening of the epoxide occurs to give an essentially equal mixture of the two γ-hydroxyacyl diastereoisomers (RS,SR)-**23** and (RR,SS)-**24** (Scheme 10) (Brown *et al.*, 1985). Compounds **23** and **24** correspond to the products of S_N2 opening of the epoxide at the least-substituted end.

Opening of racemic propene oxide with the enolate from racemic (R,S)-**1** in the presence of diethyl aluminium chloride, however, gave complex (RS,SR)-**23** as a single diastereoisomer (Brown *et al.*, 1985). Under the conditions employed transmetallation of the enolate does not occur. The formation of a single diastereoisomer under these conditions indicates complete chiral discrimination by each of the enolate enantiomers between the two enantiomers of propene oxide, despite the fact that the S_N2 opening is occurring at the unsubstituted end of the epoxide remote from the chiral centre. The relative stereochemistry within (RS,SR)-**23** was unambiguously established by a single-crystal X-ray structure analysis (Fig. 7) (Brown *et al.*, 1985). This therefore established the matched pair to be the (R)-enolate with (S)-propene oxide.

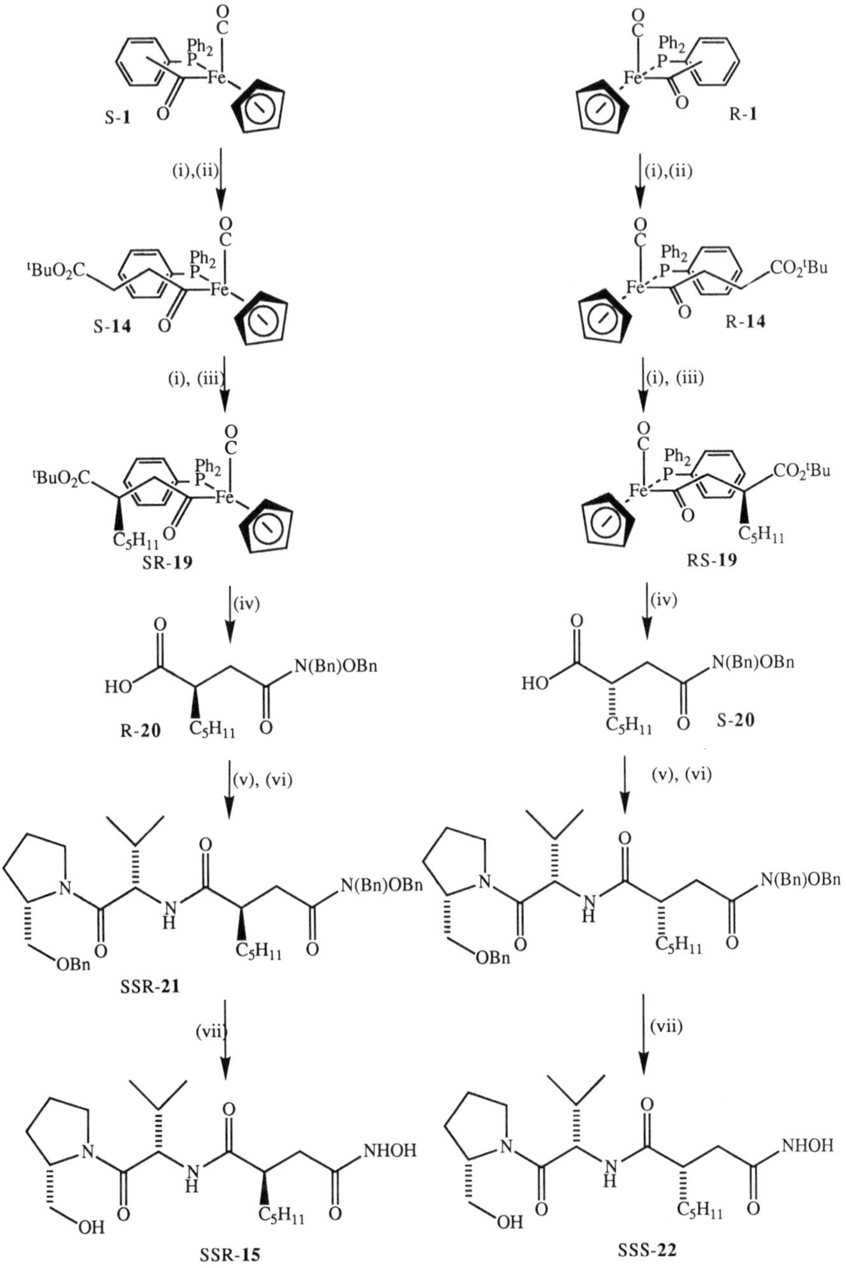

Scheme 9 Reagents: (i) BuLi, (ii) BrCH$_2$CO$_2$^{t}Bu, (iii) C$_5$H$_{11}$, (iv) Br$_2$ and HN(Bn)OBn, (v) *N*-methylmorpholine and ^{i}BuOCOCl, (vi) compound **16**, (vii) H$_2$ and Pd(OH)$_2$.

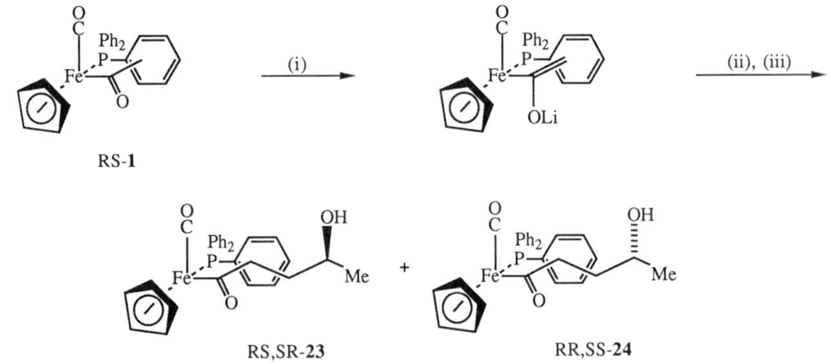

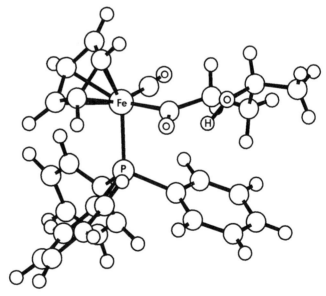

Scheme 10   Reagents: (i) BuLi, (ii) racemic propene oxide, (iii) BF₃.

Treatment of (R)-**1** with butyllithium followed by excess racemic propene oxide and excess diethyl aluminium chloride gave (R,S)-**23** as a single diastereoisomer (Scheme 11). Oxidative decomplexation of (R,S)-**23** gave (S)-4-methylbutyrolactone $((S)$-**25**). Under the same conditions starting from (S)-**1** led to the formation of (R)-4-methylbutyrolactone $((R)$-**25**).

2,4-Disubstituted butyrolactones are also available via chiral recognition

Fig. 7   X-ray crystal structure of (RS,SR)-$[(C_5H_5)Fe(CO)(PPh_3)COCH_2CH_2CH(OH)CH_3]$ (**23**).

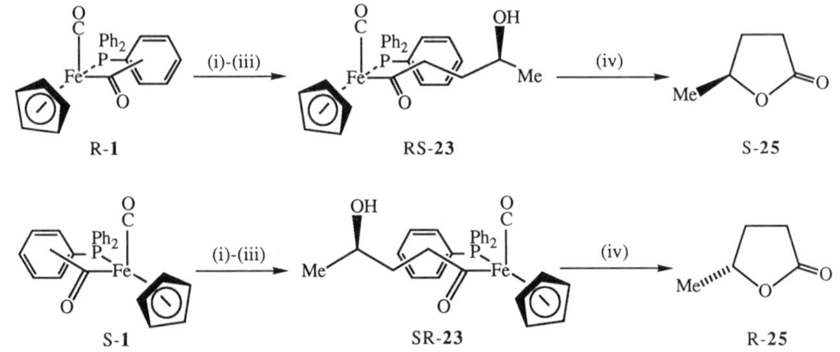

Scheme 11 Reagents: (i) BuLi, (ii) racemic propene oxide, (iii) Et_2AlCl, (iv) Br_2.

processes (Davies *et al.*, 1990). Thus, for example, treatment of the lithium enolate from (*S*)-**2** with excess racemic styrene oxide and diethylaluminium chloride gave the α-methyl-γ-hydroxyacyl complex (*S*,*S*,*S*)-**26** as a single diastereoisomer. In this reaction the α-chiral centre has been produced completely stereoselectively while the control of the γ-chiral centre results from an enantiomer recognition process (Scheme 12) (Davies *et al.*, 1990).

An authentic sample of (*S*,*S*,*S*)-**26** was prepared from (*S*)-**2** and homochiral (*R*)-styrene oxide. Decomplexation of (*S*,*S*,*S*)-**26** with bromine gave the homochiral (*S*,*S*)-*cis*-2-methyl-4-phenylbutyrolactone ((*S*,*S*)-**27**) (Scheme 13) (Davies *et al.*, 1990). The structure of (*S*,*S*)-**27** was unambiguously confirmed by a single-crystal X-ray structure analysis (Fig. 8) (Davies *et al.*, 1990). This established that the decomplexation had proceeded with retention of configuration at the γ-centre.

The epimeric homochiral *trans*-lactone was prepared from homochiral (*R*)-**2**. Addition of butyllithium to (*R*)-**2** followed by (*R*)-styrene oxide and diethylaluminium chloride gave (*R*,*R*,*S*)-**28** as a single diastereoisomer. Decomplexation produced (*R*,*S*)-*trans*-2-methyl-4-phenylbutyrolactone ((*R*,*S*)-**29**) (Scheme 13) (Davies *et al.*, 1990).

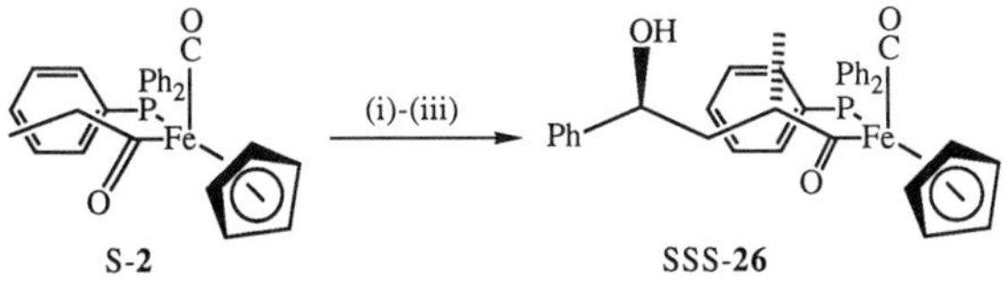

Scheme 12 Reagents: (i) BuLi, (ii) racemic styrene oxide, (iii) Et_2AlCl.

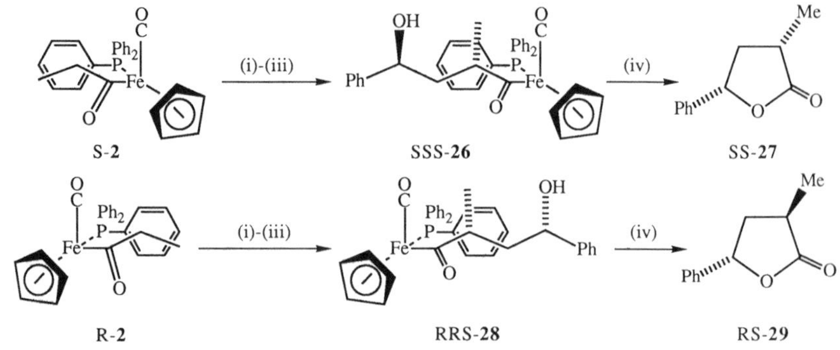

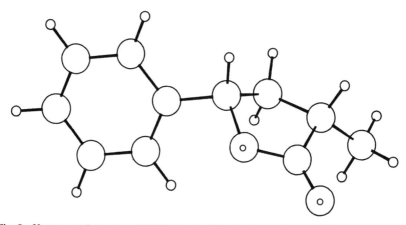

Scheme 13   Reagents: (i) BuLi, (ii) (R)-styrene oxide, (iii) Et$_2$AlCl, (iv) Br$_2$.

8 Conclusions

The reactions described above demonstrate the power of the chiral auxiliary [(C$_5$H$_5$)Fe(CO)(PPh$_3$)] in asymmetric synthesis and for chiral recognition. All the processes described involve simple alkylation reactions of iron acyl enolates. The chiral auxiliary [(C$_5$H$_5$)Fe(CO)(PPh$_3$)] provides efficient stereocontrol in many other types of reaction such as Michael additions, aldols, Diels–Alder, etc. (Davies *et al.*, 1988; Davies, 1989), and similar recognition phenomena are being investigated in these areas. In the synthesis of complex molecules it is not therefore always necessary to obtain all the fragments in homochiral form, there may be an alternative involving chiral recognition.

Fig. 8   X-ray crystal structure of (S,S)-2-methyl-4-phenylbutyrolactone (**27**).

Acknowledgements

I gratefully acknowledge the efforts of all my research collaborators whose names are listed in the references. Financial support for these projects was provided by a BP Venture Research Award from BP International, British Biotechnology, ICI Pharmaceuticals and the SERC.

References

Andrews, P. R., Carson, J. M., Caselli, A., Spark, M. J. and Woods, R. (1985). Conformational analysis and active site modelling of angiotensin-converting enzyme inhibitors. *J. Med. Chem.* **28**, 393–399.

Baird, G. J. and Davies, S. G. (1983). Stereoselective elaboration of the acyl ligand in $(C_5H_5)Fe(CO)(PPh_3)(COCHR)Li$ (R = Me,Et). *J. Organometal. Chem.* **248**, C1.

Baird, G. J., Bandy, J. A., Davies, S. G. and Prout, K. (1983). Stereochemical control and mechanistic aspects of the alkylation of $[(C_5H_5)Fe(L)(CO)$-(COCHR)-Li$^+$(L = PPh_2,PPh_2,NEt_2; R = Me,Et): X-Ray Crystal Structure of $(C_5H_5)Fe(PPh_3)(CO)(COCH(Me)Et)]$. *Chem. Commun.* 1202.

Bashiardes, G. and Davies, S. G. (1987). The asymmetric synthesis of (−)-captopril utilising the iron chiral auxiliary $[(C_5H_5)Fe(CO)(PPh_3)]$. *Tetrahedron Lett.* **28**, 5563.

Bashiardes, G. and Davies, S. G. (1988). The asymmetric synthesis of (−)-actinonin using the iron chiral auxiliary $[(C_5H_5)Fe(CO)(PPh_3)]$. *Tetrahedron Lett.* **29**, 6509.

Bashiardes, G., Collingwood, S. P., Davies, S. G. and Preston, S. C. (1989). Chiral succinate enolate equivalents for the asymmetric synthesis of alpha-alkyl succinic acid derivatives. *J. Chem. Soc., Perkin, Trans. 1*, 1162.

Bernal, I., Brunner, H. and Muschinol, M. (1988). Optically active transition metal compounds 93* X-ray determination of the structure and absolute configuration of $(+578)C_5H_5Fe(CO)P(C_6H_5)_3COCH_3)$. *Inorg. Chim. Acta* **142**, 235–242.

Blackburn, B. K., Davies, S. G. and Whittaker, M. (1989). Conformational analysis for ligands bound to the chiral auxiliary $[(C_5H_5)Fe(CO)(PPh_3)]$ in *Stereochemistry of Organometallic and Inorganic Compounds* (ed. I. Bernal), Vol. 3, p. 141. Elsevier, Oxford.

Brown, S. L., Davies, S. G., Foster, D. F., Seeman, J. I. and Warner, P. (1986). Improved stereochemical control and mechanistic aspects of the alkylation of enolates derived from $[(C_5H_5)Fe(CO)(PPh_3)COCH_2R]$. *Tetrahedron Lett.* **27**, 623–626.

Brown, S. L., Davies, S. G., Warner, P., Jones, R. H. and Prout, K. (1985). Chiral discrimination in the reaction of the enolate $[C_5H_5)Fe(CO)(PPh_3)(COCH_2)]$-Li$^+$ with monosubstituted epoxides: X-ray crystal structure of (RS,SR)-$[(C_5H_5)Fe(CO)(PPh_3)(COCH_2CH(OH)Me)]$. *Chem. Commun.* 1446.

Collingwood, S. P., Davies, S. G. and Preston, S. C. (1990). Chiral recognition in the S_N2 reaction of t-butyl 2-bromopropionate with the enolate derived from $[(C_5H_5)Fe(CO)(PPH_3)COCH_3]$. *Tetrahedron Lett.* **31**, 4067.

Cushman, D. W., Cheung, H. S., Sabo, E. F. and Ondetti, M. A. (1977). Design of potent competitive inhibitors of angiotensin-converting enzyme. Carboxy-alkanoyl and mercaptoalkanoyl amino acids. *Biochemistry* **16**, 5484.

Davies, S. G. (1989). Chiral auxiliaries. *Chem. Br.* **25**, 268.

Davies, S. G., Bashiardes, G., Beckett, R. P., Cotte, S. J., Dordor-Hedgecock, I. M., Goodfellow, C. L., Gravatt, G. L., McNally, J. P. and Whittaker, M. (1988). Asymmetric synthesis via chiral transition metal auxiliaries. *Phil. Trans. R. Soc. London, Ser. A.* **326**, 619.

Davies, S. G., Seeman, J. I. and Williams, I. H. (1986). Conformational analysis of the iron acetyl complex [(C$_5$H$_5$)Fe(CO)(PPh$_3$)(COCH)]. *Tetrahedron Lett.* **27**, 619.

Davies, S. G., Polywka, R. and Warner, P. (1990). Asymmetric synthesis of 2,4-disubstituted butyrolactones using the iron chiral auxiliary [(C$_5$H$_5$)Fe(CO)(PPh$_3$)]. *Tetrahedron* **46**, 4847.

Faucher, D. C., Lelievre, Y. and Cartwright, T. (1987). An inhibitor of mammalian collagenase active at micromolar concentrations from an actinomycete culture broth. *J. Antibiotics* **40**, 1757.

Hassall, C. H., Krohn, A., Moody, C. J. and Thomas, W. A. (1984). The design and synthesis of new triazolo-, pyrazolo-, and pyridazo-pyridazine derivatives as inhibitors of angiotensin converting enzyme. *J. Chem. Soc., Perkin. Trans. 1*, 155.

Nam, D. H., Lee, C. S. and Ryu, D. D. Y. (1984). An improved synthesis of captopril. *J. Pharm. Sci.* **73**, 1843.

Ondetti, M. A., Rubin, B. and Cushman, D. W. (1977). Design of specific inhibitors of angiotensin-converting enzyme: new class of orally active antihypertensive agents. *Science* **196**, 441–443.

Shimazaki, M., Hasegawa, J., Kan, K., Nomura, K., Nose, Y., Kondo, H., Ohashi, T. and Watanabe, K. (1982). Synthesis of captopril starting from an optically active beta-hydroxy acid. *Chem. Pharm. Bull.* **30**, 3139.

11

Sultam-directed asymmetric syntheses of α-amino acids

WOLFGANG OPPOLZER
Department of Organic Chemistry, University of Geneva,
30 Quai Ernest-Ansermet, CH-1211 Geneva 4, Switzerland

1 Introduction

Enantiomerically pure α-amino acids are of immense interest not just *per se*, but also as chiral building blocks and, last but not least, as starting materials for chiral reagents and catalysts (Williams, 1989). Here we describe practical routes to this class of compounds via π-face-selective formation of either the C_α–R or C_α–NH$_2$ bond (**A** or **B**, Scheme 1).

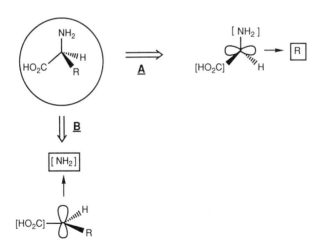

Scheme 1

CHIRALITY IN DRUG DESIGN AND SYNTHESIS
ISBN 0-12-136670-7

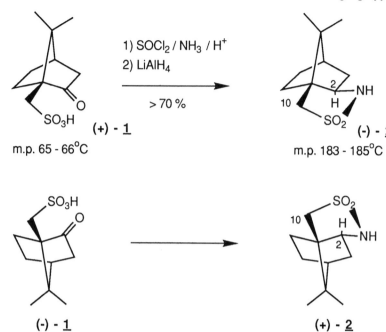

1) SOCl₂ / NH₃ / H⁺
2) LiAlH₄

$> 70\%$

(+) - **1**
m.p. 65 - 66°C

(-) - **2**
m.p. 183 - 185°C

(-) - **1**

(+) - **2**

Scheme 2

Convenient sources of chirality are bornane-10,2-sultam, $(-)$-**2** and its antipode $(+)$-**2**, accessible from inexpensive $(+)$- and $(-)$-camphorsulfonic acids in two simple operations (Scheme 2) (Oppolzer et al., 1984). Both chirophore enantiomers are commercially available in kg-quantities (Oxford Chirality, Oxford, UK).

Addition reactions to N-enoyl derivatives **I**, as well as reactions of 'enolates' (**II**) with electrophiles, proceed in high yield and with good to excellent π-face discrimination (Scheme 3). Almost all of the N-acyl products are stable and can be:

(1) readily purified by crystallization,
(2) directly analysed by ¹H-NMR and/or GC to determine their stereochemical purity, and
(3) cleaved (e.g. with LiAlH₄, LiOH, LiOOH, MeOMgI, etc.) under mild conditions without loss of the induced chirality and with easy recovery of the auxiliary (Oppolzer, 1987, 1988).

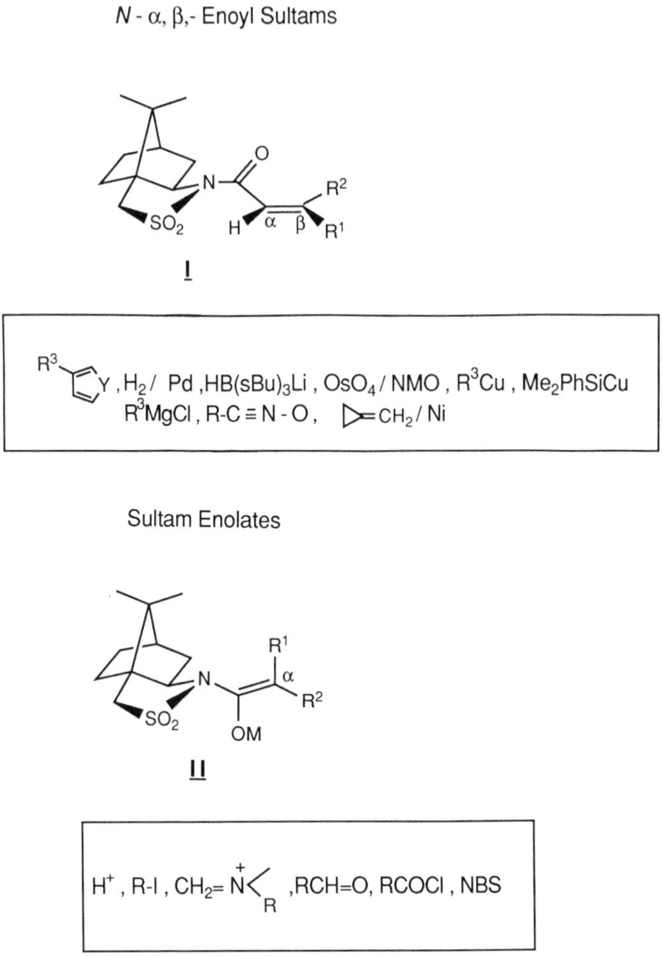

N - α, β,- Enoyl Sultams

I

$R^3\!-\!\!\backslash\!\!\!\!\!\diagdown\!\!Y$, H_2 / Pd , $HB(sBu)_3Li$, OsO_4 / NMO , R^3Cu , $Me_2PhSiCu$

R^3MgCl , R-C ≡ N - O , ▷=CH_2 / Ni

Sultam Enolates

II

H^+ , R-I , CH_2= $\overset{+}{N}\!\!<^{}_{R}$, RCH=O, RCOCl , NBS

Scheme 3

2 Alkylation of glycinate equivalents

Chiral glycine equivalents represent an attractive pivotal source for asymmetric syntheses of enantiomerically pure α-amino acids (Scheme 1, option **A**; Scheme 4) (Williams, 1989). Straightforward alkylations of glycine enolate derivatives are, however, relatively scarce and, despite their elegance, leave plenty of room for more practical and general alternatives.

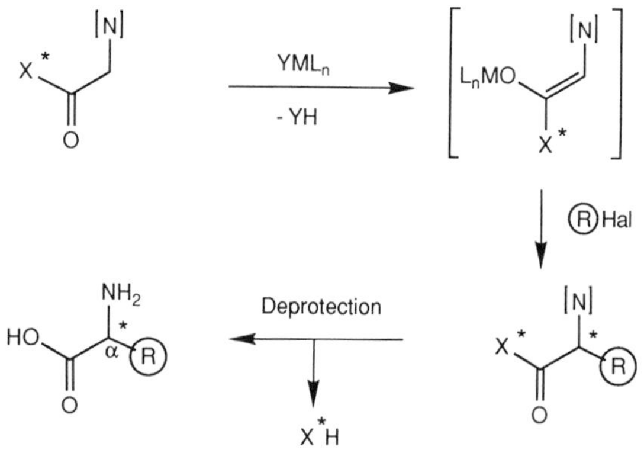

Scheme 4

Indeed, alkylation of easily available 'glycinate equivalent' (4) afforded a variety of α-amino acids (7). The crystalline, common precursor (4) reacted smoothly even with non-activated primary and secondary alkyl iodides. N-Deprotection by mild acidic hydrolysis and gentle saponification gave the readily separable sultam (2) and the free amino acids (7) in high overall yield (Scheme 5) (Oppolzer et al., 1989). Intriguingly, simple deprotonation/ alkylation of 4 at 0°C using phase transfer catalysis furnished crystallized **6b** in 77% yield without cleavage of the N-acyl moiety (Scheme 6).

3 Halogenation/azide displacement

Previously, we have shown that kinetically controlled deprotonation/ O-silylation of esters (8), addition of NBS (or NCS) and crystallization afforded diastereomerically pure α-bromo (or chloro) esters (9). Treatment of **9** with sodium azide followed by $Ti(OCH_2Ph)_4$-mediated transesterification and hydrogenolysis afforded (R)-amino acids (11; Scheme 7) (Oppolzer et al., 1986). A similar approach to amino acids (11) relies on borylation/bromination of N-acyloxazolidinones (12) and azide exchange using tetramethylguanidinium azide (Evans et al., 1987).

Scheme 8 depicts a pertinent example of synthesizing α-amino acids with induction of two stereogenic centres (at $C\beta$ and $C\alpha$). Thus, employing the sequence 1,4-addition/bromination/azidation, crotonate (15) has been converted into L-allo-isoleucine (20), an essential precursor of the psychotropic ergot peptide, epicriptine (Oppolzer and Moretti, 1986).

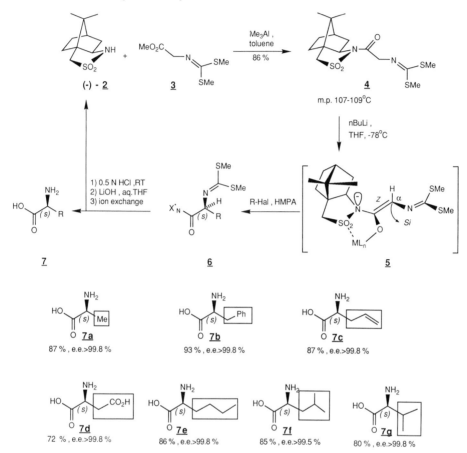

Scheme 5

Scheme 6

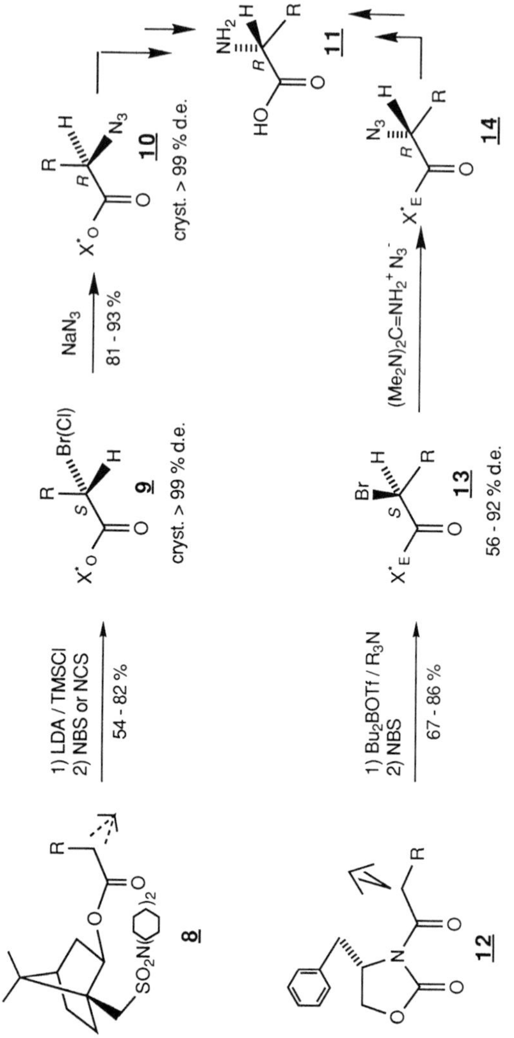

8

1) LDA / TMSCl
2) NBS or NCS
54 - 82 %

9
cryst. > 99 % d.e.

NaN₃
81 - 93 %

10
cryst. > 99 % d.e.

11

12

1) Bu₂BOTf / R₃N
2) NBS
67 - 86 %

13
56 - 92 % d.e.

(Me₂N)₂C=NH₂⁺N₃⁻

14

Scheme 7

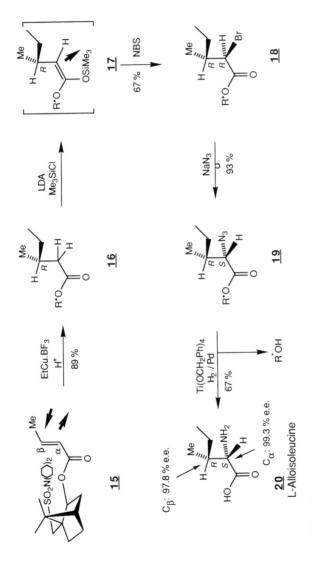

Scheme 8

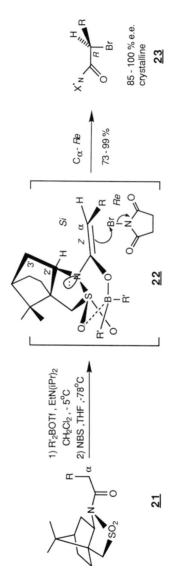

Scheme 9

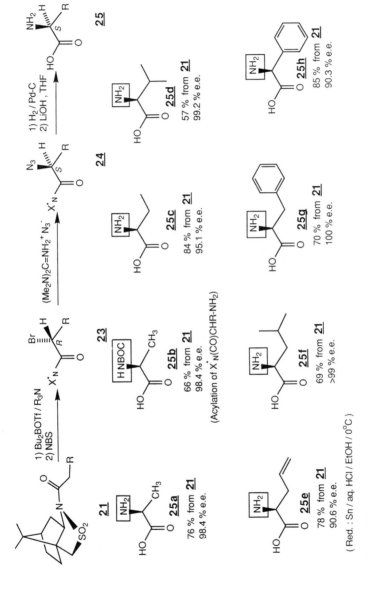

Scheme 10

Taking advantage of the more practical sultam auxiliaries (2), analogous treatment of *in situ* prepared boryl enolates (22) with NBS furnished (*R*)-bromides (23), consistent with a bromination of chelated (*Z*)-enolates (22) at their C_α–*Re* face (Scheme 9).

S_N2 displacement of the bromide with azide, followed by hydrogenolysis of the azide group and cleavage of the sultam moiety (LiOH, aq. THF, RT) furnished (*S*)-amino acids (25) in good overall yields from 21. *N*-Acylation of the primary amino group prior to the final saponification step leads to *N*-protected amino acids, e.g. to 25b (Scheme 10) (Oppolzer and Bossard, 1990).

4 Electrophilic 'amination'

Asymmetric syntheses of α-amino acids from chiral enolates by direct electrophilic C–N bond formation (Scheme 1, option **B**) have so far been restricted by the limited choice of 'amination' reagents available, *i.e.* di-*t*-butylazodicarboxylate (Gennari *et al.*, 1986; Evans *et al.*, 1986, 1988; Trimble and Vederas, 1986; e.g. Scheme 11; Oppolzer *et al.*, 1986; Oppolzer and Moretti, 1988), 2,4,6-triisopropylbenzenesulfonyl azide (Evans and Britton, 1987) and ethylazidoformate/*hν* (Loreto *et al.*, 1989).

More advantageously, 1-chloro-1-nitrosocyclohexane was used as a novel [NH_2^+] equivalent which attacked the (*Z*)-enolate (28) exclusively from the C_α–*Re* face to give (*R*)-hydroxylamine (31) on acidic workup (Oppolzer and Tamura, 1990). The nitrone intermediate (29) was identified as a [3 + 2]-cycloaddition product (30) (Scheme 12).

A variety of crystallized hydroxylamines (31) were subjected to *N/O*-hydrogenolysis (Zn/H^+) to afford amines (32) which, after saponification, gave enantiomerically pure (*R*)-amino acids in good overall yield from 21 (Scheme 13). The mildly basic removal of the sultam moiety offers several advantages such as the ready access to *N*-protected amino acids (e.g. 33h) or to α-*N*-hydroxyamino acids 36 (Scheme 14). α-*N*-Hydroxyamino acids are known as components of naturally occurring metabolites and of therapeutically interesting peptides.

1,4-Additions of organomagnesium halides to *N*-enoylsultams are an attractive alternative for obtaining chiral enolates (37), since they allow for the highly selective generation of two stereogenic centres (C_α and C_β) in one synthetic operation (Scheme 15) (Oppolzer *et al.*, 1987). Thus, the 1,4-addition/enolate 'amination' tandem 40 → 41 was the key transformation in the efficient synthesis of (*S,S*)-isoleucine (43) from *N*-crotonoylsultam (40; Scheme 16) (Oppolzer and Tamura, 1990). The potential of this approach for the asymmetric synthesis of further β-branched α-amino acids is under current investigation.

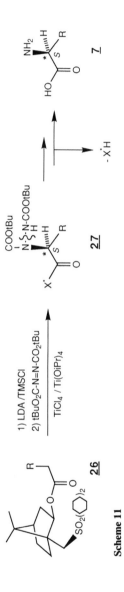

Scheme 11

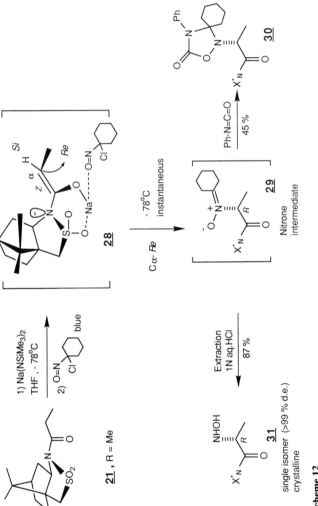

Scheme 12

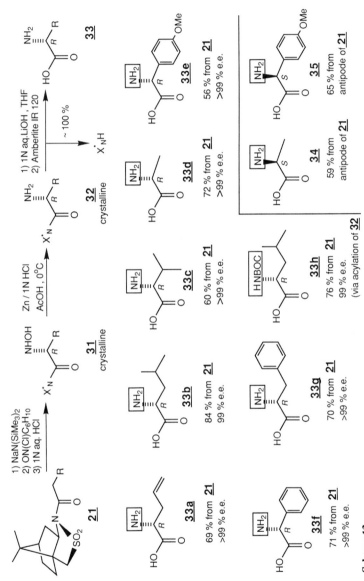

Scheme 13

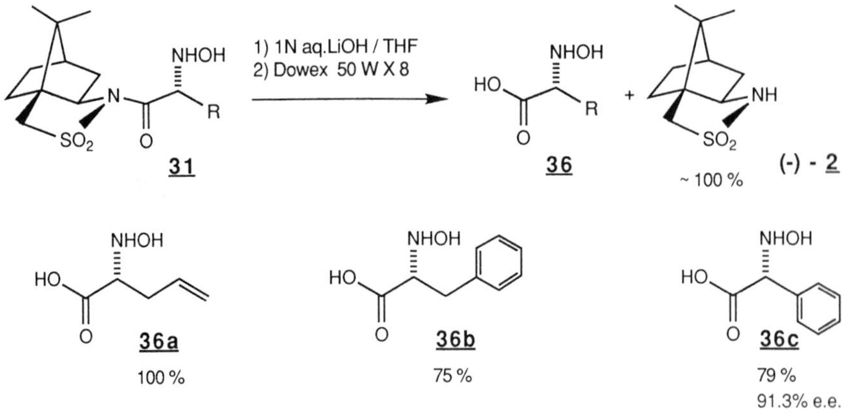
NHOH
R
N
SO2
O
31
1) 1N aq.LiOH / THF
2) Dowex 50 W X 8
HO
NHOH
R
O
36
+
NH
SO2
~ 100 %
(-) - 2
NHOH
HO
O
36a
100 %
NHOH
HO
O
36b
75 %
NHOH
HO
O
36c
79 %
91.3% e.e.

Scheme 14

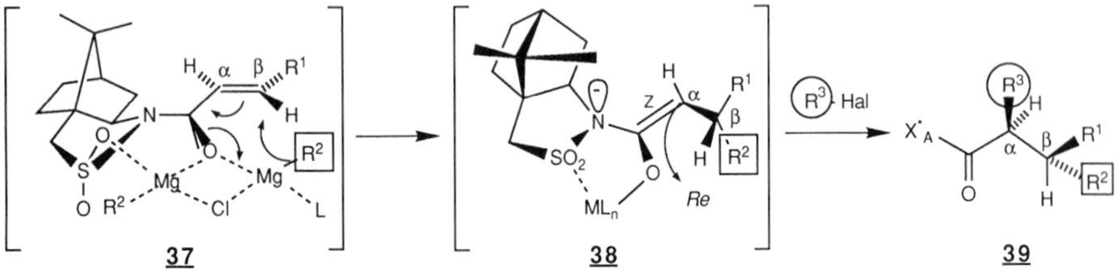
H
α
β
R1
H
N
O
S
O
R2
Mg
Cl
Mg
L
R2
37
H
Z
α
R1
β
N
SO2
ML n
O
H
R2
Re
38
R3 Hal
X*A
R3
H
α
β
R1
O
H
R2
39

Scheme 15

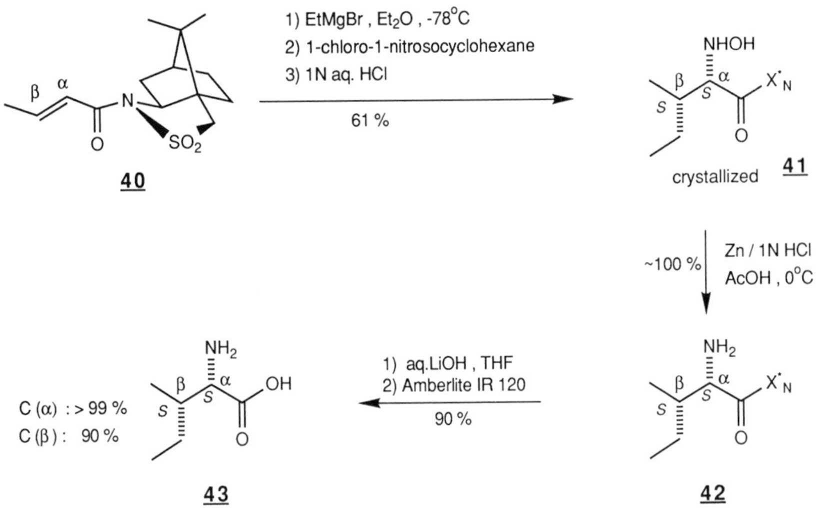
β
α
N
O
SO2
40
1) EtMgBr , Et2O , -78°C
2) 1-chloro-1-nitrosocyclohexane
3) 1N aq. HCl
61 %
NHOH
β
α
X*N
S
S
O
crystallized
41
~100 %
Zn / 1N HCl
AcOH , 0°C
NH2
β
α
X*N
S
S
O
42
1) aq.LiOH , THF
2) Amberlite IR 120
90 %
NH2
β
α
OH
S
S
O
43
C (α) : > 99 %
C (β) : 90 %

Scheme 16

5 Conclusion

Compared to a plethora of auxiliaries so far developed for asymmetric synthesis, sultams (2) are among the most practical and universal. Extensions of their utility for the synthesis of further enantiomerically pure α-amino acids are to be expected.

Acknowledgements

It is a privilege to acknowledge the crucial contributions of my coworkers R. Moretti, O. Tamura, P. Bossard, S. Thomi and R. Pedrosa. We thank the *Swiss National Science Foundation, Sandoz AG*, Basel, and *Giavaudan SA*, Vernier, for generous support of this work.

References

Evans, D. A. and Britton, T. C. (1987). Electrophilic azide transfer to chiral enolates. A general approach to the asymmetric synthesis of α-amino acids. *J. Am. Chem. Soc.* **109**, 6881–6883.

Evans, D. A., Britton, T. C., Dorow, R. L. and Dellaria, J. F. (1986). Stereoselective amination of chiral enolates. A new approach to the asymmetric synthesis of α-hydrazino and α-amino acid derivatives. *J. Am. Chem. Soc.* **108**, 6395–6397.

Evans, D. A., Ellman, J. A. and Dorow, R. L. (1987). Asymmetric halogenation of chiral imide enolates. A general approach to the synthesis of enantiomerically pure α-amino acids. *Tetrahedron Lett.* **28**, 1123–1126.

Evans, D. A., Britton, T. C., Dorow, R. L. and Dellaria, J. F. (1988). The asymmetric synthesis of α-amino and α-hydrazino acid derivatives via the stereoselective amination of chiral enolates with azodicarboxylate esters. *Tetrahedron* **44**, 5525–5540.

Gennari, C., Colombo, L. and Bertolini, G. (1986). Asymmetric electrophilic amination: synthesis of α-amino and α-hydrazino acids with high optical purity. *J. Am. Chem. Soc.* **108**, 6394–6395.

Loreto, M. A., Pellacani, L. and Tardella, P. A. (1989). Asymmetric synthesis of N-substituted α-amino esters. *Tetrahedron Lett.* **30**, 2975.

Oppolzer, W. (1987). Camphor derivatives as chiral auxiliaries in asymmetric synthesis. *Tetrahedron* **43**, 1969–2004. Erratum. *Tetrahedron* **43**, 4057.

Oppolzer, W. (1988). Metal-directed stereoselective functionalisations of alkenes in organic synthesis. *Pure Appl. Chem.* **60**, 39–48.

Oppolzer, W. and Bossard, P. (1990). In preparation.

Oppolzer, W. and Moretti, R. (1986). Enantioselective syntheses of α-amino acids from 10-(aminosulfonyl)-2-bornyl esters and di(*tert*-butyl) azodicarboxylate. *Helv. Chim. Acta* **69**, 1923–1926.

Oppolzer, W. and Moretti, R. (1988). Enantioselective syntheses of α-amino acids from 10-sulfonamido-isobornyl esters and di-*t*-butyl azodicarboxylate. *Tetrahedron* **44**, 5541–5552.

Oppolzer, W. and Tamura, O. (1990). Asymmetric synthesis of α-amino acids and α-N-hydroxyamino acids via electrophilic amination of bornanesultam-derived enolates with 1-chloro-1-nitrosocyclohexane. *Tetrahedron Lett.* **31**, 991–994.

Oppolzer, W., Chapuis, C. and Bernardinelli, G. (1984). Camphor-derived N-aryloyl and N-crotonoyl sultams: Practical activated dienophiles in asymmetric Diels–Alder Reactions. *Helv. Chim. Acta* **67**, 1397–1401.

Oppolzer, W., Pedrosa, R. and Moretti, R. (1986). Asymmetric syntheses of α-amino acids from α-halogenated 10-sulfonamido-isobornyl esters. *Tetrahedron Lett.* **27**, 831–834.

Oppolzer, W., Poli, G., Kingma, A. J., Starkemann, C. and Bernardinelli, G. (1987). Asymmetric induction at C(β) and C(α) of N-enoylsultams by organo-magnesium 1,4-addition/enolate trapping. *Helv. Chim. Acta* **70**, 2201–2214.

Oppolzer, W., Moretti, R. and Thomi, S. (1989). Asymmetric alkylations of sultam-derived glycinate equivalent: practical preparation of enantiomerically pure α-amino acids. *Tetrahedron Lett.* **30**, 6009–6010.

Trimble, L. A. and Vederas, J. C. (1986). Amination of chiral enolates by dialkyl azodiformates. Synthesis of α-hydrazino acids and α-amino acid. *J. Am. Chem. Soc.* **108**, 6397–6399.

Williams, R. M. (1989). Synthesis of optically active α-amino acids. *Organic Chemistry Series*, Vol. 7. Pergamon Press, Oxford.

Appendix: Abstracts of Posters

Contents

Mechanistic Studies on Chiral Drugs

215

Analytical Aspects

Enantioselective Synthesis

Mechanistic Studies on Chiral Drugs

Steric influences on the opioid properties of hybrid PCP/4-arylpiperidine derivatives. A. F. Casy, G. H. Dewar and Omar, A. A. Al-Deeb. *School of Pharmacy and Pharmacology, University of Bath, BA2 7AY, UK*

The pharmacological classification of phencyclidine (PCP) is unsettled. It has stimulant, depressant, hallucinogenic and analgesic properties. Like N-allylnormetazocine it binds to the σ-receptor while there is evidence of its own specific receptor [1]. Analogues of PCP which incorporate elements of the reversed ester of pethidine, e.g. **1c**, exhibit antinociceptive actions and displace [^{3}H]morphine from binding sites [2]. To probe the receptor preferences of **1c**, α- and β-3-methyl analogues have been prepared and their opioid properties compared with those of α- and β-prodine (reversed esters). Target compounds were obtained by use of the *sec*-amines (**2**) in the Strecker reaction (cyclohexanone, KCN) followed by PhMgBr. NMR features of the products confirmed retention of the stereochemistry of the precursors. Antipodes of **1a** were obtained from (R)- and (S)-**2** (α-Me). In the rat-tail-withdrawal (RTW) test ED_{50} (mg kg^{-1}) values were: *rac*-**1a** 1.0, *rac*-**1b** 2.5, (3(R)-**1a** 1.25, (3S)-**1a** > 2.5, morphine

a. R = α-Me (t to 4-Ph)
b. R = β-Me (c to 4-Ph)
c. R = H

(1)   (2)

3.15. In the tail-flick test in mice $(3R)$-**1a** was twice as active as the racemate, and its antipode almost inactive. Binding ED_{50} (nM) values were *rac*-**1a** 680, morphine 23.6, pethidine 6000, and EC_{50} values in the mouse vas deferens test were *rac*-**1a** 14.2×10^{-7}, morphine 3.95×10^{-7}. Thus stereo-SA relationships of the PCP analogues **1** mirror those of α-prodine in regard to C3 chirality ($3R$ eutomer in both series) but diverge in respect of relative geometry at C3 and C4 ($\alpha > \beta$ for **1**, $\beta > \alpha$ for prodines) [3]. Acetylation of *rac*-**1a** lowers its RTW potency to 2.5 mg kg^{-1} (acyl group essential in prodines). *Rac*-**1a** lacked affinity for the TCP receptor (Ki > 1000 nM, PCP 60) [4].

We conclude that the hybrid PCP/4-arylpiperidines **1** associate with opioid rather than PCP receptors but with a binding mode that differs from that of reversed esters of pethidine. Derivatives **1** may relate more closely to opioids in which 4-phenyl-4-piperidinol is linked through nitrogen to a $CH_2CH(H$ or Me)N(COEt)Ph chain (activity also reduced on *O*-acylation) [3]. We thank Mr K. Schellekens and Dr A. E. Jacobson for the biological data.

[1] Casy, A. F. (1989). *Adv. Drug. Res.* **18**, 177.
[2] Itzkak, Y., Kalir, A., Weissman, B. A. and Cohen, S. (1981). *J. Med. Chem.* **24**, 496.
[3] Casy, A. F. and Parfitt, R. T. (1986). *Opioid Analgesics: Chemistry and Receptors*. Plenum Press, New York.
[4] Rafferty, M. F., Mattson, M., Jacobson, A. E. and Rice, K. C. (1985). *FEBS Lett.* **181**, 318.

Ca^{2+} Sensitizing and Phosphodiesterase (PDE) Inhibiting Effects of the Stereoisomers of a Novel Positive Inotropic Thiadiazinylindolone (TDI). G. Nadler, Ph. Lahouratate and M. J. Quiniou. *Les Laboratoires Beecham, BP 58, 35762 Saint-Grégoire, France*

Experiments were carried out on new TDIs designed for positive inotropic properties (compounds **I–III**) and on the (+) and (−) enantiomers of compound **III**, i.e. compounds **IV** and **V**, respectively (obtained after deprotection of the chromatographically resolved diastereoisomeric mixture of compounds synthesized from **III** by condensation with (−)-menthylchloroformate).

The sensitization of the myocardial contractile proteins to calcium was assessed on the canine cardiac myofibrillar Ca^{2+} dependent Mg^{2+}-ATPase (MF-ATPase) [1] and on rabbit chemically skinned cardiac fibres (SF) [2] by measuring the shift of the pCa–MF-ATPase curve (at the compound's concentration of 200 μM), and of the pCa–tension curve (at 50 μM of compounds), respectively. The data were expressed as the shift in the negative logarithm of Ca^{2+} concentration required for half maximal activation (ΔpCa_{50}). The inhibition of cardiac PDE was assessed on the rabbit cardiac c-GMP inhibited soluble subtype (CGI) [3] as well as on the canine cardiac sarcoplasmic reticulum-bound (SR) [4] high-affinity c-AMP PDE.

Compound	R_1	R_2	
I	H	H	
II	CH_3	CH_3	
III	CH_3	H	(Racemate)

Results: mean n = 3 to 4

	Ca^{2+} sensitization ΔpCa$_{50}$		c-AMP–PDE inhibition IC$_{50}$ (μM)	
Compound	MF-ATPase	SF	CGI	SR
I	0.16	nt	nt	0.64
II	−0.02	nt	nt	66.00
III	0.31^a	0.13^a	0.65	0.32
IV	0.43^a	0.20^a	5.8	4.20
V	−0.13^a	−0.01	0.77	0.24

^{a} $p < 0.05$ (Student's paired t-test).
nt, not tested.

The data show that the substitution of the thiadiazine ring plays an important role in Ca^{2+} sensitization and inhibition of PDEs. Considering compound **III**, it appears that the (−) enantiomer (**V**) is mainly responsible for the PDE inhibitory effect, whereas the (+) enantiomer (**IV**) mediates the calcium sensitising effect. Such compounds could be valuable tools for the assessment of the relevance of Ca^{2+} sensitization in positive inotropism.

[1] Solaro, R. J. and Ruegg, J. C. (1982). *Circ. Res.* **51**, 290.
[2] Ventura-Clapier, R. and Vassort, G. (1985). *Pflügers Arch.* **404**, 157.
[3] Kariya, T. and Dage, R. C. (1988). *Biochem. Pharmacol.* **37**, 3267.
[4] Kauffman, R. F., Crowe, V. G., Utterback, B. G. and Robertson, D. W. (1986). *Mol. Pharmacol.* **30**, 609.

Synthesis of Isotopically Chiral [^{13}C]-Penciclovir (BRL 39123) and its use to Determine the Absolute Configuration of Penciclovir Triphosphate formed in Herpes Virus Infected Cells.

R. L. Jarvest[a], D. Barnes[b], D. L. Earnshaw[a], K. J. O'Toole[b], J. T. Sime[b] and R. A. Vere Hodge[a]. *Beecham Pharmaceuticals Research Division: [a]Great Burgh, Yew Tree Bottom Road, Epsom, Surrey KT18 5XQ, UK; [b]Brockham Park, Betchworth, Surrey RH3 7AJ, UK*

Penciclovir (BRL 39123, 9-(4-hydroxy-3-hydroxymethylbut-1-yl) guanine, **1**) is a potent and selective anti-herpesvirus agent, particularly against herpes simplex types 1 and 2 (HSV-1 and 2) and varicella zoster virus (1–3]. Currently penciclovir is undergoing clinical trials for efficacy against herpes virus infections. When HSV-1 infected cells are treated with penciclovir, high intracellular concentrations of its triphosphate ester are produced, whereas low or undetectable levels of the triphosphate are formed in uninfected cells [4]. Formation of this triphosphate is believed to be essential for the inhibition of viral DNA synthesis and hence for the observed antiviral effect of penciclovir. Phosphorylation of one of the hydroxymethyl groups of penciclovir creates a chiral centre. We have determined the stereospecificity and absolute configuration of penciclovir triphosphate formed in HSV-1 infected cells.

1 • = ^{12}C, ■ = ^{12}C
2 • = ^{12}C, ■ = ^{13}C
3 • = ^{13}C, ■ = ^{12}C

(4)

We synthesized penciclovir in isotopically chiral form by incorporating ^{13}C into one of the hydroxymethyl groups, namely compounds 2 and 3. A suitable synthetic intermediate ^{13}C-labelled ester that could be elaborated to penciclovir was subject to enzymic hydrolysis by the lipase from *Candida cylindraceae*. The recovered ester was obtained with ≥ 97% enantiomeric purity and the acid product was reesterified to the enantiomeric ester which was found to have an enantiomer ratio of 85 : 15. The absolute configuration of the enantiomerically pure ester was established by conversion to a known lactone. Reduction of the enantiomeric esters afforded isotopically enantiomeric diols which were converted to 2 and 3, respectively.

Cultured MRC-5 cells which had been infected with HSV-1 were put into a medium containing 2 or 3. The intracellular phosphates were extracted and purified by **HPLC**, collecting the peak of similar retention time to synthetic (racemic) penciclovir triphosphate. The ^{13}C NMR spectra of the triphosphates were recorded and it was found that the triphosphate derived from 2 has the ^{13}C in the CH$_2$OH moiety and the triphosphate derived from 3 has the ^{13}C in the CH$_2$OP moiety. The absolute configuration of penciclovir triphosphate produced in HSV-1 infected cells is thus (*S*) as shown in 4. It is estimated that the enantiomeric purity of the intracellular triphosphate in HSV-1 infected cells is > 95%.

[1] Harnden, M. R., Jarvest, R. L., Bacon, T. H. and Boyd, M. R. (1987). *J. Med. Chem.* **30**, 1636,
[2] Boyd, M. R., Bacon, T. H., Sutton, D. and Cole, M. (1987). *Antimicrob. Agents Chemother.* **31**, 1238.
[3] Boyd, M. R., Bacon, T. H. and Sutton, D. (1988). *Antimicrob. Agents Chemother.* **32**, 358.
[4] Vere Hodge, R. A. and Perkins, R. M. (1989). *Antimicrob. Agents Chemother.* **33**, 223.

Stereochemistry of Chiral Lipophilic Dihydrofolate Reductase Inhibitors. W. K. Chui. *Pharmaceutical Sciences Institute, Department of Pharmaceutical Sciences, Aston University, Aston Triangle, Birmingham B4 7ET, UK*

Dihydrofolate reductase (DHFR) catalyses the reduction of 7,8-dihydrofolic acid (FH$_2$) to 5,6,7,8-tetrahydrofolic acid (FH$_4$) by using NADPH as a coenzyme. FH$_4$ is used in a series of one-carbon transfer reactions which lead to the biosynthesis of DNA. Inhibition of DHFR depletes the pool of FH_4 which subsequently causes cell death. Such inhibitors have been used as antibacterial, antimalarial and antitumour agents. 1,2-Dihydro-s-triazines, which are non-classical lipophilic DHFR inhibitors, are studied in this project. It has been found that the inhibitory action of these compounds depends on the position of the substituents on the aryl ring. The *ortho* substituted triazine antifolates show reduced inhibitory activity [1]. This may be attributed to the existence of chiral atropisomers which may exhibit different affinity for the enzyme.

4,6-Diamino-2,2-dialkyl-1,2-dihydro-1-(*ortho*-substituted phenyl)-1,3,5-triazines have been synthesized by the three-component method [2]. The *ortho* substituent restricts rotation about the C–N bond causing the phenyl ring to adopt a perpendicular conformation to the triazine ring [3]. The energy barrier to rotation has been calculated by the use of molecular modelling technique. Enrichment of the enantiomeric atropisomers has been attempted by formation of diastereomeric salt and diastereomeric derivatisation. Diastereomeric atropisomers have been synthesized and studied by NMR spectrocopy. Separation of the chiral atropisomers has been achieved by the use of semi-preparative liquid chromatography. Each atropisomer is being tested for inhibitory activity against the enzyme DHFR.

[1] Kim, K. H., Dietrich, S. W., Hansch, C., Dolnick, B. J. and Bertino, J. R. (1980). *J. Med. Chem.* **23**, 1248.
[2] Modest, E. J. (1956). *J. Org. Chem.* **21**, 1.
[3] Cody, V. and Sutton, P. A. (1987). *Anti-Cancer Drug Design* **2**, 253.

Consideration of enantiomers of 3-ethyl-3-(4-pyridyl) piperidine-2,6-dione and the N-alkyl Derivatives Explains Curious Aromatase Inhibitory Activity Data. R. McCague,[1] C. A. Laughton,[2] M. G. Rowlands,[1] M. Jarman[1] and S. Neidle[2]. *Drug Development Section*[1] *and Cancer Research Campaign Biomolecular Structure Unit,* [2]*Institute of Cancer Research, Sutton, Surrey, SM2 5NG, UK*

The pyridylglutarimide 3-ethyl-3-(4-pyridyl)piperidine-2,6-dione (PG) is an inhibitor of the enzyme aromatase that converts androgens into oestrogens and is presently undergoing clinical trial for the treatment of hormone dependent breast cancer. Its enantiomers have been prepared [1] through separation of diastereoisomers obtained after appropriate alkylation of the ester formed between 4-pyridylacetic acid and Oppolzer's camphor derived secondary alcohol chiral auxiliary. Activity essentially resides in the (*R*)-enantiomer [1].

Upon alkylation of the imide nitrogen of racemic PG, the aromatase inhibitory activity profile on proceeding to successively longer N-alkyl chains is curious. Activity declines by about 30-fold in the N-ethyl-PG and then increases dramatically reaching a maximum at N-octyl-PG which is about 20-fold more potent than the parent PG [2]. This profile has been explained through molecular modelling studies where in PG the glutarimide nitrogen maps onto C2 of the steroid substrate but the N-octyl-PG binds in a different mode with the nitrogen mapping C4 of the steroid where the enzyme is thought to possess a hydrophobic pocket [3]. Testing of the enantiomers of N-octyl-PG, prepared by alkylation of (*R*)- and (*S*)-PG individually, allows this hypothesis of different binding modes to be confirmed since now, in contrast to PG, it is the *S* enantiomer that is active and *R* inactive. This study underlines the importance of considering enantiomers when comparing a drug with the natural substrate.

[1] McCague, R., Jarman, M., Rowlands, M. G., Mann, J., Thickett, C. P., Clissold, D. W., Neidle, S. and Webster, G. (1989). *J. Chem. Soc., Perkin Trans.* 1, 196.
[2] Leung, C. -S., Rowlands, M. G., Jarman, M., Foster, A. B., Griggs, L. J. and Wilman, D. E. V., (1987). *J. Med. Chem.* **30**, 1550.
[3] Banting, L., Smith, H. J., James, M., Jones, G., Nazareth, W., Nichols, P. J., Hewlins, M. J. E. and Rowlands, M. G. (1989). *J. Enzyme Inhibition* **2**, 215.

Stereomutation in 4-Arylaminoquinolines. R. J. Ife, C. A. Leach, P. J. Moore, E. S. Pepper and A. D. Shore. *Smith Kline & French Research Ltd, The Frythe, Welwyn, Hertfordshire, AL6 9AR, UK*

It has been reported that hindered 1-naphthylamines having different substituents at the N atom, give rise to a pair of enantiometric conformers [1]. We have observed similar results with 4-arylaminoquinolines. The aromatic tertiary amines SK&F 96048, 96079 and 97630 were all synthesized for testing as reversible H^+/K^+ ATPase inhibitors. The proton spectrum of SK&F 96048 shows two 'deceptively simple' triplets for isochronous protons in ring methylene groups and a similar result was observed with 97630. However, for SK&F 96079, it is clear that all protons in the two methylene groups have different proton chemical shifts. It is suggested that the reason for anisochronous methylene protons in SK&F 96079 is restricted rotation about the C(1')–N bond. Dynamic NMR at elevated temperature has been used to investigate the equilibrium between enantiomers in this class of compounds. Examples of a related group of reversible H^+/K^+-ATPase inhibitors are SK&F 97884 and SK&F 97704. In this case the rigid five-membered ring is replaced by 3-alkyryl and 4-arylamino groups with the potential for intramolecular hydrogen bonding. These two molecules also contain prochiral probes. Dynamic NMR at lower temperatures than ambient has been used to investigate enantiomerisation. Throughout the temperature range studied, the chemical shifts of the N protons in [²H]chloroform remains unchanged which supports intramolecular hydrogen bonding.

SK&F 96048 $R_1 = R_2 = H$; $R_3 = OMe$
SK&F 96079 $R_1 = Me$; $R_2 = H$; $R_3 = OMe$
SK&F 97630 $R_1 = R_2 = Me$; $R_3 = H$

SK&F 97884 $R_1 = F$; $R_2 = H$; $R_3 = CH_2OH$; $R_4 = CHMe_2$
SK&F 97704 $R_1 = R_3 = H$; $R_2 = CH_2OH$; $R_4 = CH_2CH_2CH_3$

[1] Casarini, D. and Lunazzi, L. (1988). *J. Org. Chem.* **53**, 182.

Role of a 5-Methyl Group in Dihydropyridazinone Inodilators: PDE III Activity of Enantiomers.

S. J. Bakewell, W. J. Coates, B. J. Connolly, S. T. Flynn, R. Novelli, B. H. Warrington and A. Worby. *Departments of Medicinal Chemistry and Cellular Pharmacology, Smith Kline & French Research Ltd, The Frythe, Welwyn, Hertfordshire, AL6 9AR, UK*

The role of a 5-methyl group in inodilator 4,5-dihydropyridazin-3-(2H)-ones (DHP) has been investigated by assessing the PDE III inhibitory activity of 6-(4-acetamidophenyl) derivatives. Representative results are summarized in the table. An eight-fold increase in activity was seen on introduction of a psuedo-axial 5-methyl group into DHP, but activity was decreased in the corresponding pyridazinone (P) and by a methyl substituent at alternative adjacent positions in DHP or P; the 5,5-dimethyl DHP was inactive. Enhanced activity of the 5-methyl DHP is due entirely to the $R(-)$ enantiomer; this was also true for 2-cyano-1-methyl-3-guanidino (CYGU) and 4-pyridinon-1-yl (PN) analogues. There is some evidence that the $S(+)$ enantiomers show reduced activity compared with the nor-methyl analogues.

The activity of bicyclic DHP was maintained in coplanar tricyclic DHP and P but introduction of the appropriate methyl group into tricyclic DHP did not result in the marked increase in activity seen with bicyclic DHP. Introduction of a 9a-methyl group into the indenothiadizinone did not increase activity, but the observed activity was again due to the $R(-)$ enantiomer and the $S(+)$ enantiomer was less active than the nor-methyl compound.

Reduced activity seen with the alternative methyl groups including $S(+)$-5 indicates a

X	R	R¹	R²	R³	R⁴	R⁵	PDE III IC₅₀ᵃ	PDE III IC₅₀ᵃ $R(-)$	PDE III IC₅₀ᵃ $S(+)$
C	NHCOCH₃	H	H	H	H	H	7.13		
C	NHCOCH₃	H	CH₃	H	H	H	0.9	0.69,	44%
C	NHCOCH₃	H	H	H		db	6.38		
C	NHCOCH₃	H	CH₃	H		db	97		
C	NHCOCH₃	–CH₂–		H	H	H	3.74		
C	NHCOCH₃	–CH₂–		H	CH₃	H	10.30		
C	NHCOCH₃	–CH₂–		H		db	13.40		
C	NHCOCH₃	–(CH₂)₂–		H	H	H	16.50		
C	NHCOCH₃	–(CH₂)₂–		H	CH₃	H	4.75		
C	NHCOCH₃	–(CH₂)₂–		H		db	4.76		
S	NHCOCH₃	–CH₂–		—	H	—	1.34		
S	NHCOCH₃	–CH₂–		—	CH₃	—	1.75	0.40,	6.12
C	CYGU	H	H	H	H	H	32.82		
C	CYGU	H	CH₃	H	H	H	2.84	1.78,	52.3
C	PN	H	H	H	H	H	5.09		
C	PN	H	CH₃	H	H	H	0.5	0.35,	5.25

ᵃ [Conc.] × 10⁻⁶ M for 50% inhibition of G-P ventricular PDE III, or percentage inhibition at 10⁻⁴ M.

224   Appendix: Abstracts of Posters

sterically demanding active site, while enhanced activity for $R(-)$-5-methyl substituted DHP is consistent with a specific lipophilic binding site for the methyl group [1]. However, the absence of similar enhancement of activity in the tricyclics indicates that another factor (such as damped inversion of the DHP ring) may be partly responsible for enhanced activity of 5-methyl DHP.

[1] Moos, W. H., Humblet, C. C., Sircar, I., Rithner, C., Weishaar, R. E. and Bristol, J. A. (1987). *J. Med. Chem.* **30**, 1963.
[2] [Conc.] × 10^{-6} M for 50% inhibition of G-P ventricular PDE III, or % inhibition at 10^{-4} M.

Analytical Aspects

The Use of Chiral Matrices in FAB Mass Spectrometry as an Aid in Determining Configuration. N. J. Haskins and A. P. New. *Smith Kline & French Research Ltd, The Frythe, Welwyn, Hertfordshire AL6 9AR, UK*

The use of diisopropyltartrate as a chiral FAB matrix has been reported previously [1]. Our studies have concentrated on the use of this matrix to discriminate between D- and L-amino acids and results are presented to show that more stable cluster ions are formed with the 'correct' adduct. Boric acid has been used in combination with *cis* diols to form stable cyclic borate esters [2]. Work has commenced to use this in conjunction with FAB-MS in the study of saccharides.

[1] Baldwin, M. A., Howell, S. A. Welham, K. J. and Winkler, F. J. (1987). *Proc. BMSS Conf.* **16**, 32–35.
[2] Rose, M. E., Longstaff, C. and Dean, P. D. G. (1983). *Biomed. Mass Spectrom.* **10**, 512–527.

The Determination of the Enantiomeric Excess of Fenoldopam by Inclusion Complexation using Nuclear Magnetic Resonance (NMR) Spectroscopy. J. J. Richards and M. L. Webb. *Smith Kline Beecham Research Ltd, Old Powder Mills, Tonbridge, Kent, UK*

Fenoldopam, a compound currently in development at SmithKline Beecham for the treatment of high blood pressure, contains one asymmetric centre. Some proton NMR signals due to the individual enantiomers have been obtained in D_2O after formation of an inclusion complex with β-cyclodextrin allowing the determination of enantiomeric excess to take place. One of the two benzene rings in fenoldopam is thought to be included into the cavity of the sugar molecule allowing interactions to take place within a hydrophobic environment. This method allows rapid chiral analysis of some polar molecules and salts by NMR spectroscopy.

Enantioselective Synthesis

Novel Access to Chiral Acetylenic and Allenic Amino Acids using Flash Vacuum Pyrolysis. R. A. Aitken and H. R. Cooper. *Department of Chemistry, University of St Andrews, St Andrews, Fife KY16 9ST, UK*

Several α-ethynylamine analogues of the naturally occuring amino acids (**1**) and their allene isomers (**2**) are powerful irreversible enzyme inhibitors and show promising biological activity. In an attempt to prepare these from amino acids (**3**) we have examined the flash vacuum pyrolysis (FVP) of stabilised phosphorus ylides (**4**).

R = Me, Pr^i, Bu^i
Bu^s, CH$_2$Ph

At 500°C the expected extrusion of Ph$_3$PO is accompanied by a **1,3-migration of the phthalimido group** to give allenic α-amino acid derivatives (**5**). For a range of R groups this proceeds with good retention of chirality providing a convenient potential route to allenic amino acids (**7**) and their acetylenic isomers (**6**).

Chiras™: The REACCS Database of Asymmetric Synthesis.

M. Rider,[1] G. Grethe,[1] D. Jeffrey,[1] and K. T. Taylor.[2] *Molecular Design Limited, 2132 Farallon Drive, San Leandro, CA 94577, [2]Molecular Design (UK) Limited, Southwood Summit Centre, Southwood, Hampshire GU14 0NR*

CHIRAS™ is the first comprehensive, structure-based, computer-searchable database of asymmetric syntheses. It provides rapid access to asymmetric synthesis methodology including: chiral auxiliaries, chiral pool reactions, and enzyme and microbiological mediated processes. CHIRAS™ also contains fully searchable optical yield data and specific rotations of important, optically pure starting materials. These features combine to make CHIRAS™ an invaluable and powerful tool for the design of enantioselective syntheses. This poster will illustrate the application of CHIRAS™ in asymmetric synthesis and an operational system will be available for use by delegates.

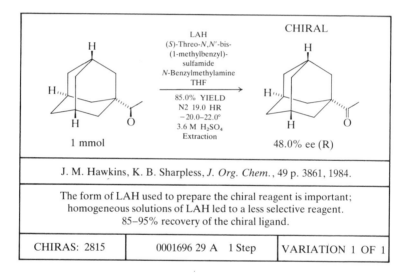

J. M. Hawkins, K. B. Sharpless, *J. Org. Chem.*, 49 p. 3861, 1984.		
The form of LAH used to prepare the chiral reagent is important; homogeneous solutions of LAH led to a less selective reagent. 85–95% recovery of the chiral ligand.		
CHIRAS: 2815	0001696 29 A 1 Step	VARIATION 1 OF 1

Chiral Recognition in the Reaction of an Inositol Triflate with the Enolate Derived from $[(\eta^5\text{-}C_5H_5)Fe(CO)(PPh_3)COCH_3]$. J. Mistry

and M. Voyle. *Department of Synthetic and Isotope Chemistry, Smith Kline & French Research Ltd, The Frythe, Welwyn, Hertfordshire AL6 9AR, UK*

The synthesis of analogues of members of the inositol cycle will be crucial in obtaining further insight into the biological importance of the cycle. The inositol triflate (1) is a common,

(1)   (2)

racemic, intermediate for the synthesis of phosphatidylinositols, which is efficiently prepared from *myo*-inositol. A kinetic resolution of this intermediate has been attempted. Treatment of the triflate with the enolate derived from optically pure $[(\eta^5\text{-}C_5H_5)Fe(CO)(PPh_3)COCH_3]$ gave the substituted inositol **2** as a single diastereoisomer in 19% yield. The starting triflate was recovered in 46% yield but was shown to have a low enantiomeric excess. This is explained by the occurrence of enantiomerically enriched products of elimination. Attempts to prevent the elimination reactions were unsuccessful. The yield of the substituted inositol **2** was increased to 29% and decomplexation was readily achieved.

Asymmetric Synthesis of α-Alkylated Tryptophan Derivatives for Incorporation with Novel CCK Ligands. G. Bourne, D. C. Horwell and M. Pritchard. *Parke-Davis Research Unit, Addenbrookes Hospital Site, Hills Road, Cambridge CB2 2QB, UK*

Cholecystokinin (CCK 26–33) (**1**) is a polypeptide distributed in mammalian central nervous system, and the gastrointestinal tract which is involved in the modulation of many physiological processes [1]. At Parke-Davis chemical research has focussed on the synthesis of 'dipeptoid' analogues of CCK [2]. Our approach [3] has led to the synthesis of α-Me–Trp–Phe–NH₂ derivatives (e.g. **2**) with micromolar affinity for the CCKB receptor, where the α-Me group stabilizes the peptide bond towards both acid and enzymatic degradation [4]. The success of this strategy prompted the need for an efficient asymmetric synthesis of α-alkylated tryptophan derivatives.

This poster describes the results of a collaborative project with Crich and Davies [5] where, for the first time, positive advantage is taken of the reactive nature of the indole group in tryptophan, to give the enolate **3** which can be alkylated with complete diastereoselectivity from the *exo* face to give either [D] or [L] α-alkyl tryptophan derivatives in good chemical yields.

26   27   28   29   30   31   32   33
Asp–Tyr(SO₃H)–Met–Gly–Trp–Met–Asp–Phe–NH₂   (1)

Boc–[D]–α–Me–Trp–L–Phe–NH₂   (2)

(3)

[1] de Belleroche, J. and Dockray, G. J. (eds) (1984). *Cholecystokinin in the Nervous System*, Ellis Horwood, Chichester.
[2] Horwell, D. C., Beeby, A, Clarke, C. and Hughes, J. (1987). *J. Med. Chem.* **30**, 729.
[3] Horwell, D. C. (1988). Peptoids from CCK-8. *Topics in Medicinal Chemistry, 4th SCI-RSC Medicinal Chemistry Symposium* (ed. P. R. Leeming) Royal Society of Chemistry Special Publication. No. 65. Royal Society of Chemistry, London.
[4] Horwell, D. C., Birchmore, B., Boden, P. R., Higginbottom, M., Ping Ho, Y., Hughes, J., Hunter, J. C. and Richardson, R. S. (1990). *Eur. J. Med, Chem.* **25**, 53.
[5] Crich, D. and Davies, J. W. (1989). *J. Chem. Soc., Chem. Commun.* 1418.

A New Chiral Synthon for the Enantioselective Synthesis of Methylcyclohexenone Derivatives. G. Potter. *Drug Development Section, Institute of Cancer Research, Sutton, Surrey SM2 5NG, UK*

We are interested in synthesizing compounds bearing the methylcyclohexenone group, present in the A ring of important steroid hormones, as potential drugs for the treatment of hormone-dependent cancers. Since these are chiral compounds it is necessary to investigate the biological activity of individual enantiomers. The utility of the tricarbonyl(4-methoxy-1-methyl-cyclohexadienylium)iron cation as a versatile synthon for constructing the methylcyclo-hexenone group has been amply demonstrated by the work of Birch [1] and Pearson and Chandler [2]. This complex can be employed in enantioselective synthesis, but the preparation of the complex in an enantiomerically pure form involves an indirect multistep approach [3]. This complex also suffers from the disadvantage of producing regioisomers upon nucleophilic attack.

The iron dienyl complex (**1**), bearing a (+)-menthoxy group in place of a methoxy group, is conveniently synthesized, and readily obtained as a single diasteriomer. Addition of a suitable nucleophile to (**1**) proceeds in an enantiospecific fashion, on the face opposite the iron atom. Nucleophilic attack also proceeds with complete regioselectivity at the methyl substituted terminus, even with hindered nucleophiles, owing to the steric bulk of the menthyl group. Decomplexation of the resultant iron diene complex followed by hydrolysis of the menthoxy diene liberates the optically pure methylcyclohexenone derivative (**2**). Due to the directness of this approach, and the prevalence of the methylcyclohexenone group in natural products, the new chiral synthon (**1**) is expected to have considerable synthetic utility.

(1)   (2)

[1] Birch, A. J. (1981). *Tetrahedron*, **37**, (Suppl. 1), 289–302.
[2] Pearson, A. J. and Chandler, M. (1980). *J. Chem. Soc., Perkin Trans. 1*, 2238–2243.
[3] Howell, J. A. and Thomas, M. J. (1985). *Organometallics* **4**, 1054–1059.

Optically Active Drugs and Intermediates from Chiral Cyanohydrins.

J. Brussee,[1] C. G. Kruse,[2] and A. van der Gen.[1] [1]*Department of Chemistry, Gorlaeus Laboratories, Leiden University, P.O. Box 9502, 2300 RA Leiden, The Netherlands.*[2] *Duphar B.V., P.O. Box 2, 1380 AA Weesp, The Netherlands*

Cyanohydrins are versatile starting materials for the synthesis of several classes of compounds such as α-hydroxyacids (-esters), vicinal diols, α-hydroxyketones, β-amino alcohols and amino acids. Using the enzyme oxynitrilase (E.C. 4.1.2.10), from almonds, we were able to prepare optically active cyanohydrins from such different aldehydes as benzaldehyde, 4-methoxy-benzaldehyde, 5-methyl furfural, piperonal, crotonaldehyde and butyraldehyde in good yield and of high enantiomeric purity [1]. Protection of the hydroxyl group with t-butyldimethylsilyl chloride (TBS-Cl) in DMF afforded stable chiral O-silyl cyanohydrins, which were shown to be excellent starting materials for a number of interesting transformations. Optically active O-protected α-hydroxyketones (acyloins) were prepared by reaction with alkyl Grignard reagents [2], followed by hydrolytic work-up. Direct reduction with $NaBH_4$ of the Grignard imine intermediates afforded N-unsubstituted β-aminoalcohols (e.g. norephedrine). Chiral induction lead to preferential formation of the erythro stereoisomers ($1R,2S$). The products were obtained in good yield and high enantiomeric excess [3]. N-Substituted β-aminoalcohols were synthesized by reductive amination of the optically active O protected acyloins (see below). $NaBH_3CN$ as reducing agent gave a fair amount of chiral induction (80–90% erythro) but separation of diastereomers remained necessary. When $Mg(ClO_4)_2$ was used as a complexing agent, imine formation was very fast and complete. Reduction of these complexed imine intermediates with $NaBH_4$ at low temperature afforded nearly quantitative yields of erythro β-aminoalcohols (e.g. ephedrine). Ethanolamines with one chiral centre could be obtained by $LiAlH_4$ reduction of O-TBS protected cyanohydrins. Remarkable is the quantitative removal of the TBS group under these conditions. Some examples of compounds obtained in optically pure form by the above methodology are presented below.

[1] Brussee, J., Loos, W. T., Kruse, C. G. and Van der Gen, A. (1990). *Tetrahedron* in press.
[2] Brussee, J., Roos, E. C. and Van der Gen, A. (1988). *Tetrahedron Lett.* **29**, 4485.
[3] Brussee, J., Dofferhoff, F., Kruse, C. G. and Van der Gen, A. (1990). *Tetrahedron* in press.

trans-1,3-Dithiane-1,3-dioxide as a Potential Chiral Acyl Anion Equivalent.

V. K. Aggarwal and R. J. Franklin. *School of Chemistry, University of Bath, BA2 7AY, UK*

The use of *trans*-1,3-dithiane-1,3-dioxide as a potential chiral acyl anion equivalent is being investigated. This material has been prepared with high diastereoselectivity (95 : 5, *trans* : *cis*) by oxidation of 1,3-dithiane with sodium periodiate. Compound (1) is highly polar and is only soluble in strongly polar solvents. However, anion reactions with aldehydes have been successfully carried out in pyridine/THF mixtures using n-BuLi as base. In this system, it is the n-BuLi-pyridine adduct that acts as the base.

Reactions carried out at −78°C are under kinetic control and adducts are formed in good yield but with low diastereocontrol (30% diasteriomeric excess (de)). Equilibration occurs with some aldehydes at 0°C to give adducts with improved diastereoselectivity (70% de) [1]. Greater diastereoselectivities are obtained using sodium and potassium counterions, under thermodynamic conditions, with bases that do not react with pyridine. For example reaction of **1** with sodium hexamethyldisilazide and benzaldehyde at 0°C leads to formation of adducts **3** and **4** in 92% de. The relative stereochemistry of the adducts was determined by recording their X-ray crystal structures.

4:96   87%

[1] Aggarwal, V. K., Davies, I. W., Maddock, J., Mahon, M. F. and Molloy, K. C. (1990). *Tetrahedron Lett.* 135.

The Stereoselective Synthesis and Analysis of Two Potential Chloride Channel Blockers. S. Richardson, D. R. Reavill, P. Camilleri, C. Dyke, and J. A. Murphy. *Smith Kline & French Research Ltd, The Frythe, Welwyn, Hertfordshire AL6 9AR, UK.*

The epithelial chloride channel has recently been the subject of a great deal of attention due to its importance in transmembrane chloride transport. Defects in the regulation of chloride channels appear to be associated with pathological conditions such as secretory diarrhoea [1] and cystic fibrosis [2]. Early evidence that N-phenylanthranilic acid acted as a reversible blocker of the chloride conductance [3] led to a search for compounds with increased activity. A survey of over 200 compounds tested for inhibition of chloride mediated short-circuit current in single isolated rabbit nephron identified NPPB(1) as the most potent [4]. The enantiomers **2a** and **2b** had different potencies when tested on the same system. Finally, racemic **3** was also tested and found to have significant activity.

(1)

(2a) R = CH_3, R^1 = H
(2b) R = H, R^1 = CH_3

(3)

To confirm the importance of enantiomeric purity on biological activity (R)- and (S)-3 were prepared using a chiral synthesis. At strategic points along the synthetic pathway diastereomeric and enantiomeric purity were determined by the appropriate HPLC technique. This methodology showed that each optical isomer of **3** could be prepared in optical purity greater than 98.5%.

[1] Fondacaro, J. (1986). *American Journal of Physiology* **250**, G1.
[2] Hwang, T. C., Lu, L., Zeitlin, P. L., Grunenert, D. C., Huganir, R. and Guggino, W. B. (1989). *Science* **244**, 1351.
Ming, L., McCann, J. D., Anderson, M. P., Clancy, J. P., Liedtke, C. M., Nairn, A. C., Greengard, P. and Welsh, M. J. (1989). *Science* **244**, 1353.
Jetton, A. M., Yankaskas, J. R., Stutts, M. J., Willumsen, N. J. and Boucher, R. C. (1989). *Science* **244**, 1472.
[3] DiStefano, A., Wittner, M., Schlatter, E., Jang, H. J., Englert, H. and Greger, R. (1985). *Pflugers Arch.* **405**, S95.
[4] Wangemann, P., Wittner, M., Di Stefano, A., Englert, H. C., Lang, H. J., Schlatter, E. and Greger, R. (1986). *Pflugers Arch.* **407**, S128.

Isopropylidine Glycerol: A Source for Versatile C_3 Chirons P. M. Smid[1] and R. J. Pryce.[2] [1]*International Bio-Synthetics, 2288EE, Rijswijk, The Netherlands.* [2]*Shell Research Ltd., Sittingbourne, Kent ME9 8AG.*

Enantiomerically pure compounds are becoming more and more important especially in the search for and development of new biologically active molecules. Various chemical and biological technologies are available to synthesize homochiral molecules. A rather new approach is through biotechnology where the capability of microorganisms to discriminate between enantiomers of chiral molecules is exploited. A particular example of the biotechnological approach is detailed in this poster. Selective oxidation of the S isomer of racemic isopropylidene glycerol (IPG) into (R)-IPG acid $((R)$-IPGA) with a specific microorganism leaves the (R)-IPG nearly untouched. International Bio-Synthetics research and development teams have developed a process for manufacturing (R)-IPG (as well as (R)-IPGA) on ton scale. Besides the process itself the poster also deals with some chemistry demonstrating the versatility of both these C_3 synthons in asymmetric synthesis.

The Enantioselective Synthesis of SK&F 95654, A Novel Cardiotonic Agent. N. H. Baine,[1] C. J. Kowalski,[1] F. Owings,[1] M. Fox[1] and M. Mitchell.[2] [1]*Smith Kline & French Research Laboratories, King of Prussia, PA, USA. Smith Kline & French Research Limited, Tonbridge, UK.*

SK&F 95654, a 6-phenyl-5-methyl-4, 5-dihydro-3(2H)-pyridazinone, is a key chiral inter-mediate to a wide variety of cardiotonic agents whose actions are based upon the selective inhibition of cardiac phosphodiesterase. A seven-step enantioselective synthesis of $R(-)$-SK&F 93505 was developed to afford a 12% overall yield of > 98% enantiomerically pure product, starting from $R(+)$-2-chloropropionic acid. SK&F 93505 was further converted to $R(-)$-SK&F 95654, an active PDE III inhibitor which holds potential for utility in the treatment of conjestive heart failure. An interesting variety of synthetic operations were carefully designed to minimize racemization of a readily enolizable chiral centre.

The Asymmetric Synthesis of Unsaturated Medium Ring Heterocycles and Applications to the Synthesis of Natural Products. N. R. Curtis, P. A. Evans, A. B. Holmes, M. G. Looney, N. D. Pearson and G. C. Slim. *University Chemical Laboratory, Lensfield Road, Cambridge CB2 1EW, UK.*

We have been interested in the Claisen rearrangement of vinyl-substituted ketene acetals (1) [1] with a view to exploiting the resulting medium ring lactones (3) in the synthesis of natural

(1) X = O
(2) X = NCOOBn

(3) X = O
(4) X = NCOOBn

(5)   (6)   (7)

products and biologically interesting target molecules. This poster describes applications of the Claisen rearrangement of (1) and (2) to produce lactones (3) and lactams (4) which can be elaborated to marine natural products such as obtusenyne (5) [2], gloeosporone (6) [3] and the potentially interesting lactam (7), respectively.

[1] Carling, R. W. and Holmes, A. B. (1986). *J. Chem. Soc., Chem. Commun.* 325.
[2] Howard, B. M., Schulte, G. R., Fenical, W., Solheim, B. and Clardy, J. (1980). *Tetrahedron* **36**, 1747.
[3] Meyer, W. L., Schweizer, W. B., Beck, A. K., Scheifele, W., Seebach, D., Schreiber, S. L. and Kelly, S. E. (1987). *Helv. Chim. Acta* **70**, 281.

Synthesis and Transformations of Some Chiral β-Lactones. B. Jackson. *Lonza A. G., 3930 Visp., Switzerland*

Wynberg and Staring [1] showed that the enantioselective cycloaddition of ketene to electron-deficient carbonyl compounds using quinine or quinidine as catalysts produces the corresponding chiral β-lactones (1). These lactones are highly functionalized and may be further transformed into useful building-blocks for EPC syntheses. In collaboration with Prof. Wynberg we have produced various chiral lactones and are also studying their transformation into other chiral compounds. Various key intermediates have been made in our laboratory and typical examples are shown in the general scheme below. Specific synthons, useful for enantioselective synthesis are presented.

[1] Wynberg, H. and Staring, A. J. G. (1982). *J. Am. Chem. Soc.* **104**, 166 and PCT Int. Appl. W O 8401,577.

Studies on the Macrolide FK506. M. Furber[1], D. K. Donald[1] and D. Hunter,[1] and A. A. Freer[2]. *Medicinal Chemistry [1]Department, Fisons plc, Bakewell Rd, Loughborough, Leicestershire LE11 0RH, UK. [2]Chemistry Department, Glasgow GQ12 8QQ, UK*

The macrolide immunosuppressant **FK506** (**1**) was subjected to an unusually mild and stereoselective Hetero–Claisen rearrangement, giving compound **2**. The expected stereochemistry, based on the familiar chair-like transition state, was confirmed by X-ray analysis.

(1)   FK506   (2)   FPL65599XX

Preparation of Chiral Building Blocks and Auxiliaries by Chromatographic Resolution on Cellulose Triacetate (CTA I). E. Francotte and R. M. Wolf. *Central Research Laboratories, R-1060.2.40, CIBA-GEIGY Ltd, CH-4002 Basel, Switzerland.*

The properties of the respective enantiomers of chiral bioactive compounds are quite generally very different. Due to increasing demand for enantio- and stereo-chemically pure substances in quantities adequate for biological tests, the interest in the chromatographic resolution of racemates on chiral stationary phases on a preparative scale has become more and more important. This method is very promising but only a limited number of preparative applications have been reported so far. In this work, we demonstrate that cellulose triacetate, **I** (CTA I), in particular, presents a number of advantages as a chiral phase for this purpose. The broad applicability and the high loading capacity of CTA I are particularly important features for preparative chromatography. Nevertheless, slight structural modifications of the racemates to be resolved can often strongly improve the resolution. This strategy has been applied to numerous practical problems and is illustrated in this work by taking as examples the chiral building blocks and auxiliaries shown below. Moreover, a systematic investigation of the influence of a substituent in *para* position of the phenyl ring for different series of aromatic compounds led to the conclusion that a large number of different interaction sites must be present in the chiral environment of the biopolymer derived stationary phase (CTA I).

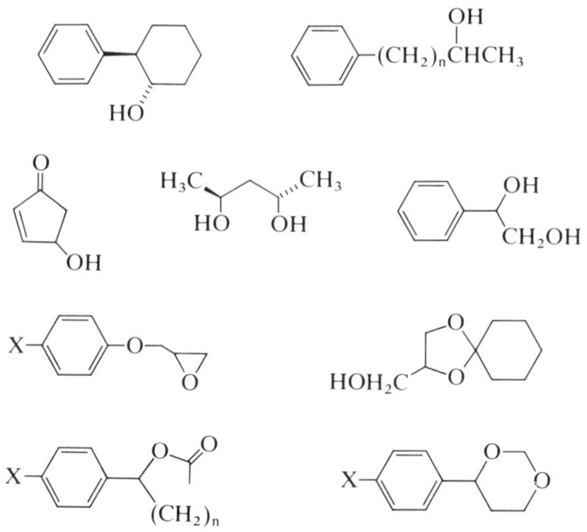

Camphorquinone: A Chiral Auxiliary. B. T. Golding,[1] W. P. Watson,[2] M. K. Ellis,[1] G. McGibbon,[1] and A. B. Maude[1]. *[1] Department of Chemistry, Bedson Building, University of Newcastle upon Tyne, NE1 7RU, UK. [2] Shell Research Limited, Sittingbourne Research Centre, Sittingbourne, Kent ME9 8AG, UK.*

The acid catalysed ketalization of D-camphorquinone with racemic 3-chloropropane-1,2-diol effects a kinetic resolution resulting in a predominate diastereoisomer. This dioxolane is separable by crystallization and is readily converted to (R)-3-chloropropane-1,2-diol and (R)-chloromethyloxirane. Diastereoselective reduction of this dioxolane followed by intra-molecular cyclization yields (1R,2S,3R,4'S)-bornane-3-spiro-2'-(1',3',7'-trioxolane) which is a protected chiral glycerol equivalent. Acidic hydrolysis of this trioxolane gives (1R,2S,2'S,4S)-2-(2',3'-dihydroxypropyloxy)-bornan-3-one, a potential precursor of sn-1,2-diglycerides and other biologically active, optically pure derivatives of glycerol. (1R,2S,3R,3S,4'S)-Bornane-3-spiro-2'-(1'3',7'-trioxolane) may also be prepared by the diastereoselective intramolecular cyclization of (1R,2S,4S)-2-(2'3'-dihydroxypropyloxy)-bornan-3-one.

Enantiomeric Synthesis of Thromboxane Antagonists. G. D. Harris, S. A. Lee, A. J. Nicholas, M. J. Smithers and A. Stocker. *ICI Pharmaceuticals, Macclesfield, Cheshire SK10 2NA, UK*

ICI 185282 (racemate)

Most of the activity resides in the (−) enantiomer of ICI 185282. Initially small quantities were obtained by classical diastereoisomeric salt resolution of the final racemate. This is wasteful since the unwanted (+) isomer, having three chiral centres, cannot easily be reused. A new synthesis has been devised in which a paraconic acid derivative is used to set up the relative *cis* stereochemistry of the aromatic group and the heptenoic acid side-chain. Resolution of the paraconic acid into enantiomers at the start of the synthesis enables enantiomerically pure material to be obtained very efficiently.

[1] Brewster, A. G., Brown, G. R. and Smithers, M. J. European Patent Application No. 177121.
[2] Harris, G. D., European Patent Application No. 142323.
[3] Lee, S. A. (1987). *Chem. Ind. (London)*. 223.

Index